Hunger and Malnutrition as Major Challenges of the 21st Century

World Scientific Series in Grand Public Policy Challenges of the 21st Century

ISSN: 2630-4856

This book series will address topics related to some of the biggest challenges facing societies around the world in the 21st century — threats such as climate change, food insecurity and malnutrition, energy and water insecurity, pandemics, conflict and violence, growing inequality and poverty, low fertility and depopulation in affluent countries, anemic economic growth and stubbornly high unemployment in much of the developed world, and rising rates of obesity and chronic diseases in developing countries. If unaddressed, these challenges have a real chance of derailing the substantial gains in living standards and quality of life achieved around the world in the last three decades.

The World Scientific Series in Grand Public Policy Challenges of the 21st Century, under the leadership of Professor Anil Deolalikar, a renowned development economist, seeks to fill this gap. It will strive to publish high-quality scientific works, including monographs, edited volumes, references, and handbooks, that address topics related to the grand challenges confronting societies around the world today.

Published

Vol. 3 *Hunger and Malnutrition as Major Challenges of the 21st Century*
edited by Raghbendra Jha (Australian National University, Australia)

Vol. 2 *Agriculture & Food Systems to 2050: Global Trends, Challenges and Opportunities*
edited by Rachid Serraj (Food and Agriculture Organization of the United Nations, Italy) and Prabhu Pingali (Cornell University, USA)

Vol. 1 *Global Challenges for Future Food and Agricultural Policies*
editor-in-chief Tim Josling (Stanford University, USA)
edited by David Blandford (The Pennsylvania State University, USA) and Katharine Hassapoyannes (European Parliament, Belgium)

World Scientific Series in Grand Public Policy Challenges of the 21st Century
Vol. 3

Hunger and Malnutrition as Major Challenges of the 21st Century

editor

Raghbendra Jha

Australian National University, Australia

World Scientific

NEW JERSEY • LONDON • SINGAPORE • BEIJING • SHANGHAI • HONG KONG • TAIPEI • CHENNAI • TOKYO

Published by

World Scientific Publishing Co. Pte. Ltd.
5 Toh Tuck Link, Singapore 596224
USA office: 27 Warren Street, Suite 401-402, Hackensack, NJ 07601
UK office: 57 Shelton Street, Covent Garden, London WC2H 9HE

Library of Congress Cataloging-in-Publication Data
Names: Jha, Raghbendra, editor.
Title: Hunger and malnutrition as major challenges of the 21st century / edited by Raghbendra Jha (Australian National University, Australia).
Description: New Jersey : World Scientific, [2018] | Series: World scientific series in grand public policy challenges of the 21st century ; Volume 3
Identifiers: LCCN 2018039245 | ISBN 9789813239906 (hc : alk. paper)
Subjects: LCSH: Food security. | Food supply. | Malnutrition. | Food policy.
Classification: LCC HD9000.5 .H834 2018 | DDC 363.8--dc23
LC record available at https://lccn.loc.gov/2018039245

British Library Cataloguing-in-Publication Data
A catalogue record for this book is available from the British Library.

For any available supplementary material, please visit
https://www.worldscientific.com/worldscibooks/10.1142/10980#t=suppl

Desk Editors: Anthony Alexander/Sylvia Koh

Typeset by Stallion Press
Email: enquiries@stallionpress.com

Preface

Hunger and malnutrition have been major global challenges for long. Addressing these challenges is crucial not just for the sake of providing a basic need — adequate nourishment to all persons — but also because there are ethical, human rights and economic arguments why these are necessary. For instance, reducing undernourishment increases labour productivity and, thus, economic growth. With undernourishment come the health and other costs of addressing the consequences of such undernourishment. However, unlike issues such as the eradication of poverty, addressing the hunger and malnutrition challenges have few fervent politically powerful advocates. The scale of the hunger and malnutrition problems could become even more challenging as global population is expected to cross 9 billion by the middle of this century.

This volume attempts to take stock of hunger and malnutrition challenges in the 21st century. This volume has chapters on thematic issues as well as deep country studies, particularly for the African countries as well as for China and India. It is to be hoped that the papers in this volume will stimulate further interest in applied research on these topics, particularly as the consequences of the evolving challenges of climate change, human conflict and increasing international protectionism, to name just three, take hold.

In putting together this volume, I have benefited much from the advice and support of a number of people. I name the most obvious of these here. The authors of the individual chapters have spared their invaluable time to contribute their excellent research to this volume. To them I am very grateful. I am also very grateful to Anil Deolalikar, the series editor for "Grand Public Policy Challenges of the 21st Century" (of which this book is a component), for his gracious invitation to contribute this volume to the series and for his unflinching support. Zvi Ruder (Senior Executive Publisher of this series at World Scientific Publishers) was very supportive throughout the process of putting together this volume. I am much obliged to Zvi for this support. Finally, I am obliged to the Arndt-Corden Department of Economics, my home in the Australian National University, for providing me with such a conducive atmosphere for my writing.

Canberra
January 2018

About the Editor

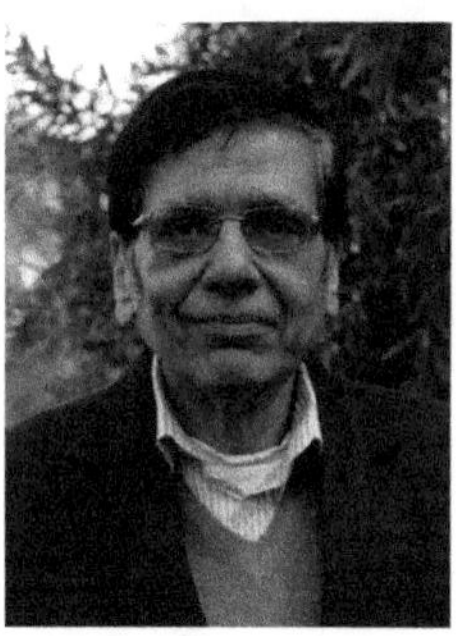

Raghbendra Jha is Professor of Economics and Executive Director, Australia South Asia Research Centre, at the Australian National University. His previous appointments include Columbia University (where he obtained his PhD) and Williams College in the US, Queen's University in Canada, University of Warwick in the UK and Delhi School of Economics, Indian Institute of Management, Bangalore and Indira Gandhi Institute of Development Research in India. He has published dozens of books/monographs and more than 150 papers in leading journals and other refereed outlets.

About the Authors

C. Peter Timmer is an authority on agricultural development, food security and the world rice economy. He served as a professor at Stanford, Cornell, three faculties at Harvard, and the University of California, San Diego, and is now the Cabot Professor of Development Studies, *emeritus*, at Harvard University. He was awarded the Leontief Prize in 2012 for advances in economic thought and delivered the 18th Annual UNU-WIDER Lecture at the UN in New York in 2014.

Peter Warr is John Crawford Professor of Agricultural Economics, Emeritus, at the Australian National University. He studied at the University of Sydney, the London School of Economics and Stanford University, where he received his PhD in economics. His current research is on the relationship between economic policy and poverty incidence in Southeast Asia.

Simrit Kaur is Professor of Economics and Public Policy and, currently, Principal of Shri Ram College of Commerce, University of Delhi. Prior to this, she was with the Faculty of Management Studies, University of Delhi. Her research interests include privatization, climate change, agricultural policy and food security. She has been a consultant for several projects and an advisor to organizations such as the Government of India, IFAD and FAO of the United Nations, and OECD.

Harpreet Kaur is an Assistant Professor, at the Department of Economics, Sri Guru Gobind Singh College of Commerce, University of Delhi, India. She has been teaching courses on statistics, mathematical economics, econometrics, macroeconomics and managerial economics. Ms. Kaur has recently submitted her Doctoral Thesis on Food Security in South Asia to the Faculty of Management Studies, University of Delhi. Her research interests include open economy macroeconomics, managerial economics, development economics and public policy.

Jing You is Associate Professor in School of Agricultural Economics and Rural Development at Renmin University of China and Visiting Fellow in the Department of Land Economy at the University of Cambridge. Her research areas are Development Economics and Applied Microeconomics, with topics on Chinese development such as poverty, inequality, labour and education.

Zekun Du is a Postgraduate student in School of Agricultural Economics and Rural Development at Renmin University of China. His research interests are in development economics and microeconometrics.

Shyam Khadka started his career in 1977 in the Agricultural Development Bank, Nepal. Since 1993 he has been with the United Nations system including IFAD, where he led India Country Programme (1997–2004) and assessment of overall development effectiveness of IFAD's portfolio of loans and grants and formulation of operational policies and strategies. In 2014, he was appointed Service Chief in the Investment Centre in FAO and since 2015 has been serving as FAO Representative in India.

Deepika Anand works as National Nutrition Expert with the FAO, India. She holds a doctorate degree in Nutrition from the University of Delhi and has also served as a faculty with the University. She has also worked as a Consultant with the World Bank, World Food Programme and World Health Organization in India. She has published several scientific papers in peer-reviewed journals and co-authored reports in nutrition and public health domain.

Nidhi Kaicker is Assistant Professor at the School of Business, Public Policy and Social Entrepreneurship, Ambedkar University Delhi. She holds a doctoral and a masters degree in management from Faculty of Management Studies, University of Delhi and a bachelors degree in Economics from St. Stephens College. Her research interests include Managerial Economics, Household Decision Making, Diets and Nutrition, and Business Valuation. She has published extensively in leading journals on these topics, and also presented her work in several international and national conferences.

Vani S. Kulkarni is a Senior Fellow in Urban Ethnography Project at Yale University and a Lecturer on sociology at the University of Pennsylvania. She holds a PhD with distinction from the University of Pennsylvania. She has received prestigious awards and has held research fellowships at Penn, Harvard and Yale. She has also been a consultant for the ADB and IFAD. Her research lies at the intersection of Global Health, Race and Caste, Gender, Identity and Inequality, Development and Democracy, and Education. She has published in several leading peer-reviewed journals. She has co-authored two books, UN reports and op-eds.

Raghav Gaiha is (Former) Professor of Public Policy, Faculty of Management Studies, University of Delhi and currently (Hon) Professorial Fellow, Global Development Institute, University of Manchester. He has been Visiting Fellow/Scholar at Harvard, MIT, Stanford, Penn and University of Cambridge. He has served as a consultant with the World Bank, ILO, FAO, IFAD, WIDER and ADB. He has coedited *The Economics of Food Securi*ty (Edward Elgar), *Diets, Malnutrition and Disease — The Indian Experience* (OUP), and *Battling Corruption: Has NREGA Reached India's Rural Poor* (OUP). In summer 2018 he will be a Visiting Scholar, Population Studies Centre, University of Pennsylvania.

Priya Rampal is a Post Doctoral Fellow at the M.S. Swaminathan Research Foundation, India. She has submitted her PhD at the Indira Gandhi Institute of Development Research, Mumbai. Her thesis focuses on the nutritional status of children, specifically, the importance of early childhood nutrition in later outcomes such as health, education and work participation. Previously, Priya worked on agriculture and livestock insurance at a research centre in Institute for Financial Management and Research.

Ranjula Bali Swain is a Visiting Professor at the Mistra Center for Sustainable Markets at the Stockholm School of Economics and a Professor of Economics at Södertörn University, Stockholm, Sweden. She is also affiliated to Uppsala University and the Center for European Research in Microfinance (Cermi) at the Solvay Brussels School of Economics and Management. Her main research interests are in environmental economics, microeconometrics and development economics.

Manoj K. Pandey is Lecturer in Economics at the Australian National University (ANU), and Visiting Lecturer at University of Papua New Guinea (UPNG) as part of ANU's partnership with UPNG and Adjunct Fellow at University of the South Pacific (USP). He has a PhD degree in Economics from ANU, an MPhil and MA in Statistics from Delhi University, and Bachelor of Arts in Statistics (Honours) from Banaras Hindu University. His previous appointments include University of South Pacific (Fiji), ANU (Australia), NCAER and IEG (India). His areas of expertise are economics of ageing, development, health, labour, food-security, gender and well-being.

Shantanu Mathur has been a development practitioner for 33 years (3 at FAO and 30 at IFAD) and currently Lead Adviser, Programme Management and Manager UN & Multilateral Partnerships (IFAD). Prior appointments include Co-Chair of Global Donor Platform for Rural Development, CGIAR Fund Council Chair of the Evaluation and Impact Assessment Committee, Vice-Chair of the CGIAR Finance Committee, and Vice Chair, GFAR. He managed the IFAD Grant programme for over 25 years and served as Head of Quality Assurance Group at IFAD. He has MA degrees from Cambridge and Delhi. And has contributed to/edited four books on rural development, research and impact assessment.

George Kararach is a Ugandan Economist, currently an Economic Affairs Officer at the Macroeconomic Policy Division, UN Economic Commission for Africa and until recently Senior Consultant, Strategy and Operations Policy Department, The African Development Bank. He holds a PhD in Economics from Leeds University, UK, and is an expert on economic reform and development with particular reference to Africa. He has published five books with major publishers including ARRF, Palgrave Macmillan, Policy Press and Oxford University Press.

Abbi M. Kedir is currently an Associate Professor/Senior Lecturer of International Business at the University of Sheffield, UK. He is an applied quantitative economist with vast experience in analyzing and modeling development issues with policy focus on economies of Africa. He has experience working as a consultant to organizations such as the World Bank, United Nations, European Commission and Department for International Development (DFID), UK.

Contents

Part I
Introduction and Thematic Issues

Chapter 1

Introduction: Hunger and Malnutrition as Major Challenges in the 21st Century

Raghbendra Jha

Professor of Economics, Australian National University, Canberra ACT 0200, Australia
r.jha@anu.edu.au

Abstract

This chapter provides an overview of the global food security challenge. It also summarizes the contribution of each of the chapters in the volume and assesses the prospects for attaining food security in the future.

Keywords: Food security, nutrition, Asia, Africa, climate change.

1. Measures of Hunger and Undernutrition

The World Food Summit (WFS) in 1996 adopted a broad definition of food security. According to this definition, food security exists when all people, at all times, have physical and economic access to sufficient, safe and nutritious food to meet their dietary needs and food preferences for an active and healthy life. This definition encompasses a wide variety of elements — temporal, spatial, quality of food and the like. A corollary of this interpretation is that lack of food security would overlap with hunger — both overt and hidden — and undernutrition and would have spillover effects onto the health and labour market performance of those affected by such insecurity. This range of issues guides my choice of contributions to this volume.

In the literature, "hunger" is said to exist when people have inadequate calorie/macronutrient intake. "Hidden hunger" is associated with inadequate intake of micronutrients such as vitamin A, riboflavin, carotene, iron, etc. When present in women and children, "hidden hunger" is an even more severe problem since adequate nutritional intake during female pregnancy and lactation is critical for development of the infant. Furthermore, adequate child nutrition is critical to the development of young children. Undernutrition, sometimes also called undernourishment, is a more generic term signifying inadequate nutritional support to ensure adequate support for work and study. Food insecurity refers to such undernutrition and can be interpreted in the sense of the WFS definition given above.

In the extant literature, at least three different measures of chronic food insecurity have been used. These are: (i) the Food and Agricultural Organization (FAO) indicator of undernourishment; (ii) inadequacy of nutrient intake as gleaned from household surveys; and (iii) childhood anthropometric measures like measures of stunting (low height for age), wasting (low weight for height) and underweight (low weight for age).

The FAO measures undernourishment as the share of people in the total population that are consuming less than the "minimum" energy requirements. This has also been called "hunger" in the literature. The FAO methodology involves the use of three key parameters: (i) the mean quantity of calorie consumption in the country calculated from the national food balance sheets, (ii) the inequality in access to these calories measured by fitting a log-normal distribution with mean dietary energy supply and the coefficient of variation as parameters and (iii) size of the country's population. The FAO then uses its measure of minimum dietary energy requirement (defined as that needed to maintain an acceptable minimum body weight, body composition, minimum sedentary physical activity and good health) to determine the extent of undernourishment.

Clearly, the FAO method has the advantage that it provides country estimates of undernourishment that are globally comparable. However, as de Haen *et al.* (2011) show, each of the three parameters underpinning the FAO methodology has been subject to severe criticism.

Further, as de Haen *et.al.* (2011) also show, results obtained from application of the FAO and other methodologies to measure the extent of undernourishment often yield inconsistent results. Naturally, this makes it difficult to be confident of the extent of prevalence of undernutrition.

The second methodology involving household surveys uses the module on expenditure (including food and non-food expenditure) incorporated into these surveys. Household food consumption is converted into nutrient equivalents, and prevailing norms of nutritional requirements are used to assess undernourishment. Compared to the FAO methodology, this approach has the advantage that it measures consumption where it actually occurs. It also permits comparison of nutrient intakes across groups of people and across regions, but not internationally. However, in many cases, per capita consumption of food is calculated by dividing aggregate household consumption by the number of people in the household or, at best, using adult equivalence scales. This ignores problems of intra-household allocation of food. For instance, Barrett (2010) argues that the mere availability of food is not enough to ensure that everyone will have access to it. Indeed, some authors have argued that the inter- and intra-household allocation of food in some countries is inefficient because females and children are often given inadequate food even when food is available. Further, since the household consumption survey is conducted during a short time span, seasonal changes in consumption patterns are not captured.

Anthropometric measures of undernutrition like stunting (low height for age), wasting (low weight for height) and underweight (low weight for age) are calculated by dividing the difference between age- and gender-specific anthropometric measures of the child and the respective median by the mean of the distribution. Thus, a normalized Z score is obtained. United Nations International Children's Emergency Fund (UNICEF) suggests that values of Z less than -2 indicate moderate undernutrition and values less than -3 indicate severe undernourishment. These measures apply to children below the age of 5, although for older children and adults the Body Mass Index (BMI) has widely been used. BMI has been defined as weight/(height)^2, where weight is measured in kilograms and height in meters.

These measures directly measure what we are most interested in and the use of alternate measures, if the results are consistent with each other, only solidifies our judgement about nutrition. These statistics, like the measures based on household surveys, allow identification of particularly vulnerable groups and regions.

That said, the use of anthropometric measures has its drawbacks as well. First, a child's weight or height is only partially linked to nutritional intake. Factors like whether the child has been exposed to disease or has access to clean water are also important in determining a child's anthropometric status. Moreover, these measures leave out other groups, particularly children above the age of 5 and adults.

Given these factors, food (in)security remains an elusive concept to articulate, let alone measure. It is not surprising, therefore, that alternative measures of food insecurity are used depending on the objective at hand. Popular indices of food insecurity used are a coping strategies index and a dietary diversity index. Barrett (2010) notes that direct hunger is individual specific and can only be measured using household-level data. He also notes the importance of household-level data in identifying particularly vulnerable groups and regions.

It is best, therefore, that efforts to get an accurate measure of malnourishment involve creating a portal containing estimates using different methods. This will provide a more complete picture of undernutrition. However, we should always keep in mind the caveat that no measure is perfect.[1]

2. The Current State of Undernutrition

The current status of undernourishment in the world is brought out by Status of Food Insecurity (SOFI) (2015) and, by and large, uses the FAO norm for estimating undernourishment.[2] This report analyses trends in

[1]For an overview of the multi-faceted issues involved in food security, see Jha and Gaiha (2016).

[2]For a general critique of the use of calorie intake for assessing undernourishment, see Srinivasan (1981). For a contrasting view, see Sahn and Stiefl (2002). See also Svedberg (2002).

undernourishment in various parts of the world in view of the fact that 2015 was designated as the terminal year for the United Nations' Millennium Development Goals (MDGs). SOFI (2015) reports a reduction in the number of undernourished from 991 million in 1990–1992 to 780 million in 2014–2016 in developing regions — a reduction of 211 million. The Proportion of Undernourished (POU) fell from 23.3% to 12.9%, a little over 1 percentage point above the MDG1c in 2015. It is claimed that 72 developing countries out of 129 have already achieved this goal. For the world as a whole, the number of undernourished persons dropped from 1.0106 billion (18.6% of the total population) in 1990–1992 to 794.6 million (10.9% of the population) in 2014–2016. Thus, for the world as a whole, MDG1c has not been achieved. The same is true of Asia where the number (percentage) of undernourished persons came down from 741.9 million (23.6%) in 1990–1992 to 511.7 million (12.1%) in 2014–2016. Africa's performance is particularly worrisome since the number of undernourished persons actually increased from 181.7 million in 1990–1992 to 232.5 million in 2014–2016; although the percentage of people undernourished came down from 27.6% to 20.0% over this period. Along the same lines, Oceania recorded an increase in the number of undernourished from 1 million in 1990–1992 to 1.4 million in 2014–2016 although the percentage of the population undernourished declined marginally from 15.7% to 14.2%. Latin America and the Caribbean met MDG1c with a drop in the number of undernourished (percentage of population) from 66.1 million (14.7%) to 34.3 million (5.5%). There was a drop in the number of undernourished in developed countries from 20 million in 1990–1992 to 14.7 million in 2014–2016. The percentage of the population undernourished remained at less than 5%.

In October 2015, the United Nations adopted a new set of Sustainable Development Goals (SDGs) to replace the MDGs. The SDGs are to be attained over a 15-year period (i.e. by 2030) and constitute 17 goals. Of these, Goal 1 (End poverty in all its forms everywhere), Goal 2 (End hunger, achieve food security and improved nutrition and promote sustainable agriculture) and Goal 6 (Ensure availability and sustainable management of water and sanitation for all) are directly linked to the subject matter of this volume.[3]

---

[3] See http://www.un.org/ga/search/view_doc.asp?symbol=A/RES/70/1&Lang=E.

3. Why Address Undernutrition

Addressing undernutrition is crucial not just for the sake of providing a basic need — adequate nourishment to all persons — but also because there are ethical, human rights and economic arguments why this is necessary. Reducing undernourishment increases labour productivity and, thus, economic growth. With undernourishment come the health and other costs of addressing the consequences (e.g. health-related costs) of such undernourishment. World Bank (2004) strongly argues the case for increasing investment in providing adequate nutrition. The social returns from such investment are very high. World Bank (2004), quoting the Copenhagen Consensus 2004, suggests that investment in nourishment may yield higher returns than investments in trade liberalization, malaria, water or sanitation. Indeed, investment in alleviating undernourishment provides the greatest opportunity to improve lives in the shortest time and at the lowest cost. However, a key consideration in assessing the incentives to invest in undernourishment alleviation is that most of the returns that flow from such investment accrue to undernourished people who are, by and large, too poor to provide a high enough return to make substantial private investment attractive. In this sense, then, the provision of public goods has a public goods component wherein there is a strong case for public investment (supported by international organizations) in this area.[4]

The ultimate aim of eradicating malnourishment is tantamount to the attainment of food security by all. Food security itself depends on the three pillars of *availability*, *access* and *utilization*. Availability is essential for access, which in turn is necessary for utilization. Accurate measurement of food security and identification of the food insecure are critical to design of policy responses.

Through much of recorded history, human beings have had short unhealthy lives because of the paucity of macronutrients (like calories, fats and proteins). This lack of *availability* has also been labelled "hunger". The consequence is the "poverty trap". whereby hunger leads to low productivity which leads to low wages and hence poverty and, in turn,

---

[4]Kakwani and Son (2016) discuss social welfare-based measures of hunger and food deprivation.

poverty leads to reduced purchasing power and hence hunger, thus completing a vicious cycle. This poverty nutrition trap has been broken in many countries largely as a result of enhanced agricultural growth and productivity. However, the problem of "hidden hunger" (lack of adequate micronutrients) persists in many countries. This leads to fatigue, lack of resistance to disease, cognitive disability, etc. Appropriate diet following from high agricultural productivity has also broken this "hidden hunger" and the consequent "poverty nutrition trap" in many countries. But poverty nutrition traps (particularly with respect to micronutrients) still do exist in some developing countries, e.g. see Jha *et al.* (2009a) for the case of rural India.

Even if sufficient food is available, it does not automatically follow that everyone will have access to adequate amounts of safe food. Much depends on inter- and intra-household allocation of food. In some South Asian and African countries, it is alleged that there is a bias against provision of adequate food to women and girl children even when adequate food is available. Alderman *et al.* (1995) and Bobonis (2009) typify some of the vast literature which has argued that unitary models of the household that assume that allocation within a household is altruistic and dictated by individual needs are not substantiated by empirical evidence and that a model of bargaining within the household is more appropriate. Even subsidized food through public distribution systems is not immune from such biases. Basu and Das (2015) analyze the reported bias against the poor in India's Targeted Public Distribution Scheme (TPDS), particularly in states where the TPDS functions well.

Evidence about what contributes to the pattern of intra-household preferences is provided by Quisumbing and Smith (2007). The most significant difference seems to be by gender. Birth order of the child with or without interaction with the gender, relationship to the household and age of the household member all seem to matter. Such a bias in household allocation affects not only the nutritional status of females in the household but also the economic growth prospects of the country. Thus, World Bank (2001) shows that if in the 1960s the countries of Sub-Saharan Africa and South Asia had the same gender differences as the East Asian countries and closed this gap at the same rate as East Asia did, their GDP growth rates would have been 0.5–0.9% higher per year. Moreover, the status of women (including their nutritional attainment) has a strong impact on the nutritional, health and education status of the children in the household. Hence, when the bargaining power of women in the household improves, the nutritional, health and education prospects for the next generation improve.

Thus, future policy must be sensitive to this fact and design the allocation of food subsidies accordingly, e.g. by transferring this subsidy to the bank account of the wife or partner of the male "head" of the household. There is need to end formal discrimination using appropriate legislation, targeting credit towards women entrepreneurs, targeting food and cash transfers towards women, providing support for childcare and providing enhanced support for female participation in the labour market.

Finally, merely having access to the food does not necessarily imply that food will be *utilized*. Much could be lost due to wastage and other factors. Thus, enhancing food processing and storage become key ingredients of a strategy to reduce waste and smoothen consumption of food over time.

4. Ensuring Availability, Accessibility and Utilization

These themes are developed in this volume. There are chapters on improving the availability of food and the trade-offs that may exist among increasing different types of food. The book also deals with problems affecting the distribution of food and, in particular, the role that international trade can play in this area. Models of access to food are also discussed as well as the methods and technologies of food utilization.

So far as food *availability* is concerned, there are pressures on both the demand and supply sides. On the demand side, the world's population is likely to rise to 8 billion by 2030 and more than 9 billion by 2050. However, with population growth in China already tapering off and India's population growth continuing to decelerate, there is likely to be a plateauing of the total world population around the 9.4 billion mark expected in 2050. In addition, rising incomes in many countries in the developing world mean that food consumption patterns will go through a transformation with more emphasis placed on high-quality diets.

Another significant issue confronting future food availability is the increasing shift from grain to the production of bioenergy. In light of recent rises in fuel prices, liquid biofuels have been increasingly produced for use in automotive and other machines. What the FAO calls first-generation liquid biofuels are manufactured from a range of crops that are specific to particular regions. In the temperate regions, rapeseed, corn and other cereals are used as biofuel feedstock. In the tropical regions, cane sugar, palm oil and, to a lesser degree, soybeans and cassava are used.

Among the biofuels, those derived from food crops are in the most advanced stage of development and are, hence, of particular concern since many governments are looking at biofuels to reduce dependency on petroleum products. In this context, Senauer (2008) argues that higher food prices due to increase in biofuel production could result in a sharp rise in the number of hungry people in the developing world. This increase in the incidence of hunger is likely to be highest in the urban areas of developing countries since many of the rural poor are subsistence farmers.

In addition, Senauer provides evidence that biofuel use has led to an increase in the extent of Greenhouse Gas (GHG) emissions. Conversion of natural ecosystems to agricultural use creates a "carbon debt" by releasing into the atmosphere CO_2 stored in the natural biomass and undisturbed soil.

Hence, on both these counts, there is a strong case for reducing the production of biofuels for mass consumption.

5. Implications of Change in Dietary Patterns

Parallel to this, there is increased consumption of foods with high sugar and fat content, which has implications for obesity and, further down the line, for non-communicable diseases and other health issues. This dietary transition is already taking place at a rapid rate and has several costs attached to it. Popkin *et al.* (2001), for example, discuss the health implications of the shift in dietary intakes towards higher fat and lower carbohydrate content in India and China.

Change in dietary patterns, following rapid increases in income, along an Engel curve type of response function imply the increased consumption of milk, other dairy products, fresh fruits and vegetables and, in particular, meats. This shift in dietary patterns has serious implications for agricultural resource use and GHG emissions. In this context, Eshel *et al.* (2014) show that the environmental costs for each calorie consumed are approximately the same for dairy, poultry, pork and eggs. However, beef production requires 28, 11, 5 and 6 times more land, irrigation water, GHG and Nr (reactive nitrogen and nitrogen fertilizer), than the average of the other livestock derived foods listed above. Hence, a rapid and sustained move to livestock-based products, particularly beef, would imply considerable stress on resources and lead to substantial increases in GHG emissions. Thus, a program of consumption taxation of these products to dissuade their sustained increased consumption may become an attractive policy option. Indeed, policies to reduce livestock-based consumption have the potential to reduce the environmental costs of food production quite considerably.

Alongside the increase in consumption of foods with high sugar and fat content, an additional concern is the persistence of inadequate micronutrient intake — particularly by women and children. There are strong biological arguments for women, particularly those who are pregnant or lactating, to have sufficient micronutrient intake. If children, particularly those who are younger than 2 years, have inadequate micronutrient intake, they may remain affected for life.

From the supply side, the increased demand for food and change in the structure of food demand will translate into increased competition for water, energy, arable land, etc. At the same time, the effects of climate change, particularly those affecting rainfall patterns and natural disasters, could affect agricultural productivity. This underscores the importance of developing and harnessing new technologies to ensure adequate food supplies at affordable prices. Even so, it would be necessary to protect vulnerable groups from spikes in food prices and high food price volatility. Furthermore, sufficient food needs to be made available to all, thus not just the quantum of food production but also its composition and distribution are important. The preservation of the biodiversity and ecosystem of the world is important for ensuring future food security.

Addressing this combination of emerging demand and supply issues amounts to a formidable task for global policymakers. To quote Godfray *et al.* (2010) "This challenge requires changes in the way food is produced, stored, processed, distributed and accessed that are as radical as those that occurred during the 18th- and 19th-century Industrial and Agricultural Revolutions and the 20th-Century Green revolution" (p. 812). More likely the challenge is even greater — given its scale.

6. Addressing the Anticipated Increase in Food Demand

World Bank (2008) reports that given current projections for world population in 2050, an extra 70–100% more food will be required. Between 2000 and 2030 alone, cereal production would have to increase by nearly 50% and meat production by 85%. Keating *et al.* (2014) report that between 2010 and 2015, food demand will increase by between 45% and 71%. Between 2010 and 2050, the energy deficit is likely to be 127×10^{15} kilocalories. Meeting this additional demand will lead to considerable strain on food systems and calls for very sharp increases in agricultural land productivity. Such increases will have to be sensitive both to the needs of the most vulnerable/food insecure and to the requirement that such increases in productivity be sustained.

Cassman (1999) and others have quantified a "yield gap", defined as the difference between realized productivity and the best that can be achieved using the best of current technology, seeds, etc. Such yield gaps exist for many crops and many countries. For instance, Cassman (1999) estimates this yield gap in the case of rice to be about 40% in the case of Southeast Asia. Hence, there exists considerable scope for expanding food output. A host of technical and institutional factors are among the reasons for the low yield of foodgrains. For instance, farmers may not have access to the best technology, knowledge and skills or finance may not be available and/or available only at high rates of interest.

Indeed, literature on the "yield gap" has increased astronomically (http://www.yieldgap.org/) Demand and supply projections to 2050 under Business as Usual (BAU) scenario reveal the extent of the shortfall of food. Keating *et al.* (2014) argue that there is no silver bullet for fixing this problem and suggest the use of a complex 14-pronged strategy to meet this shortfall. The 14-pronged strategy can be classified into three groups: (i) reducing demand, (ii) filling the production gap and (iii) avoiding losses. Keating *et al.* (2014) argue that reducing demand consists of (a) reducing food waste from farm to consumer, (b) reducing overconsumption in human diets, (c) reducing the livestock component of human diet and (d) developing "smart" biofuel policies and/or technologies. Filling the production gap would involve (a) expanding the land resources used for agricultural production, (b) expanding the use of water and irrigation resources, (c) greater use of aqua-culture on land or ocean, (d) increasing the yield in existing crops, (e) developing farming systems that use land and water more intensely and (f) improving the genetic content of crops. Finally, strategies that avoid losses in current and future production potential include (a) developing pest resistance and ensuring biosecurity, (b) addressing soil and water degradation, (c) minimizing the impact of climate change on food production and (d) adapting food production systems to the impacts of climate change when such change is unavoidable.

The pursuit of such a coordinated set of policies requires concerted policy at the national, regional and international levels. In addition, such a policy is needed to augment food output as well — an issue to which we now turn.

7. Increasing Food Production

A key aspect of food production is that it is highly site-specific. Some regions of the world have failed states that are incapable of executing policies. Those states that are capable of carrying out policies designed to enhance food output need to strike a balance between investing in economic growth as a means to boost agriculture and investing in agriculture to boost economic growth. In countries which have a high share of their GDP originating in agriculture, there is no conflict between the two, but in countries that want to make a distinct transition out of agriculture in order to sharply increase per capita GDPs such a conflict does exist. Even if it is deemed desirable to invest in agriculture, there could be another trade-off between investing resources into regional and national infrastructure, such as roads and ports, and investing in local social and economic capital. High costs because of poor quality and/or unavailability of seeds, lack of credit and other marketing and intermediating costs, and inadequate access to food markets may also reduce incentive for food production and lead to the creation and/or enlargement of yields gaps.

Furthermore, the yield gap does not stay constant, and maintaining a low yield gap would require continuous increases in productivity. This underscores the need for continued investment in innovation and research.

Even if food production and agricultural growth go up, this will not necessarily translate into increased nourishment and reduced poverty. We need to understand the specific channels through which these changes can take place. Bresciani and Valdes (2007) investigate four important transmission channels: rural labour markets, farm incomes, food prices and linkages to other economic sectors.

Improving domestic infrastructure, particularly roads and communications, and increasing international trade could improve market access and thereby provide incentives to augment food production and reduce yield gaps. But unrestrained global trade in food could bypass the most vulnerable communities.

Furthermore, environmental costs of good production, storage and transport are often pretty steep (Pretty *et al.*, 2005). As Stern (2007) argues, food production has important externalities such as the emission of methane and nitrous oxide (more harmful than CO_2 emission) which are not incorporated into the price of food. Agricultural operations involve nutrient run-offs from soil, water shortages due to over extraction and the like. Hence, although it is possible to design strategies for reducing or closing the yield gap, the environmental impacts of such strategies are uncertain. Hence, addressing hunger and food insecurity requires action across a wide spectrum of areas including energy, water supply, land use, seas, the ecosystem and biodiversity. Integrating action along all these lines is a key requirement and a major challenge for policymakers (Foresight Project, 2011).

8. Biotechnology to Combat Hunger

Genetically Modified (GM) crops are often touted as one of the principal technological breakthroughs that could reduce hunger in the future. However, the adoption of GM technology has also been a very divisive issue between two broad camps — the pro-GM American group and the anti-GM European lobby. GM seeds are often hailed as "miracle seeds" by their advocates, indeed one of the principal means to avoid the quasi-Malthusian future that the world might face given current population growth and food output projections.

Herring (2007) reviews the debate between the two sides and emphasizes the point that the scientific evidence behind GM technology is still quite scant so that a definite judgement about the alleged disadvantages of GM technology (e.g. soil degradation, excessive use of fertilizers, etc.) cannot be made.

Apart from this, farmers in developing countries are subject to a variety of risks resulting from, *inter alia,* droughts, floods and other natural calamities. Hence, the GM debate has got very charged and has become quite personal (Miller and Kershen, 2014).

As Herring (2007) argues, it is ironic that although people are generally supportive of genetically modified pharmaceuticals, they are reluctant to adopt GM crops. Indeed, field crop trials of GM crops have been burnt and GM science itself has been called "imperialistic" science. There are widely divergent views on who bears the costs and reaps the benefits of GM technology.

Notwithstanding the above, there is a case for persisting with GM technology — at least to the extent that science endorses it (Basu and Qaim, 2007). Concurrently, there is a case for intensive R&D activity into GM technology and the provision of financial incentives to carry out such research. GM technology offers a potential window of opportunity for sharply augmenting food yield and needs to be pursued.

Nevertheless, as Timmer (2003) notes, biotechnology by itself will not provide a complete solution to the problem of global hunger, particularly in a world in which the rich nations subsidize their agriculture so intensively. But the need to accelerate agricultural growth remains. Biotechnology could improve the yield of basic grain crops, enhance output growth in degraded and hostile environments and improve yields of non-grain crops. Further, since GM crops require typically fewer inputs than other crops they reduce the cost of production, *ceteris paribus,* and the (micro) nutrient content of food can be enhanced by biofortification.

Moreover, the path to greater adoption of biotechnology is fraught with uncertainty because the science is uncertain and many issues remain unresolved. Further, it is not clear which technology will be most profitable and, as argued above, the politics of adoption of this technology has not yet been sorted out.

9. Access to Food

In the terminology of Sen (1982), the problem of ensuring food adequacy as discussed above is a "technological approach" to the food problem. While demand and supply of food are essential ingredients in a strategy of assuring food security, Sen argues that there is a second approach —the "society-focused" approach which is of the view that political economy has a significant role to play in assuring food supply. The strongest argument in favour of this approach is that in recent times, although per capita availability of food has actually gone up there are large pockets of hunger and deprivation. Indeed, as shown at the beginning of this chapter, the number of hungry people could be increasing. Thus, food availability per capita is a very poor indicator of hunger or starvation. In fact, only when food is distributed equally among everyone can food availability per capita be considered a good indicator of hunger.

Since this has never been the case, a person's entitlement to food depends broadly, *inter alia*, on the remuneration they can get by selling their labour and how they can convert this remuneration into food purchases. Thus, hunger can exist or even increase without a rise in food prices. Sen's entitlement approach is group-specific, whereas the technological approach is aggregative.

Thus, according to Sen, food policy should anticipate needs, be ready to provide relief and generate entitlements for the hungry on a sustained basis. If it was possible, the simplest way to achieve these would be to supply free food. However, this will be expensive, if not also fiscally irresponsible. A more focused policy would be to subsidize food for the poor. If large-scale rural unemployment is also present, a third way would be to provide food for work. Such work might include the digging of irrigation canals and providing other rural infrastructure. These programs presuppose the existence and maintenance of a large stock of food grains. However, the efficiency of such policies have had more than their fair share of inefficiencies and wastage.[5]

Such considerations directly lead to the importance of avoiding acute food scarcity — sometimes leading to a famine. Unfortunately, such quasi-Malthusian outcomes are not just a relic of the past. Starvation, even the acute type exemplified by famines, does not mean that there is not enough food to eat. What matters is that people do not have enough food to eat (Sen, 1981). Sen considers two factors to be responsible for the occurrence of famines. The first is the endowment of skills, labour and capital that people have to trade. The second is the terms on which this endowment can be converted into food. Not having enough of the former is a "direct entitlement failure," and the latter a "trade entitlement failure." This approach is strengthened by the work of Ravallion (1997). He argues that when economies are under stress there are several severe market and institutional failures. In such situations, an exogenous shock can result in the kind of consumption stress that famines involve. Using estimates of multiple determinants of starvation, Ravallion reinforces Sen's entitlement approach as an explanation for famines.

While the entitlements approach has much to credit it with, there exists an alternative explanation (emphasizing inadequate availability) for the occurrence of famines. The most significant contribution to this alternative approach is O'Grada (2009). Unlike Sen, O'Grada argues that shortage of food is a very significant contributor to the occurrence of famines and provides evidence in support of this from a number of severe famines, including the Great Bengal Famine of 1943 and other severe famines. Hence, both the availability of food and the entitlement to food need to be taken into account when addressing acute food scarcity.

Famines, however, are not one-off events. Following a famine, there are long periods of acute malnutrition which often translate into stunting of children and have other deeper anthropometric consequences (Noland *et al.*, 2001; Kloos and Lindtjørn, 1994). Thus, while preventing the

---

[5] However, the evidence on the efficacy of these policies in reducing hunger is mixed. See, for example, Jha *et al.* (2013) for the case of India.

occurrence of acute food scarcity and famines is of extreme importance, attending to the after-effects of such acute food shortage is also a pressing concern.

10. Nutrition and the Role of Economic Growth

A large literature has grown up around examining the relationship between economic growth and poverty reduction and has, by and large, found that economic growth does lead to poverty reduction. Since the poverty line in many developing countries is based on nutritional intake, it is natural to extend this question to inquire whether economic growth also reduces undernourishment. Smith and Haddad (2002) studied child nutrition data from a large number of countries and came to the conclusion that income growth has a very strong impact on child nutrition. They come to the conclusion that substantial reduction in child undernutrition over the period 1990–2004 can be attributed to income growth. However, it is also important to ensure that a substantial portion of the incremental income accruing from economic growth be allocated to the alleviation of child undernutrition.

The beneficial effects of economic growth on child nutrition do not necessarily extend to adult undernutrition. In the case of India and some other countries, there is evidence to suggest that undernourishment in the general population has actually increased with rising income (Deaton and Drèze, 2009; Smith, 2013). Part of the explanation for this phenomenon lies in the shift in tastes towards more tasteful (rather than more nutritious) food with rising incomes (Behrman and Deolalikar, 1989; Jha *et al.*, 2009b) and the rising relative price of nutrients (Gaiha *et al.*, 2013).

11. Food Price Crises and How to Deal with Them

Timmer (2010) is of the view that food price crises are rare but regular events, occurring once every 30 years or so and are often unique events. The two most recent crises (1972–1973 and 2007–2008) had completely different origins. The former was caused primarily by an increase in petroleum prices, whereas the latter was largely a rice market phenomenon. Rice is the staple diet for most Asians, a huge chunk of humanity, and most Asian countries aim to be self-sufficient in rice. Hence, the rice market is very thin with very small quantities (compared to other food items) in international markets. Thus, disruptions to international trade in rice cause sharp increase in the level and volatility of rice prices in the short run and, more often than not, pressure for government intervention to stabilize prices.[6] Price rises also stimulate domestic production. Hence, there is a market as well as a government response.

At this stage, it is pertinent to ask how far the government response has been able to shield domestic consumers from rise in international food prices. Domestic, not international, prices affect consumer welfare, and the magnitude of the domestic response will help us understand the feedback effects to global demand and supply which will ultimately affect international prices. Dawe (2008) was the first to examine the extent to which the surge in world food prices during 2007–2008 was transmitted to domestic prices. He discovered that Asian countries were more likely to stabilize rice prices than wheat, but wheat price stabilization was still quite substantial in many countries. This is not surprising since rice, not wheat, is the major staple crop in Asian countries. The actual increase in domestic prices in large Asian countries was smaller than that in international prices. This degree of change varied considerably. Hence, there could be a short-term role for government to stabilize domestic prices.

An expanded view of this issue is taken by Anderson *et al.* (2013) who examine the impact on poverty of government intervention to stabilize

---

[6]The impact of such interventions on poverty in individual countries would depend on whether most of the poor are net sellers or consumers of grain. In the short run before adjustments in purchases can be made, the impact of food price increases on households is the product of the proportional change in the real price of a particular food item and the household's net purchase of that food. For net buyers of food, we would expect this impact to be large since the largest item in the household consumption basket is food. However, there is empirical evidence to suggest that most households in poor countries are rural and earn their living from farming. For these people, a rise in food prices could well augment income. In any case, food shares of total consumption expenditure alone are highly imperfect indicators of the welfare impact of food price rises. At the very least, these need to be augmented by the shares of household income obtained from the sale of food. Ivanic and Martin (2008) show that the short-run impact of food price rises in most cases is to raise the poverty head count ratio as well as the poverty gap.

prices. They find that, on balance, impediments to free trade in food grains in the aftermath of a food price shock have not helped in poverty reduction. A key reason for this is that such pre-emptive action by national governments overlooks the feedback effect of such action on international prices. Hence, part of the challenge for alleviating hunger in the 21st century is the smooth functioning of international trade in food. This is particularly important in light of the sharp increases in Preferential Trade Agreements (PTAs) and the role that trade in agricultural products performs in these PTAs.

Furthermore, and as highlighted by Timmer (2010), the role of politics during food price crises needs to be underscored. The building of international political consensus on how to address food price crises and prevent abrupt imposition of quotas and/or export bans should be emphasized.

Another point to be noted from Timmer (2010) is that current prices are not a good guide for what future prices will be like. Hence, it becomes difficult to find benchmarks for considering whether and when a food price crisis has occurred or is likely to occur. In this context, Bobenrietha *et al.* (2013) developed stock-to-use ratios for food grains which are shown to be actually consistent with the actual price series. Useful as this analysis is, more work needs to be done to quantify critical values for stocks beyond which a crisis can be said to occur. Furthermore, just as in standard forecasting exercise, confidence bands for the stock-to-use ratios need to be developed.

In this context, Toye (2009) considers whether the free market can be considered an adequate mechanism for redressing economic distress arising from rising food prices. The 2007–2008 food price crisis affected many commodities including wheat, rice, maize, butter and milk, poultry, meat and palm oil, among others. Reasons for the sharp rise in food prices in 2007–2008 included a rise in the price of oil, a drought in Australia, rising food demand (particularly from China), increased biofuel production and increased speculation which exacerbated existing price increases. But there is no reason to believe that these factors have caused some kind of structural break in these time series. In particular, speculation could work to rapidly dampen prices when such prices are on a downward trajectory. Bad weather events, like a drought, should be considered stochastic events and do not necessarily cause a change in the trend of prices.

However, sustained increases in income, notwithstanding stabilizing populations, should see a change in the demand structure for cereals and may amount to a structural break sometime in the future. Rising food prices will have deleterious effects on the poor, particularly those who are net buyers of food. To address these issues, the "invisible hand" of the market will need government support, including national governments, supported by the international donor community, devoting more resources to the targeted relief of the poor in developing countries; increasing the investment in the agricultural sector, focusing more on irrigation, rural roads, research and education; removing all obstacles to free trade in food; and eliminating distortionary biofuel subsidies.

Another vital element in the food delivery debate is the fact that an increasing amount of food will be delivered to consumers by supermarkets. This requires considerable overhaul of supply chains including agricultural modernization, migration of workers from the rural to the urban sector and emergence of urban industrial centres. Hence, economies will have to be prepared for the structural transformation that this will entail.

In particular, small farmers may lose out to supermarket supply chains once this structural transformation takes place. This has the potential of increasing food insecurity among small and marginal farmers and agricultural labourers. This underscores the importance of developing social safety nets and absorbing labour in alternative occupations.[7]

In this context, it is useful to inquire whether food aid can play a role in buttressing nutrition in developing countries. A classic contribution in this area is Mellor (1980). He argues that in the face of large calorie deficiencies, food aid can play a significant role in augmenting nutrition. Sometimes, this effect needs to be supplemented through rationing schemes and food for work programs targeted towards the poor.

[7] Jha (2014) shows in the case of India that despite the country's strong performance in economic growth its social safety expenditures are below those of countries with similar, even, lower GDP per capita in Purchasing Power Parity terms.

The consequent drop in food prices can have a dampening effect on food production which can be ameliorated through financial aid for higher procurement prices.

However, in real life food aid has rarely worked this well. Food aid should be countercyclical to domestic production in the recipient country, whereas it has often been pro-cyclical. This amounts to a misdirection of food aid. Furthermore, food aid has often been directed towards countries where the donor country has a strategic interest — not necessarily towards the country with higher nutritional deficiency. Furthermore, there are questions about the efficacy of food subsidy and food work programs in many of the developing countries towards which such food aid has been directed.[8]

12. Addressing Global Hunger

Finally, we come to the core issue of the prospects for addressing global hunger. A report commissioned by the UK Government Office for Science (2011) argues persuasively that hunger is the "antithesis of development". Thus, the alleviation, if not the elimination of hunger, must be a principal focus for research and policy for academics and policymakers. Addressing the risks that accompany widespread hunger (e.g. increased morbidity of children, higher incidence of disease, stunting, etc.) should also be given high priority.

While hunger is a condition that prevails today, food insecurity is relevant over time and is, hence, more pervasive than hunger. Undernutrition, particularly the inadequate access to micronutrients, can be debilitating for women and children.

In the regions most afflicted with hunger and food insecurity, i.e. Africa and South Asia, agricultural production needs to be augmented by

---

[8] Jha and Gaiha (2012) show that India's National Rural Employment Guarantee Program (NREGP) has not performed adequately with respect to the provision of 100 days of employment to each person in the rural sector who seeks employment under this scheme. Similarly, Jha *et al.* (2013) show that India's TPDS, which is central to the provision of food security, has had a chequered record at best despite huge public subsidies to support this program.

the harnessing of technologies, institutions, infrastructure and markets. In general, agricultural growth is associated with higher rates of poverty reduction in many poor countries. Hence, an all-out effort to improve agricultural growth and productivity is needed. Furthermore, since empirical evidence suggests that women are better providers within the household, the empowerment of women within the household and society is a must for addressing food insecurity and hunger. Such efforts could improve economic access to food for all. These efforts need to be complemented with efforts to empower women.[9] Empirical evidence suggests that increases in GDP from agriculture have a much larger impact on the expenditures of the poorest sections of the population. Thus, there is room for optimism that agriculture can help ameliorate global hunger.

In addition to supplementing the efforts to revamp agricultural productivity, this chapter advocates that governments commit to making the elimination of poverty and hunger central to any program of agricultural expansion. These policies should be supplemented with a strong effort to empower women. Their role in agricultural growth and their access to safe and adequate food should be assured by public policy (see footnote 9).

Effective social protection schemes should be designed to ensure that adequate food supplies reach the most vulnerable sections of society and lagging regions.[10] However, considerable attention needs to be paid to the design and continuous evaluation of such social safety nets as their efficacy cannot be taken for granted.

Finally, it should be understood that since hunger is a silent scourge on humankind, its eradication does not have a natural advocacy group. Public policy, civil society organizations and the like have an important role to play to ensure that the eradication of hunger gets the central focus it deserves.

---

[9] There is another aspect of assuring food availability, i.e. food wastage and food storage, which deserves emphasis. Estimates for the Indian economy reported in a BBC news item indicate that about 40% of fresh fruits and vegetables go waste. This amounts to about $7 billion annually. In addition, poor maintenance of food stocks by the Food Corporation of India leads to substantial grain loss.

[10] Jha (2014) shows in the case of India that despite the country's strong performance in economic growth, its social safety expenditures are below those of countries with similar, even, lower GDP per capita in Purchasing Power Parity terms.

13. Summary of Chapters in the Volume

The literature surveyed above is concerned with a long list of topics, and covering all or even most of which would be difficult in one volume. Hence, this volume concerns itself with key thematic and region specific issues. This volume is divided into three parts. The first part titled "Introduction and Thematic Issues" consists of three chapters. This introductory chapter is followed by a chapter on "The Political Economy of Food-based Social Safety Nets: Lessons from Indonesia's Experience Managing Food Security". Timmer examines possible ways of resolving the dilemma between ensuring high prices for farmers so that they have incentives to produce more and assuring food security and price affordability for consumers who are poor and unable to afford the resulting market prices. In this intriguing chapter, Timmer provides a history of how Indonesia has developed social safety nets to address this issue and articulates the fundamental question whether high producer prices which lead to domestic food security are the price that has to be paid to ensure political stability. A corollary of this argument is that protection of poor consumer groups would require efficient food safety nets. Timmer examines the performance of these safety nets for the case of rice in Indonesia.

Income and prices have traditionally been accepted as major drivers of food demand. However, recent waves of globalization could have led the sharp structural changes in the relationship between food demand, income and prices. In the next chapter of this volume, Peter Warr explores the evidence on two such possible demand shifters: urbanization and the ageing of the population. Both of these factors are known to affect food supply but could as well affect food demand. Warr surveys the literature on the relevance of these two factors to the demand for food, and finds that both urbanization and ageing raise the demand for energy-dense foods that take less time to prepare than traditional foods, and reduces the demand for hard-to-prepare staples. These effects are quantitatively higher in the case of urbanization as compared to ageing. This chapter thus provides important information for predicting future food demand.

Chapter 4 authored by Simrit Kaur and Harpreet Kaur examines conflicts and climate change as correlates of food security using fixed-effects panel data regression analysis over the period 1991–2014 for South Asia. The econometric analysis reveals that both conflicts and climate change worsen the already precarious food security situation in South Asia. In fact, the impact is even greater when prolonged conflicts are considered. Analyzing conflict–climate interactions, food insecurity appears to worsen further with temperatures deviating from their pre-structural break averages, when considered along with prolonged armed conflicts. The chapter concludes by recommending policies addressing food insecurity, conflicts, and climate change adaptation and mitigation.

The second part of this volume examines food security issues in the two Asian giants of China and India. Chapter 5 titled "The Chinese Dual Malnutrition: Facts, Challenges and Perspectives" by Zing You and Zekun Du reviews the dual burden of malnutrition — under- and overnutrition in terms of overweight and obesity facing Chinese children. Child nutrition and health have improved dramatically over the past three decades with less than one out of ten children being undernourished. However, income growth has induced excessive intake of fat and proportionately less protein and carbohydrates. About 15% of children are overweight or obese. Overnutrition appears to be a new threat to child development. Together with remaining undernutrition, it adds to the double burden of child malnutrition, challenging the government's blueprint of "healthy China" by 2030. The government has made great efforts in fighting against undernutrition, while overnutrition has not raised enough attention or action.

Chapter 6 titled "Food Security: The Indian Story" by Shyam Khadka and Deepika Anand succinctly reviews the progress in addressing long-standing problems of undernutrition in India. They begin by overviewing the current nutritional scenario in India and the strong nutritional transition that has taken place with economic development. Changes in dietary consumption patterns are reviewed and key determinants of nutritional outcomes are identified. Like many other economic variables, nutritional outcomes exhibit substantial spatial variation over India. The chapter identifies the districts in India experiencing the most severe undernutrition so that they could be targeted for policy intervention. The authors discuss the role of pro-nutrition agriculture in alleviating undernutrition, the emerging challenge of obesity and overweight in some sections of the population and outline the prospects for nutritional enhancement in India.

Chapter 7 titled "Is Variety the Spice of Life? India's Nutrition Experience" by Nidhi Kaicker, Vani Kulkarni and Raghav Gaiha revisits an important controversy in the analysis of calorie intake in India, viz., a decline in calorie intake in India in recent decades despite high economic growth. Deaton and Drèze (2009) had attributed this decline to lower calorie "requirements, due to improvements in sanitation, health, and more sedentary life styles". This chapter builds on the analyses of Behrman and Deolalikar (1989) and Jha *et al.* (2009a) who show that calorie elasticities are substantially less than food expenditure elasticities wherein food variety *per se* is valued. Using household-level data for 1994–2012, this chapter shows that diet diversification is associated with higher costs of calories mainly because of reliance on more expensive calories. This analysis also confirms that higher costs of calories and greater affluence are associated with reduction in calorie intake.

Chapter 8 titled "Food Security, Agriculture and Female Malnutrition in India" by Priya Rampal and Ranjula Bali Swain investigates the key linkages between maternal and child nutrition in India and underscores the important role that women play in agrarian economies. It reviews the nutritional status of women and children in India noting the fact that attaining nutritional adequacy is more important for them as compared to male adults. The role of agricultural remedies in attending nutritional deficiencies of women and children as well as social and public health policies such as adequate provision of water, sanitation and health are also discussed. The 2016 National Policy for Women and other programs being carried out by government agencies and self-help groups are also discussed. The chapter ends with some insightful policy recommendations.

Part III of the book reviews food security and nutritional issues in Africa. Chapter 9 titled "Africa's Food Insecurity and its Determinants" by Manoj Pandey examines progress of food insecurity in Africa and its determinants. He uses fixed-effect panel data regression approach to analyze annual data between 1990 and 2016 for 59 African countries. Key findings are that expansion of food production and agricultural output are strongly associated with reduced prevalence of undernourishment, depth of food deficit and prevalence of food inadequacy. While a higher aggregate income growth is associated with improved food security, rising rate of inflation and faster population growth have opposite effects. Remittances received by countries help to reduce prevalence and depth of food insecurity. Though not very consistent, better access to electricity, improved water sources and better road infrastructure are significant factors associated with better food security. The results add to the growing evidence on the importance of food self-sufficiency, rising aggregate and agricultural growth that could compensate for negative effects of rising rate of aggregate inflation and population growth.

Chapter 10 is titled "Agricultural Research Technology and Nutrition in Sub-Saharan Africa" and is authored by Raghav Gaiha and Shantanu Mathur. The chapter examines the relationships between agricultural research, technology and nutrition in Sub-Saharan Africa (SSA), drawing upon a rich and insightful literature. Given low productivity of African agriculture compared to the rest of the world, large increases in agricultural productivity are possible. This is central to the problem of reducing hunger and poverty in Africa, particularly SSA. These productivity gains are possible and could accrue where governments allocate the necessary resources to agricultural research and development. In SSA, however, public investment in agriculture is still far lower than what is needed. This is worrisome given that hunger in SSA has grown faster than in the rest of the world. This chapter carries out an assessment through a review of a large number of studies that have examined the factors determining adoption of innovative agricultural technology, their benefits and the underlying mechanisms, sustainability of the benefits, empowerment of women farmers and child nutrition, and prospects of youth employment in agriculture and elsewhere. A case is then made out for greater investment in agricultural research.

Chapter 11 titled "Rethinking Agricultural Transformation and Food Security in Africa" by Abbi M. Kedir and George Kararach notes two key tendencies in African agriculture in relation to food security. These tendencies are a rapidly rising population implying a rising demand for food. The other feature is one where farmers in African countries are subject to a variety of risks resulting from, *inter alia*, droughts, floods and other natural calamities that undermine agricultural productivity and robust food production. After a review of food security and its importance in development, this chapter discusses the role of technology and research in the transformation of African agriculture and food security, respectively. The fifth part discusses lessons from within and outside Africa on successful technology and research, and explores various policy options including the role of technology and research, trends in agricultural R&D expenditure, capacity challenges in agricultural technology research (both physical and human), political economy of biotechnology and the role of technology and food security. The benefits of African regional integration from the recently proposed WTO agricultural trade policy reforms (e.g. not complete but partial and reluctant removal of subsidies by rich countries) are also evaluated.

The final chapter (Chapter 12) of the book, authored by George Kararach and Abbi M. Kedir, is titled "Nutrition, Health and Productivity in Africa: Evidence from Ethiopia". This chapter is particularly relevant since Ethiopia has faced major food insecurity problems over the last four decades — with a significant recent drought affecting millions of households, adversely impacting nutritional attainment. It becomes critical to understand the effect of such nutritional shortfall on productivity and, more generally, on human capital investment. Formal quantitative analysis of this phenomenon is hampered by the paucity of data. This chapter examines fairly large individual-level data on nutrition and other relevant variables such as schooling, gender of the individual, schooling of parents, location and ethnicity. Using a rich panel data collected through the Ethiopian Urban Household Survey, the authors conduct a detailed analysis of a measure of nutrition/health, its determinant and its effect on productivity (i.e. wage), controlling for endogeneity and heterogeneity of nutrition returns. The econometric analysis is conducted in the context of both panel data and quantile regression models and covers all major cities of Ethiopia. Several pertinent policy conclusions are also advanced.

Acknowledgement

I would like to acknowledge with gratitude Raghav Gaiha's long-standing collaboration with me on the topic of food security.

References

Alderman, H., Chiappori, P., Haddad, L., Hoddinott, J. and R. Kanbur (1995) "Unitary versus Collective Models of the Household: Is It Time to Shift the Burden of Proof?" *The World Bank Research Observer*, Vol. 10, No. 1, pp. 1–19.

Anderson, K., Ivanic, M., and W. Martin (2013) "Food Price Spikes, Price Insulation, and Poverty", Policy Research Working Paper 6535, The World Bank.

Barrett, C. (2010) "Measuring Food Insecurity", *Science,* Vol. 327, pp. 825.

Basu, A. and M. Qaim (2007) "On the Adoption of Genetically Modified Seeds in Developing Countries and the Optimal Types of Government Intervention", *American Journal of Agricultural Economics*, Vol. 89, No. 3, pp. 784–804.

Basu, D. and D. Das (2015) "Social Hierarchies and Public Distribution of Food in Rural India", *The Journal of Development Studies*, DOI:10.1080/00220388.2015.1075975.

Behrman, J. and A. Deolalikar (1989) "Is Variety the Spice of Life? Implications for Calorie Intake", *The Review of Economics and Statistics*, Vol. 71, No. 4, pp. 666–672.

Bobenrietha, E., Wright, B. and D. Zeng (2013) "Stocks-to-Use Ratios and Prices as Indicators of Vulnerability to Spikes in Global Cereal Markets", *Agricultural Economics*, Vol. 44, Supplement, pp. 43–52.

Bobonis, G. (2009) "Is the Allocation of Resources within the Household Efficient? New Evidence from a Randomized Experiment", *Journal of Political Economy*, Vol. 117, No. 3, pp. 453–503.

Bresciani, F. and A. Valdes (eds.) (2007) *Beyond Food Production: The Role of Agriculture in Poverty Reduction.* Cheltenham, UK: Edward Elgar.

Dawe, D. (2008) "Have Recent Increases in International Cereal Prices Been Transmitted to Domestic Economies? The Experience in Seven Large Asian Countries", ESA Working Paper No. 08-03, FAO.

De Haen, H., Klasen, S. and M. Qaim (2011) "What Do We Really Know? Metrics for Food Insecurity and Undernutrition", *Food Policy*, Vol. 36, pp. 760–769.

Deaton, A. and J. P. Drèze (2009) "Food and Nutrition in India: Facts and Interpretations", *Economic and Political Weekly*, Vol. 14, No. February, XLIV.7. Available at: http://www.princeton.edu/~deaton/downloads/Food_and_Nutrition_in_India_Facts_and_Interpretations.pdf.

Eshel, G., Shepon, A., Makov, T. and R. Milo (2014) "Land, Irrigation Water, Greenhouse Gas, and Reactive Nitrogen Burdens of Meat, Eggs, and Dairy Production in the United States", *Proceedings of the National Academy of Sciences*, Vol. 111, No. 33, pp. 11996–12001.

Foresight Project (2011) "The Future of Food and Farming", *Final Project Report.* London: The Government Office for Science.

Miller, H. I. and D. L. Kershen (2014) "Wealthy Activist Vandana Shiva is a Poor Advocate for the Poor", *Forbes Magazine*, Vol. July.

Gaiha, R., Jha, R. and V. S. Kulkarni (2013) "Demand for Nutrients in India: 1993 to 2004", *Applied Economics*, Vol. 45, No. 14, pp. 1869–1886.

Godfray, C., Beddington, J., Crute, I., Haddad, L., Lawrence, D., Muir, J., Pretty J., Robinson, S., Thomas, S. and C. Toulmin (2010) "Food Security: The Challenge of Feeding 9 Billion People", *Science*, Vol. 327, pp. 812–818.

Government Office for Science (2011) *Prospects of Eliminating Hunger, Final Project Report.* London: HM Government.

Herring, R. (2007) "The Genomics Revolution and Development Studies: Science, Poverty and Politics", *Journal of Development Studies*, Vol. 43, No. 1, pp. 1–30.

Ivanic, M. and W. Martin (2008) "Implications of Higher Global Food Prices for Poverty in Low-Income Countries", Policy Research Working Paper 4594, The World Bank.

Jha, R., Gaiha, R. and A. Sharma (2009a) "Calorie and Micronutrient Deprivation and Poverty Nutrition Traps in Rural India", *World Development*, Vol. 37, No. 5, pp. 982–991.

Jha, R., Gaiha, R. and A. Sharma (2009b) "Modelling Variety in Consumption Expenditure on Food in India", *International Review of Applied Economics*, Vol. 23, No. 4, pp. 503–519.

Jha, R. and R. Gaiha (2012) "NREGS: Interpreting the Official Statistics", *Economic and Political Weekly*, Vol. 47, No. 40, pp. 18–22.

Jha, R., Gaiha, R., Pandey, M. K. and N. Kaicker (2013) "Food Subsidy, Income Transfer and the Poor: A Comparative Analysis of the Public Distribution System in India's States", *Journal of Policy Modeling*, Vol. 35, No. 4, pp. 887–908.

Jha, R. (2014) "Welfare Schemes and Social Protection in India", *International Journal of Sociology and Social Policy*, Vol. 34, No. 3–4, pp. 214–231.

Jha, R. and R. Gaiha (2016) *The Economics of Food Security* (in two volumes). Cheltenham: Edward Elgar.

Kakwani, N. and H. Son (2016) *Social Welfare Functions and Development: Measurement and Policy Applications*. London: Palgrave Macmillan.

Keating, B., Herrero, M., Carberry, P., Gardner, J. and M. Cole (2014) "Food Wedges: Framing the Global Food Demand and Supply Challenge Towards 2050", *Global Food Security*. Available at: http://dx.doi.org/10.1016/j.gfs.2014.08.004.

Kloos, H. and B. Lindtjørn (1994) "Malnutrition During Recent Famines in Ethiopia", *Northeast African Studies*, New Series, Vol. 1, No. 1, pp. 121–136.

Mellor, J. (1980) "Food Aid and Nutrition", *American Journal of Agricultural Economics*, Vol. 62, No. 5(Proceedings Issue), pp. 979–983.

Noland, M., Robinson, S., and T. Wang (2001) "Famine in North Korea: Causes and Cures", *Economic Development and Cultural Change*, Vol. 49, No. 4, pp. 741–767.

O'Grada, C. (2009) *Famine: A Short History*. New Jersey: Princeton University Press.

Popkin, B., Horton, S., Kim, S., Mahal, A. and J. Shuigao (2001) "Trends in Diet, Nutritional Status and Diet-related Noncommunicable Diseases in China and India: The Economic Costs of Nutrition Transition", *Nutrition Reviews*, Vol. 59, No. 12, pp. 379–390.

Pretty, J., Ball, A., Lang, J. and L. Morrison (2005) "Farm Costs and Food Miles: An assessment of the full cost of the UK weekly Food basket", *Food Policy*, Vol. 30, No. 1, pp. 1–19.

Quisumbing, R. and L. Smith (2007) "Intrahousehold Allocation, Gender Relations, and Food Security in Developing Countries", in *Case Study #4-5 of the Program: "Food Policy for Developing Countries: The Role of Government in the Global Food System"*, eds. Per Pinstrup-Andersen and Fuzhi Cheng, Cornell University (In collaboration with Søren E. Frandsen, FOI, University of Copenhagen Arie Kuyvenhoven, Wageningen University, Joachim von Braun, International Food Policy Research Institute).

Ravallion, M. (1997) "Famines and Economics", *Journal of Economic Literature*, Vol. 35, No. 3, pp. 1205–1242.

Sahn, D. and D. Stifel (2002) "Robust Comparison of Malnutrition in Developing Countries", *American Journal of Agricultural Economics*, Vol. 84, No. 3, pp. 716–735.

Sen, A. (1981) "Ingredients of Famine Analysis: Availability and Entitlements", *The Quarterly Journal of Economics*, Vol. 96, No. 3, pp. 433–464.

Sen, A. (1982) "The Food Problem: Theory and Policy", *Third World Quarterly*, Vol. 4, No. 3, pp. 447–459.

Senauer, B. (2008) "Food Market Effects of a Global Resource Shift Toward Bioenergy", *American Journal of Agricultural Economics*, Vol. 90, No. 5, pp. 1226–1232.

Smith, L. and L. Haddad (2002) "How Potent is Economic Growth in Reducing Undernutrition? What Are the Pathways of Impact? New Cross-Country Evidence", *Economic Development and Cultural Change*, Vol. 51, No. 1, pp. 55–76.

Smith, L. (2013) "The Great Indian Calorie Debate: Explaining Rising Undernourishment during India's Rapid Economic Growth", IDS Working Paper, Vol. 2013, No. 430.

SOFI (2015) *The State of Food Insecurity in the World*. Rome: Food and Agricultural Organization. Available at: http://www.fao.org/3/a-i4646e.pdf.

Srinivasan, T. N. (1981) "Destitution: A Discourse", *Journal of Development Economics*, Vol. 8, No. 1, pp. 3–19.

Stern, N. (2007) *The Economics of Climate Change*. Cambridge: Cambridge University Press.

Svedberg, P. (2002) "Undernutrition Overestimated", *Economic Development and Cultural Change*, Vol. 51, No. 1, pp. 5–36.

Timmer, P. (2003) "Biotechnology and Food Systems in Developing Countries", *Journal of Nutrition*, Vol. 133, No. 11, pp. 3319–3322.

Timmer, P. (2010) "Reflections on Food Crises Past", *Food Policy*, Vol. 35, No. 1, pp. 1–11.

Toye, J. (2009) "Development with Dearer Food: Can the Invisible Hand Guide Us?" *Journal of International Development*, Vol. 21, No. 3, pp. 757–764.

World Bank (2001) "Engendering Development", Policy Research Report 21776, Washington DC.

World Bank (2004) *Repositioning Nutrition as Central to Development: A Strategy for Large Scale Action*. Washington DC: The World Bank.

World Bank (2008) *World Development Report: Agriculture for Development*. Washington DC: World Bank.

Chapter 2

The Political Economy of Food-based Social Safety Nets: Lessons from Indonesia's Experience Managing Food Security*

C. Peter Timmer

Cabot Professor of Development Studies, Emeritus, Harvard University, Cambridge, MA 02138, USA
ptimmer63@gmail.com

Abstract

Food security has a long history in Indonesia, stretching back to efforts by royal rulers to ensure reliable availability of rice to their subjects. The Dutch colonial powers followed more of a *laissez-faire* approach until the Great Depression in the 1930s, when they were forced to take

*This chapter grows out of more than four decades as a policy analyst and advisor in Indonesia, and builds on an earlier paper for the World Bank that was an attempt to understand how Indonesia managed to stabilize rice prices for a quarter of a century, from 1973 to 1998, and then instituted a food-based social safety net in place of a stabilization policy. Author was involved personally over this entire time period, so much of what is reported in this paper draws on direct experience.

over the rice economy to prevent widespread hardship. The Indonesian government largely followed in the Dutch footsteps, but devoted even more resources to keeping rice prices stable. The world food crisis in 1972/73 caused the government to devote substantial policy attention and economic resources to increasing rice production in an effort to achieve self-sufficiency. This goal has been increasingly elusive after it was reached temporarily in the mid-1980s.

Ever since, the debate over food security in Indonesia has been focusing on two different dimensions of this issue — urban and rural. The urban approach is the widespread, inclusive economic growth that brings the great mass of the population above a meaningful poverty line. Also, stable rice prices in key urban markets are really a guarantee of food security to a rising share of the population (as many rural workers move to urban jobs).

Two reinforcing factors eliminate rural poverty — migration to urban opportunities and stimulation of farm incomes (beyond the impact of higher productivity) for the remaining rural population via higher commodity prices. This approach necessitates a reasonably wealthy urban middle class that willingly pays for the higher food prices and a progressively smaller and more productive agricultural workforce, i.e. a successful structural transformation. Japan, South Korea and Taiwan are countries that have followed this path.

But if farmers (especially, in Asia, rice farmers) become a very potent voting bloc in newly democratic societies, while many poor households still remain, in both rural and urban areas, the poor cannot outvote a coalition of urban middle-class households who want to guarantee supplies of rice in their local markets and farmers who want higher rice prices as a way to compensate for the loss of economic competitiveness in the production of labor-intensive crops (especially rice). This is the Indonesian story, but it also resonates in countries like Malaysia, the Philippines, Thailand and even China. Poverty is dealt with politically by distributing rice directly to poor households, and much of this chapter discusses Indonesia's experience with public rice distribution.

Keywords: Price stability, food security, structural transformation, rice economy, food logistics agency.

1. Introduction

Guaranteeing that food is available on a reliable and regular basis to all citizens is part of the "mandate of heaven" under which all Asian rulers are empowered, democratic or authoritarian. Indonesia is no exception. Its rulers have tried to maintain ready access to affordable rice since at least the 17th century. For most of its history, the main social safety net in Indonesia has been a public guarantee that rice would be available in urban markets at affordable (and stable) prices. If some citizens were too poor to be able to access this market-priced rice, they suffered, or were helped by local community organizations. The State's obligation extended only to affordable rice at stable prices in urban markets. When the State failed in this obligation, it often lost power.

This Asia-wide pattern is centuries old, but it would have resulted in only a minority of urban households being food secure unless further steps were taken. There are several possible logical pathways beyond the paradigm of stable rice prices in urban markets as the main approach to food security in Asia. One would be widespread, inclusive economic growth that brings the great mass of the population above a meaningful poverty line, so that stable rice prices in key urban markets really are a guarantee of food security to a rising share of the population (as many rural workers move to urban jobs).

Rural poverty is eliminated by two reinforcing factors — migration to urban opportunities and stimulation of farm incomes (beyond the impact of higher productivity) for the remaining rural population via higher commodity prices, an approach that is widespread in all developed countries. This approach is highly popular as a political strategy and has uniformly been rewarded by electoral success for parties that follow it. To work, however, this approach needs a reasonably wealthy urban middle class that willingly pays for higher food prices, and a progressively smaller and more productive agricultural workforce, i.e. a successful structural transformation. Japan, South Korea and Taiwan followed this path.

A second approach starts the protection of agriculture much earlier in the historical process of structural transformation, when farmers (especially, in Asia, rice farmers) become a very potent voting bloc in newly democratic societies. Many poor households remain, in both rural and urban areas, but they are not enough to outvote a coalition of urban middle-class households who want to guarantee supplies of rice in their local markets, and farmers who want higher rice prices as a way to compensate for the loss of economic competitiveness in the production of labour-intensive crops (especially rice). This is the Indonesian story, but it also resonates in Malaysia, the Philippines, Thailand and even China.

How can politicians reconcile high rice prices (to "ensure" food security via increased rice production) with the existence of a substantial proportion of households unable to afford that rice? The answer is obvious, both politically and logistically. Distributing rice directly to poor households (despite how ineffective the actual delivery system might be) is a political winner. And for the food logistics agency, previously charged with stabilizing rice prices around a long-run trend in world prices, the reality of high domestic rice prices sharply reduces the need for those services. A new mandate, to procure rice at high prices from farmers and deliver it at subsidized prices to poor households, is also a new lease on life. This new approach, now well established as the political norm in Indonesia, has emerged from a sequence of food crises over several centuries.

2. Ten Crises that Shaped Indonesia's Approach to Food Security

(1) The Indonesian sultanates rule with a "mandate from heaven: rice for the people". Sultan Amangkurat I prohibited the export of rice from Java in 1655 in response to a drought that sent rice prices up by 300%.

(2) The Dutch took over the rice economy of the Netherlands East Indies in March, 1933, in response to collapsing rice prices in the region. Rice milling, inter-island and international trade in rice, and price formation were all tightly controlled by government agencies, most of them newly formed for the task. These actions reversed earlier Dutch policy that allowed free trade and market prices to dictate rice production and price formation.

(3) The collapse of the Sukarno government in 1965–1966, after a decade of spiraling inflation and repeated shortages of rice in urban markets, gave the new Suharto government a mandate for stability, a mandate it eagerly seized as a political endorsement of military control. A food logistics agency (BULOG) was established to control rice prices, with a head who reported directly to the president, and with a line of credit at subsidized interest rates from the Central Bank.

(4) The world food crisis in 1972–1973 caught the Indonesian government, and BULOG, unprepared. After several years of price stability, rice prices spiralled out of control and the government quickly tried to arrange emergency imports from a world rice market that completely disappeared for nearly a year. The response, once control was regained late in 1973, was to formulate plans for greater attention to agricultural development, to increasing productivity of the rice sector and to keeping rice prices stable.

(5) Surpluses are just as hard to manage as shortages. The collapse of commodity prices in world markets in the mid-1980s, including for rice, again caught BULOG unprepared for the new contingencies. A major re-evaluation of how to define and maintain food security in Indonesia was commissioned. A new focus on poverty came to the fore with the realization that surplus rice could be distributed as part of a social safety net. By 1991, BULOG had implemented a trial programme of "Special Market Operations (OPK)" to deliver rice directly to drought-stricken villages as a poverty-relief effort.

(6) The focus on disposing of rice surpluses caused BULOG to lose track of its actual stock situation in mid-1994. A drought caused rice production to fall, BULOG did not respond when stocks were depleted early in 1995 before the new rice harvest started in March, and a rice crisis was in the making. President Suharto replaced the head of BULOG and the new head ordered emergency imports that arrived just in time to keep rice prices from getting out of control. Knowing what to do makes all the difference, but "business as usual" was a failure. Still, by August, 1996, it was possible for the *Jakarta Post* to report a story (based on an interview with me) that "BULOG to limit itself to poverty alleviation", a recognition of the changing dynamics in the rice economy.

(7) The Asian financial crisis in 1997–1998 caused Indonesia to lose control of its macroeconomy. An important lesson was learned: it is impossible to stabilize rice prices when the macroeconomy and exchange rate are out of control. Out of the macropolitical chaos emerged a new OPK, the "Special Market Operations" that BULOG implemented to deliver rice to poor households. This programme almost immediately became the largest element in the country's shift to targeted social safety nets as it gave up its effort to stabilize prices.

(8) Democracy also emerged in 1998 out of the chaos after the Asian Financial Crisis, and the political economy of food security in Indonesia took entirely new directions. High rice prices as a conscious political choice of policy in 2004–2006 became the dominant approach, with quite significant impact on the poor. RASKIN (*Beras untuk Orang Miskin*), the OPK programme re-labelled as "rice for the poor", became the political "answer" to the problems for food security caused by high rice prices. Although "rice self-sufficiency" had long been a key objective of Indonesia's drive for food security, stable rice prices had always trumped the desire to restrict imports. That political calculus changed in the first half of the 2000s.

(9) Indonesia was quite successful in getting through the 2007–2008 world food crisis, partly because its domestic prices were already high. When the Minister of Trade announced a ban on rice *exports* early in 2008, the world rice market took little notice — Indonesia has never been a significant rice exporter. But domestic consumers and traders were reassured that ample supplies were available and there was no panicked hoarding of the sort seen in the Philippines and even urban markets in Vietnam. Stable domestic prices, even if very high, were a political winner for Susilo Bambang Yudhoyono's (SBY's) second Presidential campaign in 2009.

(10) BULOG ran out of rice in 2015–2016, the worst *El Niño* year on record. Some officials in the new Jokowi government tried to order imports in a timely fashion, even recalling publicly the fall of the Suharto government over spiraling rice prices during the previous worst *El Niño* in 1997, when imports were also delayed. But rice imports had become political dynamite, and the contracts were delayed or cancelled. Rice prices spiralled, BULOG had to cut back deliveries to Raskin recipients, and once again the country learned that "rice self-sufficiency" is not food security. Nascent efforts to reform the Raskin program, even to convert it to cash in urban settings and rural areas with good market infrastructure, were put on hold.

Crises focus the mind, and political action. Interpreting the long-run impact of these repeated food crises over nearly four centuries of Indonesian history is a matter of judgement, of course, but at least three phases in the evolution of policy approaches to food security are visible to this observer. First, stabilizing rice prices in urban markets has long been the political touchstone of legitimacy. Second, a strategy of pro-poor growth, building on the potential to improve rural labour productivity via broad-based agricultural development, brought the rural poor into the political calculus of food security. And third, perhaps prematurely, the country moved explicitly to a targeted, food-based social safety net as the offset to a political strategy of buying the votes of rice farmers via high rice prices. This strategy utilizes Raskin, the State-funded programme of rice distributions to the poor that began officially during the Asian Financial Crisis in 1998 (when the Suharto government fell as well and a new democratic government took over). Each of these phases is discussed in turn.

3. Phase 1: Rice Price Stabilization in Indonesia

Why did Indonesia attempt to stabilize rice prices for very extended periods of time? The long perspective encourages a related question about institutional learning: "how?" The motivation issue is important because it drives the search for effective mechanism design that permits rice prices to be stabilized in a cost-effective manner. With the "why" question answered, the "how" question becomes clearer.

A bit of autobiography. Virtually everything I know now about food policy comes from my experience in Indonesia since 1970. I like to think I left behind a legacy of informed analysis of the key food policy issues that played out over my four decades of very active engagement in the country (and region), but none of that analysis would have been forthcoming, much less useful, without the constant questioning from key policy makers of "what to do?" Their questions constantly drove the analysis. But their questions were always about "how". No one in Indonesia at the time, policymakers, academics, journalists, or the "man in the street", ever doubted that stable rice prices were not just a "good thing", but essential to political stability and economic growth. Rice was, as the influential student newspaper *Harian KAMI* put it in late 1967, "the barometer of the economy".

No modern economist would have a clue as to what that means. But for a young advisor to the government in the 1970s (and later as a more experienced analyst), figuring out how to stabilize rice prices was the quintessential core of development. Without stable rice prices, there would be no government; without a government, there would be no development. Given the history of other countries in Asia that had managed rapid economic growth — Japan, South Korea and Taiwan — that seemed like a compelling argument at the time, and still does.

So, for what it's worth, here is my take on why rice price stabilization was so important to policy makers in Indonesia over many decades, and how we tried to do it. This was very much "learning by doing," and my own academic base more or less forced me to ask, "*why* is this so important, and *how* do we do it efficiently?" It took several years after I arrived in Indonesia for me to even understand that rice price stabilization was not "desirable" within the mainstream paradigm of trade economics — there are actually "gains to trade" from price instability. I have spent several decades trying to reconcile that "cognitive dissonance" with both my day-to-day activities in Indonesia and my academic career at Harvard, where I tried to explain to students why stable rice prices were so important and how to manage the stabilization process.

3.1. *The Motivation for Rice Price Stabilization in Indonesia: A Brief Overview*[1]

Food security as a political concept requires an operational definition. In most Asian countries this has taken the form of domestic price stability relative to world prices, thus requiring state control over trade flows in rice. In order to minimize the need to resort to trade at all, and to avoid the uncertainties in the international price of rice, self-sufficiency has also become a popular objective, the more so as countries become rich enough to afford the protection implied by measures needed to implement policies that achieve greater degrees of self-sufficiency.

A further impetus towards greater domestic rice production has been the fear of food shortages in urban areas, which evoke a universal and visceral reaction. Governments are held accountable for provisioning cities at reasonable costs, and citizens have repeatedly demonstrated their

---

[1]This material draws especially on Timmer (1995), which was an effort to distill lessons from 25 years of personal involvement in the process of stabilizing rice prices in Indonesia.

capacity to bring down governments that fail in this obligation.[2] It is acute food shortages — not the average level of food prices — that induce anti-government panics, however. Food shortages are simply the mirror image of sharp price rises.

Indonesia provides a particularly vivid case study of policy initiatives designed specifically to stabilize the domestic price of rice — using imports or domestic production to avoid food shortages — with a careful analytical debate paralleling the policy actions. The role of trade versus domestic production as the basis for food security has been analyzed and discussed in a surprisingly open and articulate manner since the beginning of the Suharto government in 1967.[3]

The proximate definition of food security in Indonesia has always revolved around price stability, especially for the price of rice, the country's primary food staple. The analysis that underpinned this approach never focused only on the static and partial equilibrium consequences of changes in rice prices. Instead, an effort was made, even well before computable general equilibrium models became a standard tool of policy analysis, to consider dynamic and economy-wide ramifications of price policy, the distributional consequences for farmers and consumers, and the role of other commodities in the rice stabilization program.

3.2. *Is Food Security Ensured Through Self-sufficiency in Rice?*

Self-sufficiency in rice and other foodstuffs such as sugar and soybeans has been a consistent (if often rhetorical) objective of Indonesian agricultural policy since the beginning of the New Order regime in 1967 (Timmer, 1975). Because of fluctuations due to weather (especially *El Niño* events), diseases and pests, rice production in Indonesia is unstable and in any particular year can be above or below the trend in rice consumption. In order to stabilize the rice economy from production

[2] The revolutions in Tunisia and Egypt in 2011 are only the latest examples. See Kaplan (1984) for a fascinating historical account of the relationship between urban masses and their rulers with respect to provisioning of basic foodstuffs.

[3] An early summary of the analytical debate is in Timmer (1990).

instability, as well as from sharp fluctuations in world prices for rice, BULOG, the Indonesian Food Logistics Agency, was charged to operate a floor and ceiling price policy using domestic buffer stocks as the balance wheel to smooth out year-to-year fluctuations in production and consumption. The goal was to keep rice consumption on a smooth trend despite unstable rice production. The primary policy instrument for stabilizing rice *consumption* is the stabilization of rice *prices,* which has been BULOG's most important task.[4]

Successful stabilization of rice prices between a policy-determined floor and ceiling price requires an active and on-going *analytical capacity* — to determine the appropriate levels for the floor and ceiling price each year — that is directly linked to the political (and budgetary) decision-making process. Indonesia developed this capacity gradually through the early 1970s and 1980s, relying initially on foreign experts and eventually on local analysts, many of whom had returned from foreign academic training. Much of this analytical effort is now in the public record.

From the late 1960s until the early 1980s, imports of rice were used routinely by BULOG, as the balance wheel between supply and demand in its defence of a floor price and ceiling price for rice. The world food crisis in 1972–1973 stimulated serious efforts to increase rice production, and the long-sought goal of rice self-sufficiency was achieved in the mid-1980s. Thus, the balancing role of international trade was superseded by the problems of managing domestic buffer stocks as the sole mechanism for balancing seasonal and annual differences between production and consumption.[5]

---

[4] This approach works well when incomes are reasonably stable, but fails when there is an economy-wide collapse, as in 1998. See Timmer (2010) for further discussion of the macro setting for successful rice price stabilization.

[5] President Suharto's determination to avoid rice imports took international trade as a balancing mechanism off the policy agenda. Indeed, Indonesia was supposed to be "self-sufficient" in rice — after all, FAO had given him a gold medal in 1985 for that achievement. By the early 1990s the President's economic advisors had convinced him that "self-sufficiency on trend" was a more appropriate policy objective, and limited imports again became operationally feasible, although obtaining permission from the President remained difficult and BULOG was no longer able to count on imports for short-run supply management. The political difficulty in arranging for rice imports remains to this day.

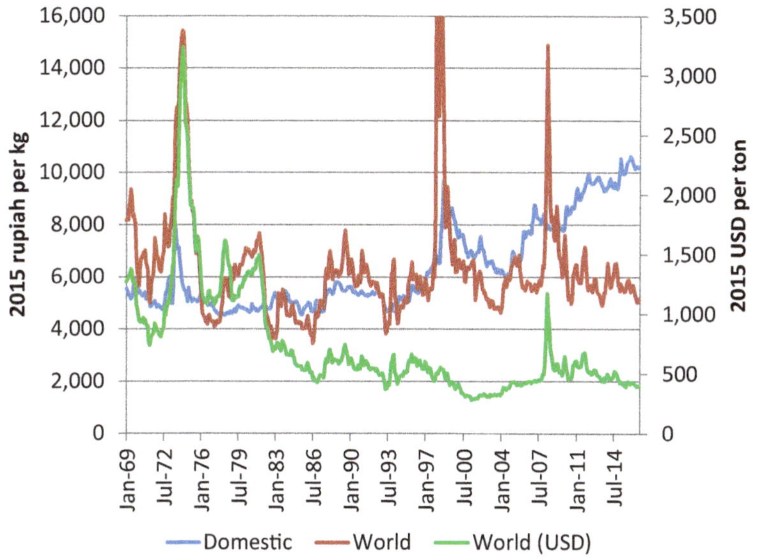

Figure 1. Real rice prices in Indonesia, domestic (Rp) (blue), imported from World (Rp) (red), and imported from World (USD) (green).

Source: Courtesy of David Dawe.

Figure 1 shows clearly that BULOG was quite successful in stabilizing rice prices from late in 1973, when it regained control of domestic prices after a good rice harvest, until the Asian Financial Crisis in late 1997. For the statistically minded, Table 1 presents the comparative evidence by time period using the coefficient of variation (CV, or the standard deviation of monthly prices divided by the mean of prices). The reference for stability of domestic prices is what is happening to world prices. As Table 1 shows, domestic rice prices have always been somewhat more stable than world prices, but the relative stability is especially striking for the Suharto era from January, 1969, to right before the Asian Financial Crisis in July, 1997. During this time period, when BULOG was most successful in its logistical operations, the domestic CV is less than a third of the world CV. The comparison would be even more striking if it ran from late 1973, after BULOG regained control of the Indonesian rice economy (and "learned its lesson…") until mid-1977.

Table 1. Real Rupiah prices.

	I. Whole period (January 1969 to July 2014)	II. Suharto pre-1998 AFC (January 1969 to July 1997)	III. Post Suharto (January 1999 to July 2014)	IV. Post 2007/8 food price crisis (November 2008 to July 2014)
Mean				
Domestic	5132.91	4303.20	6562.17	7490.28
World	4760.10	4452.22	4988.76	4928.22
Standard deviation				
Domestic	1263.43	410.94	943.61	563.05
World	1591.70	1448.70	1042.13	684.18
Coefficient of variation				
Domestic	0.25	0.10	0.14	0.08
World	0.33	0.33	0.21	0.14

Source: Courtesy of Peter Warr.

After 1998 (and the establishment of democracy), BULOG has not been very successful at stabilizing rice prices, but high rice prices seem to be the political objective rather than stable or efficient prices. It is also worth pointing out that there was a sharp spike in 1998 in "world" rice prices as measured in real Rupiahs, a spike that does not appear when world rice prices are measured in US dollars. The difference, of course, is that the Asian Financial Crisis caused the Indonesian Rupiah to collapse. It is impossible to stabilize domestic rice prices in the middle of a complete meltdown of the economy and political system.

3.3. *Lessons from Indonesian Experience*

A key element of government involvement in reaching self-sufficiency is through the *level* of rice prices maintained in the domestic economy.

Other things being equal, a higher level of rice prices will increase rice production, decrease rice consumption and make self-sufficiency easier to achieve. It has often been said that Indonesia can always be self-sufficient in rice at some price; the issue is whether consumers can maintain satisfactory levels of rice consumption as well. But domestic rice prices do not exist in a vacuum. In particular, their level relative to the trend of prices in the world market and relative to the costs of inputs to farmers (especially fertilizer prices) strongly influences the efficiency with which consumers and producers allocate the scarce economic resources of the society.

Stabilization itself is also an element in domestic production and its contribution to food security. The short-run policy issue is the level of BULOG stocks considered appropriate for maintaining stable rice prices. With infinite stocks, prices can be kept completely stable, but both economic theory and experience dictate that a finite stock level cannot defend price stability under all circumstances.[6] Accordingly, an important trade-off exists. Larger buffer stocks permit a longer period of stable prices, but at costs that rise exponentially with the size of the buffer stock. Smaller stocks require that prices fluctuate more, but with substantial cost savings. The only escape from this apparent dilemma is to add a degree of freedom to the system by permitting supplies to move into or out of the country as an additional balance wheel, once stocks are drawn down or warehouses filled up. As noted, a rigid definition of "self-sufficiency" removed the operational role for imports for a number of years. Still, this experience in trying to understand the value of additional stocks in the Indonesian context of coping with self-sufficiency was valuable after the world food crisis in 2007–2008 in understanding the value of additional stocks at a global level (which must be self-sufficient by definition). See Timmer (2014b) for a review of different approaches to valuing grain reserves.

Three elements of government policy interact to create the economic environment for self-sufficiency in rice, and its subsequent role in food

[6] See Williams and Wright (1991) for a sophisticated analysis of the limits to price stabilization with finite stocks.

security: (1) public investments in rice production to maintain it on the trend of rice consumption — mostly in rice research and extension, irrigation facilities and rural roads; (2) the establishment of a domestic level of rice (and fertilizer) prices that reflects their long-run opportunity costs in world markets — a substantial, market-wide fertilizer subsidy in the mid-1980s was a major factor in boosting rice production to self-sufficiency and the debate over fertilizer subsidies continues even today and (3) stabilization of domestic rice prices through market interventions using buffer stocks as a balance wheel — and imports when politically feasible.

Each of these elements has powerful efficiency effects individually, as well as direct impact on the state budget, and these effects make each component a separate, important policy issue. But the interconnections among the three elements make it impossible to set policy for one without having a substantial impact on the others. *Consistency among all three elements is essential* in the long run if substantial resources are not to be wasted. Achieving this consistency is clearly the most difficult aspect of designing a policy to assure food security at the macro level.

3.4. *The New Policy Debate: Price Stability at What Price?*

Price stabilization has remained an important policy objective during surpluses and deficits, but the financial costs,[7] feasible levels of prices and general policy thrust with respect to the agricultural sector are sharply different when the rice economy is in surplus and the main political

[7]Relatively little is known publicly about the financial costs of BULOG's activities to stabilize rice prices. The best estimate is for 1991, a year when BULOG was actively managing the price stabilization effort solely on the basis of its domestic buffer stock. For that year, the full financial costs of BULOG's rice activities were $233 million, which amounted to 0.11% of total GDP, and about 1.2% of the National Budget. See Pearson (1993) for more details.

problem is maintaining the floor price for rice farmers, and when it is in deficit and urban prices are rising. Because of the high costs of storing rice in the tropics, the finite size of stocks, and the sharply limited role for imports for political reasons, wider margins between the floor price and ceiling price have become a *de facto* balance wheel as well, but these wider margins call in question the implicit assumption that food security and price stability are synonymous.

Indonesia made a policy decision in 2004 to raise domestic rice prices significantly above world prices (by preventing imports). When shortages started to emerge in mid-2006 and domestic prices rose quickly, a vigorous and open debate took place over the impact of the rice import ban, and how to arrange imports in a timely fashion to prevent further price increases and harm to the poor. By early December, 2006, *The Jakarta Post* ran a "Headline" story where I argued that "Banning rice imports [is] 'not the right option.'"

A paper prepared for the Minister of Trade at the time presented options for managing the impending rice crisis by arranging emergency rice imports. She immediately requested Presidential permission to start the import process. An *INPRES* was issued on December 9, 2006, authorizing imports. Unfortunately, there was enough political and bureaucratic opposition to prevent rice imports from arriving until late February, which was far too late to prevent a sharp spike in rice prices in December 2006 and January/February 2007. A significant increase in poverty was subsequently reported from SUSENAS data collected in March 2007. This increase in poverty was directly caused by the decision to restrict rice imports and keep domestic rice prices well above world prices (Warr, 2011).

This episode was repeated late in 2015 and early in 2016 as the severe *El Niño* impacted rice production in Indonesia (despite claims by the Ministry of Agriculture that rice production actually increased). Attempts to import rice were thwarted by domestic political interests and prices rose more than 50% in just 3 months. Stabilizing rice prices as the foundation of Indonesia's food-based social safety net is clearly a thing of the past.

4. Pro-Poor Growth and Food Security: The Inclusion of Rural Households as the Second Phase in a Food-Based Social Safety Net[8]

Only 60 years ago, Indonesia was one of the poorest countries in Asia. The story of its poverty and poverty reduction is a story of the political and economic eras that determined the nation's development trajectory: colonial rule and exploitation; authoritarian rule, coupled with sustained growth, then dramatic collapse; and, most recently, democracy accompanied by economic flux and tentative stabilization. At independence in 1945, dislocated by Japanese occupation during World War II after years of exploitative Dutch colonialism, the vast majority of Indonesia's population was impoverished. By 1993, however, with poverty reduced to 14% of the population and annual economic growth at more than 7%, Indonesia was ranked along with a handful of other East Asian countries as a High-Performing Asian Economy (World Bank, 1993) and lauded for its astonishing transformation. In order to understand this remarkable turnaround it is necessary to develop an understanding of the key factors that drove the change in livelihoods of some 100 million Indonesians.[9] This section tells the extraordinary story of poverty reduction and economic growth that has occurred since Indonesia emerged from colonial rule.

[8]This section draws on Chapter 2, "A History of Growth and Poverty Reduction", in *Making the New Indonesia Work for the Poor: A Poverty Assessment,* conducted by the World Bank in 2006. I was the main author of Chapter 2. See Timmer (2004, 2010) for further discussion of the links between a strategy of pro-poor growth based on agricultural development and a stable food system.

[9]Indonesia provides global lessons that the development profession has built on: "Indonesia is the original home of the dual economy. Boeke's experience during the Dutch colonial administration of Java led him to identify two types of economic agents, 'rational' and 'traditional' — with almost entirely separate spheres of economic activity" (Boeke, 1946). Lewis (1954) built his Nobel-Prize-winning model of the dual economy with unlimited supplies of labour on the behaviour of such agents (Timmer, 2005, p. 15).

4.1. *A Troubled History and Chronic Poverty*

For the duration of the 350-year period of Dutch colonial rule, the trade and tax regime favoured Dutch extraction of income with dire consequences for the Indonesian population. Analysis provided by Van der Eng and interpreted by Timmer (2005) enables an examination of growth, the severity of poverty (through a comparison of the annual food energy intake measured in kcals), and the income elasticity of consumption over the past century. The record shows marked variability in both the rate of economic growth and how well it was connected to the poor over a series of political and economic epochs. During the 19th century, growth in consumption was negative, estimated at –0.34 kcal/year — the second-lowest in Indonesia's measured history — while the index of pro-poor growth (IPPG)[10] was only a fraction of the long-term average, illustrating the severe disconnect between the poor and the modest economic growth that occurred during this period. In the mid- to late-19th century, similar to most other regions of Southeast Asia, the historical record of Indonesia was one of severe poverty (Timmer, 2004).

The collapse of export prices and disastrous economic management in the 1920s resulted in the lowest growth rate and least pro-poor growth period in Indonesia's recorded history. At the beginning of the 20th century, when Dutch public opinion influenced the management of the colonies, a more developmental approach, known as "ethical policy", was implemented for a brief period. The policy brought significant benefit to the economy (growth reached 1.63% per year) and to the poor (food

[10]A crude "index of pro-poor growth" IPPG shown in Table 2 is based on an analytical relationship between the overall incidence of poverty and the observed, average income elasticity of demand (based on regression analysis of the long-run time series data). The income elasticity of food energy (calories) for the entire period from 1880 to 1990, estimated to be 0.313, is used as the long-run base, scaled to one (in bold). It is multiplied times the long-run growth rate in per capita incomes, 0.89% per year, to generate the long-run average Index of Pro-Poor Growth (IPPG) of 0.89. The income elasticity for each separate epoch is then scaled relative to the long-run average, and multiplied times the growth rate in per capita incomes, to generate the IPPG for each epoch. Note that the IPPG incorporates both the growth and the distributional dimensions of pro-poor growth, and this index is thus a country-specific version of Equation (1) in "Concept Paper on Operationalizing Pro-Poor Growth," World Bank (2004).

intake increased an annual average of 1.39 kcal). But this internal investment in the country lasted for only a brief period. The collapse of world prices for export commodities in the 1920s, and the abysmal economic management of Indonesia[11] during the Great Depression resulted in the lowest growth and rate of pro-poor growth in any period before independence. It is true that by then the colonial authorities had built a significant network of irrigation and transport facilities, but there was very little investment in educating the nation's population. According to national survey data, only 3.5% of the population was attending school of any kind in 1939, compared with 26.7% in 1995. Poverty increased significantly during the period of World War II and the subsequent struggle for independence, which only reached closure with final acceptance by the Dutch in 1949. The tumultuous global period spanning the Great Depression, the Pacific War, and the fight for independence (1925–1950), saw a marked deterioration in per capita income growth rates (–2.42%) and a negative rate of pro-poor growth (–2.57%). (Table 2).

After independence, during the period when the Indonesian nation was being built, weak and inward-looking policies resulted in an increase in poverty rates. By the early 1960s, similar to other post-independence states, poverty had fallen in the postwar recovery and Indonesia was muddling along with modest growth and weak but quasi-democratic governance. After Sukarno imposed "guided democracy" in 1959, however, the situation deteriorated sharply. Adopting an inward-looking development policy and severely neglecting agriculture, Indonesia was "a prime exemplar of the dangerously degenerative consequences of weak governance and a sickly economy" (McIntyre, 2003). Incomes fell dramatically and the hyperinflation of 1965–1966 had an adverse impact on the entire population as the poverty rate increased rapidly and the economy collapsed.[12] Probably 70% of the population was absolutely poor by 1966.

[11] The Dutch forced the Netherland East Indies, the Dutch colonial name for Indonesia, to stay on the Gold Standard well after their regional competitors, including the Japanese, devalued.

[12] At 2.37, the IPPG is surprisingly high during the Sukarno era, when economic policy is widely regarded to have been a disaster. But a combination of a modest recovery from the quarter century of depression and wars, with average per capita incomes rising 1.5%

Table 2. Long-term patterns of pro-poor growth in Indonesia.[13]

Time period	Annual growth in income per capita (%/yr)	Annual growth in consumption (kcal) (%/yr)	Income elasticity of consumption for kcal	Index of pro-poor growth (IPPG)*
Dutch colonial exploitation 1880–1905	0.33	−0.34	0.051 **0.165**	0.05
"Ethical Policy" under the Dutch 1905–1925	1.63	1.39	0.878 **2.805**	4.57
Depression, Pacific War, and fight for independence 1925–1950	−2.42	−0.78	0.333 **1.064**	−2.57
The Sukarno era, including the "Guided Economy" 1950–1965	1.46	0.68	0.509 **1.626**	2.37
The "New Order" regime of Soeharto 1965–1990	3.45	2.10	0.595 **1.901**	6.56
Long-term averages 1880–1990	0.89	0.22	0.313 **1.000**	0.89

Note: * See text and footnote 10 for the definition of IPPG and an explanation of how it is calculated and interpreted.
Source: Timmer (2005).

Hunger was widespread (Timmer, 2003). Unsurprisingly, in 1968, with no hint of the future, Myrdal (1968) observed in *Asian Drama*... "no economist holds out any hope for Indonesia".

4.2. *A Period of Growth and Rapid Poverty Reduction*

The trajectory of growth and poverty transformed dramatically under the New Order government of President Suharto. Starting in 1968, for three

per year, and large average income elasticity for food energy, suggest that what growth there was actually reached the poor.

[13] Details of the regressions are provided in Timmer (2005), along with a full explanation of the analytical relationship between the overall incidence of poverty and the average income elasticity of demand for food energy.

remarkable decades, Indonesia's GDP grew an average of 7.4% per annum. As a result, in 1997 Indonesia's per capita income reached US$906, more than quadruple the 1968 level. When compared with previous periods in Indonesian history, the quarter century from 1965 to 1990 saw an annual growth of caloric intake of 2.1% a year, 50% higher than the next best epoch in 1905–1925 and almost 10 times the long-term average. The index of pro-poor growth reached 6.56 for the period 1965–1990 — the highest in Indonesian history — 7 times the long-term average and nearly half as large again as the next best epoch in 1905–1925.

The story of Indonesia's poverty reduction is first and foremost a story of sustained pro-poor growth. From 1970 onwards, large and sustained reductions in poverty in Indonesia have only occurred during periods of sustained economic growth: the more rapidly the country's economy grew, the more rapidly poverty was reduced; slower growth always resulted in slower reduction in poverty; and the greater the economic crisis, the more severe was the setback. Over these three decades, each percentage point of growth resulted in a 0.3% reduction in poverty.

The pro-poor performance for these three decades was based on a conscious strategy that combined rapid economic growth with investment and policies that ensured growth reached the poor. The strategy integrated the macroeconomy with the household economy by lowering the transactions costs of operating in markets. This strategy also effectively combined efforts to increase human capabilities and increase demand for the output from poor households, including their labour (conceptualized in Figure 2). It was designed and implemented by highly skilled economic planners (the "technocrats") outside the political sphere, but at the direct urging of President Suharto. Huge investments were made in the expansion of education, family planning and health; transactions costs fell markedly through the construction of roads and other infrastructure that enabled the poor to be connected to the growth process; and, sound macroeconomic management was (from the late 1970s) accompanied by a competitive exchange rate.

Good exchange-rate management enabled Indonesia to stimulate an export-led economy and labour-intensive growth, ensuring the poor were connected into the country's growth. Between 1976 and 1978, income distribution deteriorated sharply as the real appreciation of the rupiah reduced the profitability of tradable goods production, especially in agriculture (Warr, 1984). Although the regional and commodity dimensions of

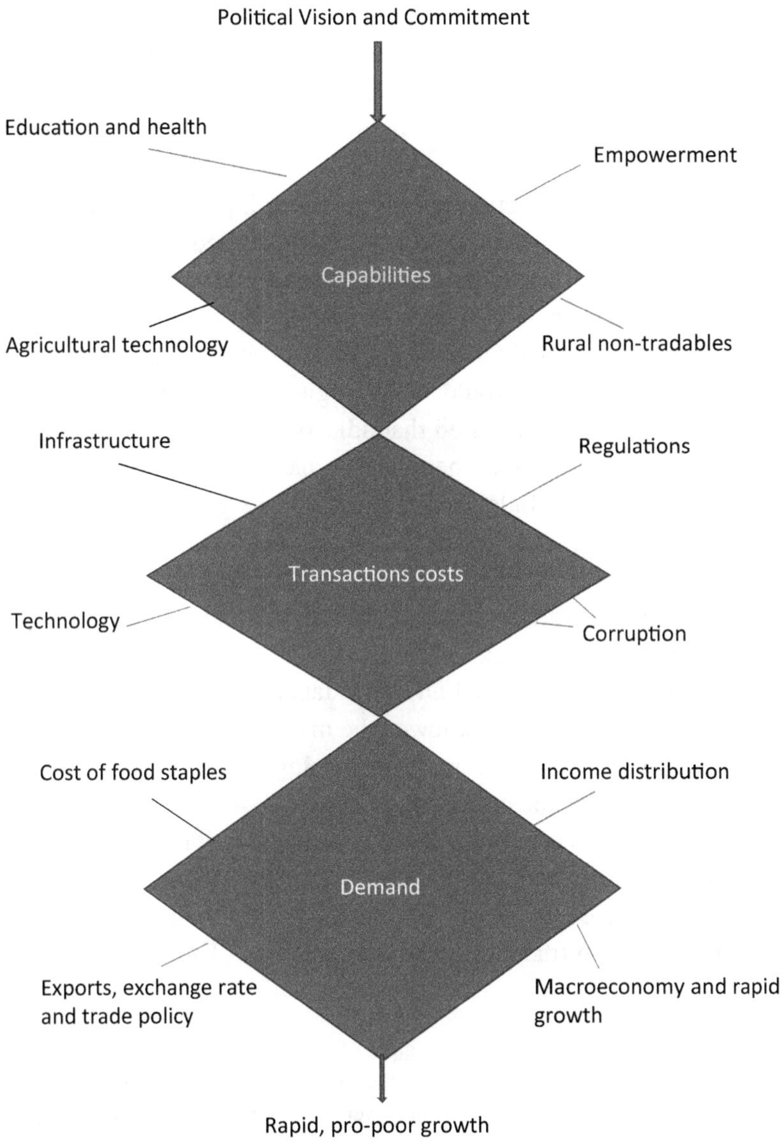

Figure 2. The road to pro-poor growth.

Source: Timmer (2004).

poverty masked its economic roots, during the mid-1970s there was a growing awareness of income inequalities and severe poverty in rural areas. The technocrats took a highly strategic approach to what was then diagnosed as "Dutch Disease" and, in November 1978, devalued the rupiah, to the surprise of financial markets.

Tradable goods production rapidly recovered, particularly in the agriculture sector. After 1978, poverty rates again started to decline assisted by a significant recovery in the share of income (19.9% in rural areas), garnered by the bottom 40% of the distribution. By the end of the decade, the poverty headcount had fallen to 28.6%. Despite this, the national Gini coefficient reached what would be its highest point for the rest of the decade. The government ensured that adjustments were made in the decade that followed. By 1983, when the international oil boom slowed and commodity prices fell, Indonesia restructured its economy and policies with devaluation and trade openness. Agriculture continued to grow and rice prices were kept stable. Simultaneously, the government pursued aggressive exchange rate protection, devaluing first in 1983 and again in 1986 (Hill, 1996; Thorbecke, 1995).

The fortuitous "push" in FDI from Japan and the "pull" from the attractive climate in Indonesia allowed the manufacturing sector to become a significant employer of the poor, increasing wages by the end of the 1980s. This growth in the commercial sectors created a boom in the non-tradable economy[14] where most of the poor make a living (Timmer, 1997, 2002). As the export economy boomed in the late 1980s and early 1990s, and overall GDP grew by nearly 7% annually, roughly half of that growth was made up of non-tradable goods and services (Timmer, 2004).[15] The

---

[14]The two commercial sectors are the "engines of growth" because of their potential for rapid productivity gains. Connecting them to the "non-tradable" sector, however, is the key to a high "elasticity of connection" between overall economic growth and rapid poverty reduction. Unless demand from rising incomes in the commercial sectors spills over to this non-tradable sector, the poor tend to be left out of the growth process. See Table 4 for data on the "poverty elasticity of economic growth" over time. Much of the variance in this elasticity is explained by changes in real rice prices.

[15]There is little scope for productivity gains in the non-tradable sector. To raise incomes there, higher wages are needed in tradable sectors, along with flexible labour markets. National income accounts, however, are not kept according to this distinction — hence, the data are more impressionistic.

reform of trade policy was accompanied by targeted investment — made possible by the massive oil windfall — in sectors that benefited the poor. Sound macroeconomic management was strongly supported by investment in sectors that benefited the poor — education, health, family planning, and infrastructure — enabling the poor to benefit from the oil windfall at the household level.

To enhance tradability and boost agricultural productivity, the government focused on the development of physical infrastructure and facilities throughout the country. The oil windfall also supported the development of widespread and large-scale investment in infrastructure assets. Up until 1994, the government was spending 30% of its development budget on infrastructure, i.e. 2.3% of GDP. The expansion of the road network was particularly significant. In 1977, local roads (mostly farm-to-market roads) totalled 8,500 km and rose in a 30-year period to 31,900 km by 1998. The transformation of Indonesia's network of highways took off and accelerated in the 1970s, expanding at 8.3% annually between 1970 and 1998. This, together with the massive investment in trucks, radically transformed Indonesian capacity to move goods to ports and around the country in just two short decades. The impact on transaction costs was significant.

4.3. *The Financial Crisis in 1997–1998*

The crisis and recovery showed that the price of rice is the most important determinant of poverty at the household level in Indonesia. Price stability matters to the poor (Timmer, 2004). Rice prices are important for poverty alleviation, not only in terms of their short-term direct benefits on the poorest quintiles but also because they play a key role in the structural transformation of the agricultural sector and the economy as a whole. In agriculture, low rice prices encourage farmers to diversify crops by making it cheaper to put rice in the market while reducing the incentives to plant rice when the market price is low. The result is a move towards crops that give the poor higher-profit margins. In Indonesia, artificially high rice prices have slowed down the crop diversification process, as well as investments in non-farm rural activities (Timmer, 2004).

Households also cut back their spending, resulting in a significant increase in malnutrition. This had both long- and short-term impacts on human and household assets: health, education and savings. Part of the long-term impact of the crisis can be seen in rising levels of malnutrition among children under 5 years of age. The malnutrition rate among these children followed a downwards trend until 2000. Malnutrition in Indonesia reached a low of 23% in 2000, but subsequently increased to almost 26% by 2003.[16]

During the economic contraction the government developed and extended a number of formal safety net programs. The *Jaringan Pengaman Sosial* or JPS Social Safety Net programs, known until then for their patchy record, were extended to help protect the chronically and transitory poor from the impacts of the crisis. Initially, these crash programs were directed to urban areas throughout the country but were also intended to reach rural areas where harvest failures were causing massive hardship. The JPS programs had four goals: (i) to ensure the poor could obtain food at affordable prices; (ii) to create employment; (iii) to preserve access to social services such as health and education and (iv) to sustain local economic activity through regional block grants and small-scale credit programs (Sumarto *et al.*, 2001). Evidence highlights the mixed effectiveness of the various programs (SMERU, 2004). While the scholarships programme had a positive impact by keeping children in school, and the health-card programme showed improved access of the poor to public health facilities, the Raskin (subsidized rice for the poor) programme saw higher levels of capture by higher quintiles (see further discussion in Section 5).

5. Managing Raskin: Poverty and Politics

This section seeks to understand the actual impact of targeted rice distributions on the welfare of poor households and determine the efficiency of

[16] Block *et al.* (2004). The rise in malnutrition levels seems to have been caused by a combination of several effects, including the impact of changes in the relative prices of rice, cassava and cooking oil (a carry-over from the depreciated real exchange rate after the crisis and government policy towards rice imports), and the presence of a cohort effect resulting from underweight children born during or just after the crisis of 1998. Not all this can be attributed to the crisis. Research has also shown that the use of infant feeding supplements as a substitute for breastfeeding, the incidence of which has increased by almost 10% over the past few years, is associated with a significant increase in malnutrition levels, while the rate of utilization of Posyandu services, already in decline long before the reversal of the malnutrition trend, has no statistically significant effect on malnutrition levels.

BULOG operations in procuring, storing and distributing rice to these households. Both dimensions have received considerable attention over the past decade and a half, although none of the studies discusses the politics behind the rice-based social safety net. A quick summary of these high-quality studies is all that is attempted here.

Four studies in particular serve as effective summaries of the state of understanding of Raskin's impact on poverty alleviation during and after the Asian Financial Crisis in 1998. The first, carried out in the immediate aftermath of the crisis by the architects of the OPK, was published in 2001 (Tabor and Sawit, 2001), although their quantitative evidence used in the evaluation only went through the end of 1999. This early evaluation is by far the most positive report on the costs and benefits of what ultimately became known as the Raskin programme.

In 2006, the World Bank carried out a substantial poverty assessment, in which the Raskin programme was evaluated as one of several Indonesian social safety nets designed to help poor households. The main focus of this major research project was to understand the main pathways out of poverty for Indonesia's poor rural households, but it also focused on "making growth work for the poor". The report was heavily influenced by the on-going project at World Bank headquarters on pro-poor growth (in which Indonesia served as the poster child).[17]

By 2012, a follow-up report on Raskin by the World Bank had become increasingly hostile to the poor targeting, high costs, and lack of accountability of the program. This report relied heavily on existing studies, especially from SMERU and local universities, to document the lack of impact of Raskin deliveries of rice to the poor. The availability of panel data from SUSENAS was especially damning, as little of the Raskin rice could be seen in household consumption data.

Following on the 2012 World Bank report, BAPPENAS requested World Bank assistance for a "Business Process Review" of Raskin, with the official intent to identify inefficiencies in the logistical operations of BULOG in its Raskin procurement and distribution system. The study was carried out by Deloitte/Monitor on behalf of a steering committee that

---

[17] I was the author of the Indonesian case study for the project. See Timmer (2005, 2007a, 2007b).

included all of the bureaucratically interested official Raskin parties, and which was chaired by BAPPENAS.[18]

Their four evaluations are briefly summarized below. It is important to recognize that all four of these reports relied heavily on the available ongoing research into the cost-effectiveness of the Raskin programme. SMERU has long been the gold standard of this research, and its work is cited heavily. But other Indonesian researchers also contributed significantly to our understanding of how well Raskin works in reaching poor households in a cost-effective manner. A concluding section discusses the political economy of this evolving record.

5.1. *Tabor and Sawit Evaluation of OPK in 2001*

The Tabor and Sawit's evaluation of OPK was conducted at the request of BULOG, which cooperated fully with the two senior consultants who had helped design OPK in the aftermath of the Asian Financial Crisis and loss of control over domestic rice prices. The very positive tone of the evaluation stems from two factors: (1) the OPK programme was compared with a general rice price subsidy that the government attempted in the immediate months after the crisis broke in late 1997 — the targeted subsidy was considerably more cost-effective and (2) both authors had been actively engaged in helping BULOG "troubleshoot" the teething problems in OPK's early implementation, and there was a palpable sense of relief that the programme was clearly working pretty well.

> The government's initial reaction to the deteriorating food security situation in 1997 and 1998 was to impose sweeping controls on food trade and marketing and to use public grain stock releases to hold down food prices. From mid-1997 to mid-1998, trade and price controls were used to maintain domestic food prices at 50 to 60 per cent of prevailing import parity prices. Food price subsidies for fiscal 1998/1999 were initially budgeted at Rp 4 trillion but eventually reached Rp 12 trillion,

[18]I served as a consultant to the Deloitte/Monitor team, with the support of both BAPPENAS and the World Bank.

> the equivalent of 12.4 per cent of government development outlays and just under 2 per cent of GDP.
>
> Faced with a widening gap between domestic and international food prices, large quantities of rice and other basic foodstuffs were smuggled out of the country. Rather than sell rice at distress prices, farmers withheld rice from the markets and urban traders ran down their stocks. As supplies became more scarce, domestic rice prices rose by nearly 50 per cent from May to August of 1998, triggering a near-panic in several urban markets.
>
> By August 1998 the government abandoned its general food price subsidy policy. A targeted rice subsidy program (Operasi Pasar Khusus [special market operation], or OPK program) was mounted to protect the food security of low-income households. Under OPK, eligible households are allowed to buy ten (later twenty) kilograms of rice per family per month at a subsidized price of Rp 1,000 per kilogram from the government.
>
> The introduction of OPK was just one of many changes that were to sweep Indonesia's food markets in 1998 and 1999. In September 1998 the government announced that BULOG (the National Food Logistics Agency) would confine its domestic procurement activities to rice and would dispose of its non-rice food stocks. In September the government also announced that trade in foodstuffs would be liberalized, including rice. This was implemented in November 1998, ending BULOG's long-standing rice import monopoly. In January 2000 rice imports were fully liberalized, and a 30 per cent specific import duty was applied to imported rice. This dismantling of BULOG's broad-based food trade monopoly and price stabilization authority implies that, by default, the OPK targeted rice subsidy program has become the government's single most important policy instrument for protecting food security. Taken together with the liberalization of food markets, the attempt to target rice subsidies to the poor represents an important innovation in government's food security tool kit.

It is not possible to review the full details of the Tabor and Sawit evaluation, as it is full of data and careful analysis of all features of the programme. They note the attention the programme has received by other evaluators:

> The OPK program has been extensively monitored and evaluated, both by the program implementers and by independent NGO and university evaluators. The independent monitoring and evaluation reports reveal

> a number of common implementation problems, the most important of which are: (i) that the BKKBN welfare criteria were not designed specifically to identify food insecure households and that villagers often define food insecurity differently from the way in which program managers would define it (SMERU, 1998; Sumarto *et al.*, 2000; Wiebe, 1998); (ii) there is a tendency in some beneficiary villages to redistribute the rice more widely amongst both poor and near-poor families, hence diluting the impact on the very poor (Rachman *et al.*, 1999; Sumarto *et al.*, 2000); (iii) that operational costs have been insufficient to meet the high transport costs to some Outer Island regions (State Ministry for Food and Horticulture Affairs, 1999); (iv) that some food insecure families are not eligible to participate in the program (Tim-JPS, 1999); (v) that the program was not well socialized by the government and understood by the poor population (Tim-JPS, 1999) and (vi) that urban coverage was very low (*Pusat Pengembangan Agribisnis*, 1998).

Despite these difficulties, the authors conclude on a very optimistic note:

> A targeted food subsidy program should become the cornerstone of any effort aimed at providing social protection for Indonesia's food insecure households. Although the OPK program was launched in wake of the El Niño drought and during the first year of the monetary crisis, it should not be considered as an anti-crisis program per se. Rather, it should be seen as the main "food security" pillar of an evolving social protection system that is constantly improved to help ensure that the poor can afford to meet minimal nutrition norms.
>
> The OPK program should certainly not be the "only" pillar of a national food security system. Broad-based rural development, food supplementation for underweight children, nutrition education, vitamin and micro-nutrient supplementation, enhanced village storage, and healthy diet diversification efforts are also important components of a national food security effort.
>
> The OPK program demonstrates that the government of Indonesia can deliver targeted food subsidies in a reasonably cost-effective fashion. That the program has been mounted as quickly as it has and is quite cost-effective reflects positively on the government's logistics capabilities. That OPK generates significant economic and nutritional benefits

> (relative to program costs) implies that a public investment in targeted food security has considerable economic merit.
>
> In theory, income transfers can be provided in cash instead of in kind, and indeed some of the social safety net programs are operated on a cash transfer basis. The main advantage of using rice-based subsidies rather than some form of cash grant or food stamp schemes is: (i) rice is widely consumed by the poor, and whether there was or was not a subsidy program, food insecure households would spend a large part of their income buying rice; (ii) a rice-based income transfer leaves both a commodity-based and financial accounting trail that can be readily monitored and evaluated; (iii) eligible beneficiaries will demand provision of the commodity for which they must make a co-payment; and (iv) the OPK program's operational costs are relatively modest compared to the overall fiscal transfer. These costs would probably be in the same range as those of a food stamp type scheme, but with considerably less risk of fraud and corruption.

Subsequent implementation of the OPK programme, and its slight reorganization as Raskin (Rice for the poor) in 2002, did not bear out this optimistic evaluation. Three factors intervened: First, despite the dismissal by Tabor and Sawit of Indonesia's rice stabilization programme because it failed in 1997 and 1998 (note that stable rice prices are not part of a broader food policy in their conclusions), a return to more normal rice prices after 2000 also brought a return of government efforts to stabilize rice prices, efforts which sometimes conflicted with the logistical needs for Raskin rice; (2) BULOG was converted from a State-Owned Enterprise with reporting responsibilities to the Cabinet to a "Perum", a private company that could be asked to take on public tasks for a negotiated fee. Raskin became BULOG's primary public task, but its private status permitted it to become much less transparent in its financial and logistical operations and (3) the "big-bang" decentralization of political power radically changed the ability of centrally-funded and directed organizations to carry out activities at the local level. At a minimum, these activities, such as rice distributions to the community level, became much more complicated to administer. Often, local administrators were simply interested in other priorities than getting cheap rice to their constituents. As we shall see, all three factors played increasing roles in the cost-effectiveness of BULOG's implementation of the Raskin programme.

5.2. *World Bank Evaluation of Raskin in 2006*

Attention turned quickly to how well targeted the safety net programmes were in an environment of budgetary tightness. As part of a general effort by the World Bank to help Indonesian policy makers understand how to "make the new Indonesia work for the poor", an extensive poverty assessment was undertaken in 2005 and 2006, in which special attention was paid to the various social safety net programmes that had been introduced after 1998. The conclusion was that targeting had been quite poor, including for Raskin.

> Historically, program targeting in Indonesia has not been particularly strong. Evidence from various targeted programs shows that targeting performance of most safety net and poverty programs has been low. The under-coverage error — the proportion of the first quintile of households that are not included in the program — is generally over 50 percent. Similarly, the leakage error — the proportion of beneficiaries who are classified as non-poor or above the bottom quintile — is around 50 to 70 percent. Several elements of safety net program design explain the reasons for less-than-efficient targeting of the poor.

5.2.1. *Where has all the Raskin gone? Improving the effectiveness of the subsidized rice distribution programme*[19]

With coverage of 57% of the poor, the Raskin (*beras miskin*) programme has been one of the most important components of the government's social protection system. Introduced as the *operasi pasar khusus* (OPK) programme in mid-1998 at the peak of the crisis, Raskin delivers subsidized rice to poorer households. However, it has been criticized for weak targeting and excessive leakages.

Under the Raskin programme, the National Logistics Board (BULOG) planned to distribute about 2 million tons of subsidized rice to some 8.3 million households in 2005. Each selected household is supposed to

[19]This section draws on a special "Spotlight" on inefficiencies and leakages at the end of Chapter 6, "Making Social Protection Work for the Poor," in World Bank (2006).

have received 20 kg of rice per month at the subsidized price of Rp 1,000 per kg. The rice is purchased by BULOG from wholesalers at a price determined annually by presidential decree (Inpres) using a budget allocation from the government to BULOG to cover the cost of the subsidy. The price paid to BULOG for each kg of rice in 2005 was Rp 3,351 per kg, equivalent to a 2005 budget allocation of Rp 4.7 trillion. The compensation programme associated with the removal of the fuel subsidy in 2005 added a further Rp 765 billion to the 2005 Raskin budget.

5.2.2. *The poverty targeting of the Raskin programme*

Raskin reaches more than half of the poorer households in the country, making it an important instrument of social protection. However, it delivers rice to far more non-poor households than poor households, such that only around a quarter of all recipient households are classified as poor. Table 3 shows that, of the Rp 4.7 trillion allocated to the programme in 2005, only about one-fifth was actually received by the poor. The bulk (52%) went to the non-poor and more than a quarter of the money went to BULOG to cover operational running costs.

5.2.3. *Leakages in the Raskin programme*

The three types of leakages in Raskin are lost rice, "lost" money and high mark-up prices.

Lost rice: BULOG distributes rice to distribution points in villages and sub-districts throughout the country, and leakages of rice occur at various levels in the distribution process. Comparing official administrative data on amount of rice distributed with the data from household surveys on the

Table 3. Distribution of the Raskin subsidy to the poor, the non-poor and BULOG.

Subsidy received by the non-poor	52%
Operating Costs and BULOG profit	28%
Subsidy received by the poor	20%

Source: World Bank staff calculations.

Table 4. Poverty elasticity of growth over time.

	Annual % change in per capita income	Annual % change in poverty index	Poverty elasticity of growth
1967–1976	5.48	–6.0	–1.09
1976–1980	6.37	–8.1	–1.27
1980–1984	4.23	–6.8	–1.61
1984–1987	2.69	0.7	–2.60
1987–1990	6.66	–4.6	–0.81
1990–1993	5.41	–4.6	–0.85
1993–1996	5.23	–6.2	–1.19
1996–1999	3.25	9.9	–3.05 (+)
1999–2002	2.49	–8.2	–3.29

Note: The Poverty Elasticity of Growth (PEG) is calculated as the ratio of the percentage reduction in the headcount poverty index relative to the percentage change in per capita incomes (in US$ PPP) from the World Bank Data Base on Pro-Poor Growth.
Source: Timmer (2005).

amount actually received by households, about 18% of the rice seems to have gone missing, suggesting that the welfare losses from corruption may be so large that they offset the potential welfare gains of the program. An updated estimate of leakages calculated in 2006 using the same methodology found that more than 30% of rice went missing between BULOG's warehouses and the households receiving it from November 2003 to January 2004.

This loss is equivalent to 164,000 tons of rice valued at Rp 433 billion (US$43 million). However, there is a wide variation in leakage by province: the greatest leakage is in Banten, where more than 75% of the Raskin was lost, and in another six provinces the leakage rates were over 50%. However, in six other provinces less than 10% of the rice went missing.

In addition, rice never reaches the poor in some areas because of the allocation mechanism used at the village level. In theory, rice is only supposed to be given to pre-welfare and welfare households (according to the BKKPN's classification of households). However, in some places allocations are given out to all village members, or by alternative non-transparent allocation mechanisms. As a result, the amount received by households is typically much less than 20 kg. Surveys suggest that sometimes it can be as little as 5–6 kg, greatly diluting the benefit to poor households.

"Lost" money: Distribution of the rice from the village (desa) or outside Java at the sub-district (kecamatan) level down to households is conducted by teams of village officials. The media have reported cases where village heads collected money from poor households and never paid BULOG for the rice received. However, a lack of transparency in the amounts of rice allocated to sub-districts or villages undermines the ability of poor communities to hold BULOG and village officials accountable.

The poor pay more

In many cases, the poor were asked to pay more than the Rp 1,000 per kg amount mandated by the programme in 2005. On average, Raskin recipients had to paid an extra 19% "operational costs" or some Rp 30.5 billion (US$3 million) between November 2003 and January 2004. The highest average mark-up was observed in Jakarta, where recipients paid Rp 2,900 for Raskin rice — almost 3 times the official price.

5.2.4. *Reforms are needed to make Raskin work for the poor*

It would be wrong to abolish Raskin, but some critical reforms should be considered.

(1) Identifying clear lines of accountability within BULOG is a key first step in stemming losses. It is crucial to clarify responsibilities and penalties associated with corruption in programme implementation. The creation of an investigative team at the highest level could send a message that corruption will be seriously punished by BULOG's senior management.
(2) Improving transparency regarding rice allocations and benefit amounts would increase community participation in the distribution process and reduce leakages at the village level. In addition, formalizing the rules regarding the operational costs for distributing the rice would give certainty to the Raskin selling price, avoiding misuse and mark-ups.

(3) Independent monitoring should be encouraged. In this context, the government could undertake a study to identify the districts in which most leakages occur and try to pinpoint the biggest holes in the system. Understanding the incentives of officials involved in the programme would also be useful in tackling the underlying causes.

(4) Involving the private sector in the distribution process. Most villages in Indonesia are well served by private rice traders. It therefore makes little sense for BULOG to play the same role as the private sector. If distribution costs were benchmarked by locality, then the private sector could compete for this business through a transparent bidding process. Thus, BULOG could devote its resources to managing and monitoring the performance of private operators rather than implementing the programme itself. Only in remote areas where no private operators were willing to undertake distribution for a reasonable cost should BULOG continue to deliver rice directly.

World Bank Evaluation of Raskin in 2012[20]

A special study of Raskin was conducted in 2012 in response to rising criticism of the Raskin programme in the media and among local policy analysts: The first two and last points of the Executive Summary are quite explicit on the reforms needed if Raskin was going to continue as the country's main targeted poverty program:

> **Poor households in Indonesia benefit from stable prices and tools which help safeguard food expenditure…**
>
> Food is the largest single category of expenditure for poor households and instability in food prices, especially rice prices, threatens progress in poverty reduction. A well-timed, well-targeted, and effectively managed in-kind transfer could supplement poor household income as well as keep price increases in check.

---

[20]This is taken from the Executive Summary of the World Bank (2012) Evaluation of the RASKIN Program.

> **... but Raskin will not effectively deliver either service without a major overhaul.**
>
> Raskin does not effectively accomplish either of the above goals for poor households because of overlapping weaknesses in design, operation, and oversight. In order to be an effective expenditure of public revenues that contributes to Indonesia's social safety net, Raskin needs *at a minimum* to accomplish reforms in
>
> (1) targeting, allocation, and local-level distribution so that vulnerable households benefit from low-cost access to a significant benefit;
> (2) oversight and monitoring of Raskin policies and outcomes below the regional distribution points and
> (3) socialization and dissemination of program goals, outcomes, financial performance, and delivery schedules. ...
>
> **Without a comprehensive overhaul, Raskin should consider focusing on price stabilization only.**
>
> The current Raskin does not deliver a substantial benefit to poor and vulnerable households and has not attempted to substantially improve its service for those households. Raskin may instead be more effective as a market-targeted, supply-side intervention that keeps local markets for rice "thick", with as many buyers and sellers as possible. If Raskin were reliably delivering rice to existing markets, the current lack of local-level oversight of outcomes could be tolerated and all households with market access would still derive benefits from low and stable prices and a functioning market in rice.

Although not widely distributed, this report was quite influential in reform-minded segments of the government, and led fairly quickly to an action program to make Raskin more effective, or even to convert it into a cash transfer programme.

5.2.5. *Deloitte/Monitor "Business Process Review" (BPR) of Raskin*

The Deloitte/Monitor "Business Process Review" of Raskin was initiated by Bappenas with technical assistance from the World Bank. Although the final report was submitted in early 2015, its reception was muted by the change in government and the rice crisis that emerged from mishandling the impact of the *El Niño* drought. Excerpts from the draft Executive Summary below provide clear guidance on what the team thought needed to be done to make Raskin a cost-effective programme.

> The Subsidi Beras bagi masyarakat berpendapatan rendah (Raskin, with a new name adopted in 2012: subsidized rice for low-income communities) program provides rice to poor and near-poor Indonesians. BULOG purchases and delivers rice to distribution points throughout the archipelago, while local governments manage rice from distribution point to beneficiaries. As the largest social assistance program targeted to poor households, Raskin is a key component of the Indonesian government's support for food security.
>
> The Tim Koordinasi (Tikor) Raskin Pusat identified potential challenges with the efficiency and effectiveness of Raskin service delivery, including low quality of delivered rice, distribution delays, leakage of rice, inadequate coordination and monitoring, and perceived poor program cost/benefit ratio.
>
> As identified with input from an expert group meeting (EGM), the Republic of Indonesia should begin utilizing near-cash transfers [also known as the electronic benefits transfer or EBT] in areas of high retail infrastructure (mostly urban areas) and embark on a concerted effort to improve the continued delivery of rice in areas of limited retail infrastructure (mostly rural areas). In the future, as retail infrastructure expands throughout the archipelago, so should the use of EBT also.
>
> The implementation will require a concerted effort and due to the complexity and/or size of investment will require support from the Tikor and other key stakeholders. In total, 9 interrelated initiatives have been identified to improve processes throughout the entire supply chain. It is estimated that the entire project will take up to 5 years to fully implement, however, multiple initiatives will be completed along the way providing value in a shorter time-span. The total implementation cost has been estimated at a high level to range from 600 billion to 1.2 trillion IDR for all initiatives.

The full text of the draft provides extensive data and analysis on the Raskin programme. But as noted at the beginning of this section, there is no discussion of the politics behind the programme, or how to build political support for the recommended changes. Since the submission of the Deloitte/Monitor report in 2015, the Jokowi government has moved gradually to a cash-transfer programme in a number of trial regions, with the intent to phase out rice distributions almost entirely by 2019.[21]

6. The Political Economy of Food-Based Social Safety Nets

The evolution of food security strategies from stabilizing rice prices in urban markets, to incorporating poor rural households through pro-poor economic growth, and ultimately to targeted social safety nets that start out life as food-based but which ultimately end up as cash transfers, would seem to parallel the broader structural transformation of an economy (Timmer, 2017). The rising political influence of farmers as they become a smaller share of the workforce, and their production a smaller share of the economy, has long been a paradox to economists (Lindert, 1991; Timmer, 2015). Behavioural economics now provides a reasonably persuasive explanation for this paradox because the gap in labour productivity between farmers and workers in the rest of the economy often rises during the early stages of a successful structural transformation, and this rising gap induces significant political tensions which politicians can "buy off" by supporting higher farm incomes (Timmer, 2014a).

The obvious question thus becomes, "is high price protection for rice farmers in Asia the necessary price to be paid for political stability that fosters rapid economic growth?" Economists have long been reluctant to go very far down this path, as it specifically rejects "efficient" policies for ones that are politically motivated. But the historical record is pretty clear, at least for the Asian countries that have managed rapid economic growth and a successful structural transformation (Timmer, 2016). My WIDER lecture on the political economy of managing structural transformations concluded as follows:

> A way must be found to make markets work to deliver long-run growth. No alternative exists to organizing economies around market-based

[21] See Timmer *et al.* (2017) for a discussion of these recent changes.

transactions if societies are to reach their goals of greater material welfare and broad political freedom. Markets produce both. But markets also fail in important social tasks. Responsible governments must find a way to prevent those failures through careful regulation and to fix them when innocent workers and consumers cannot participate in the promises of market outcomes.

Thus, finding a way for governments to deliver effective and efficient safety nets as both a moral and political imperative — to allow markets to deliver on these promises — becomes the essence of policy-making. Governments, like the poor, live in the short run. Their vision and strategic design for inclusive, long-run growth must survive the day-to-day challenges of managing power. 'Stability' would seem to be essential to building this bridge between short-run political imperatives and long-run performance — stability in food prices, in the macroeconomy, in the political arena. Within a reasonably stable environment, competitive politics then offer a mechanism for the political economy of food security to meet these challenges (Timmer, 2015, p. 47).

References

Boeke, J. H. (1946) *The Evolution of the Netherlands Indies Economy.* New York: Institute of Pacific Relations.

Block, S. A. *et al.* (2004) "Macro Shocks and Micro Outcomes: Child Nutrition during Indonesia's Crisis", *Economics and Human Biology*, Vol. 1, No. 2, pp. 21–44.

Deloitte/Monitor Consulting Group (2014) *World Bank Raskin BPR Project.* Phase 3: To-Be Report (Draft), Jakarta.

Hill, H. (1996) *The Indonesian Economy Since 1966: Southeast Asia's Emerging Giant.* Cambridge: Cambridge University Press, Cambridge, UK.

Kaplan, S. L. (1984) *Provisioning Paris: Merchants and Millers in the Grain and Flour Trade during the Eighteenth Century.* Ithaca: Cornell University Press.

Lewis, W. A. (1954) "Economic Development with Unlimited Supplies of Labor", *Manchester School of Economics and Social Studies*, Vol. 22, pp. 139–191.

Lindert, P. H. (1991) "Historical Patterns of Agricultural Policy", in *Agriculture and the State: Growth, Employment, and Poverty in Developing Countries*, ed. C. P. Timmer. Ithaca, NY: Cornell University Press, pp. 29–83.

McIntyre, A. (2003) "Indonesia as a Poorly Performing State?" Australian National University. Processed.

Myrdal, G. (1968) *Asian Drama: An Inquiry into the Poverty of Nations.* New York: Pantheon Books.

Pearson, S. R. (1993) "Financing Rice Price Stabilization," *Indonesian Food Journal,* Vol. IV, No. 7, pp. 83–96.

Pusat Pengembangan Agribisnis (1998) *Evaluasi operasi pasar khusus di DKI Jakarta: Hasiltinjauan lapan tahap II* [Evaluation of the OPK Program in Jakarta: Phase II Report]. Jakarta.

Rachman, L., Pujihastuti, U., Sabarinah, S. and D. Sukandar (1999) *Deskripsi hasil evaluasi pelaksanaan operasi pasar khusus beras* [The Results of the Evaluation Studies of the OPK Rice Program]. Jakarta: State Ministry for Food and Horticulture Affairs.

SMERU Research Institute (1998) *Results of a SMERU Rapid Field Appraisal Mission:Implementation of BULOG's Operasi Khusus in Five Provinces.* Jakarta.

SMERU (S. Sudarno, A. Suryahadi and W. Widyanti) (2004) "Assessing the Impact of Indonesian Social Safety Net Programs on Household Welfare and Poverty Dynamics", SMERU Working Paper.

State Ministry for Food and Horticulture Affairs (1999) *Special Market Operation (OPK) Information Package.* Prepared for the IBRD SSNAL Appraisal Mission.

Sumarto, S., Suryahadi A. and L. Pritchett (2000) *Safety Nets and Safety Ropes: Comparing the Dynamic Benefit Incidence of Two Indonesian "JPS" Programs.* Jakarta: Social Monitoring and Early Response Unit.

Sumarto, S., Suryahadi, A. and L. Pritchett (2001) "Safety Nets and Safety Ropes: Comparing the Dynamic Benefit Incidence of Subsidized Rice and Public Works Programs in Indonesia", Paper for presentation at the Vulnerability and Poverty Workshop, Third Asian Development Forum, Bangkok, June 12–14.

Tabor, S. R. and M. H. Sawit (2001) "Social Protection via Rice: The OPK Rice Subsidy Program in Indonesia", *The Developing Economies,* Vol. XXXIX-3 No. 9, pp. 267–294.

Thorbecke, E. (1995) "The Political Economy of Development: Indonesia and the Philippines", The Frank H. Golay Memorial Lecture. Cornell Southeast Asia Program. NY: Ithaca.

Tim-JPS (1999) *Kebijaksanaan pokok dan penyempurnaan program-program jarring pengaman sosial tahun anggaran 1999/2000* [Key Policies and Programmatic Improvements in the Social safety net program for budget year 1999/2000]. Jakarta: Sekretarin Tim Pelaksana.

Timmer, C. P. (1975) "The Political Economy of Rice in Asia: Indonesia", *Food Research Institute Studies*, Vol. 14, No. 3, pp. 197–231.

Timmer, C. P. (1990) *Food Price Stabilization: The Indonesian Experience with Rice*. Paper prepared for the Asia/Near East Bureau of the United States Agency for International, Harvard Institute for International Development, One Eliot Street, Cambridge, MA 02138, under USAID Contract No. DAN-4084-Z-00-8034-00.

Timmer, C. P. (1995) "Food Security and Rice Price Stabilization: An Essay in Honor of Bustanil Arifin", in *Beras, Koperasi dan Politik Orde Baru* [*Rice, Cooperatives and New Order Politics*]. Jakarta, Indonesia: Ministry of Cooperatives and Small-Scale Enterprises, pp. 326–351.

Timmer, C. P. (1997) "How Well do the Poor Connect to the Growth Process?" Harvard Institute for International Development for the USAID/CAER Project.

Timmer, C. P. (2002) "Agriculture and Economic Growth", in *The Handbook of Agricultural Economics*, Vol. II, eds. B. Gardner and G. Rausser. Amsterdam: North-Holland, pp. 1487–1546.

Timmer, C. P. (2004) "The Road to Pro-Poor Growth: The Indonesian Experience in Regional Perspective", *Bulletin of Indonesian Economic Studies*, Vol. 40, No. 2, pp. 177–207.

Timmer, C. P. (2005) "Operationalizing Pro-Poor Growth. Indonesia", Country Study for the World Bank, Draft chapter.

Timmer, C. P. (2007a) "How Indonesia Connected the Poor to Rapid Economic Growth", in *Delivering on the Promise of Pro-Poor Growth: Insights and Lessons from Country Experiences,* eds. T. Besley and L. Cord. London: Palgrave MacMillan and the World Bank, pp. 29–58.

Timmer, C. P. (2007b) "A Historical Perspective on Pro-Poor Growth in Indonesia," in *Determinants of Pro Poor Growth: Analytical Issues and Findings from Case Studies*, eds. M. Grimm, S. Klasen and A. McKay. London: Palgrave MacMillan, pp. 164–190.

Timmer, C. P. (2010) "Reflections on Food Crises Past", *Food Policy*, Vol. 35, No. 1, pp. 1–11.

Timmer, C. P. (2014a) "The Political Economy of Food Security: A Behavioral Perspective," in *Handbook on Food: Demand, Supply, Sustainability and Security*, eds. R. Jha, R. Gaiha and A. Deolalikar. Cheltenham: Edward Elgar, UK, pp. 22–40.

Timmer, C. P. (2014b) "What are Grain Reserves Worth? A Generalized Political Economy Framework", in *Trade, Development, and Political Economy in East Asia: Essays in Honour of Hal Hill*, Chapter 13, eds. P. Athukorala,

A. A. Patunru and B. P. Resosudarno. Institute of Southeast Asian Studies (ISEAS), Singapore, pp. 235–248.

Timmer, C. P. (2015) *Managing Structural Transformation: A Political Economy Approach*, 18th Annual WIDER Lecture, Helsinki, Finland.

Timmer, C. P. (2016) "The Role of Agriculture in 'Catching Up:' A Gerschenkronian Perspective", in *Diverse Development Paths and Structural Transformation in the Escape From Poverty*, eds. M. Andersson and T. Axelsson. Oxford University Press, Oxford, UK, pp. 68–92.

Timmer, C. P. (2017) "Food Security, Structural Transformation, Markets and Government Policy", *Asia and the Pacific Policy Studies*, Vol. 4, No. 1, pp. 4–19.

Timmer, C. P., Hastuti and S. Sumarto (2017) "The Evolution and Implementation of the Raskin Program in Indonesia", Draft chapter for a World Bank Project Evaluating Food-Based Safety Nets in a Number of Countries.

Warr, P. G. (1984) "Exchange Rate Protection in Indonesia", *Bulletin of Indonesian Economic Studies*, Vol. XX, No. 2, pp. 53–89.

Warr, P. G. (2011) "Food Security vs. Food Self-Sufficiency: The Indonesian Case", *The Indonesian Quarterly*, Vol. 39, No. 1, pp. 56–71.

Wiebe, F. (1998) *OPK Field Notes*. Jakarta: Harvard Institute for International Development.

Williams, J. C. and B. D. Wright (1991) *Storage and Commodity Markets*. Cambridge: Cambridge University Press.

World Bank (1993) *The East Asian Miracle: Economic Growth and Public Policy*. New York: University Press.

World Bank (2004) "Concept Paper on Operationalizing Pro-Poor Growth", Washington DC.

World Bank (2006) "Making the New Indonesia Work for the Poor: A Poverty Assessment", Jakarta, Indonesia.

World Bank (2012) "Evaluation of Raskin Rice Subsidy Scheme", Jakarta, Indonesia.

Chapter 3

Structural Shifters in the Global Demand for Food: Urbanization and Ageing

Peter Warr

John Crawford Professor of Agricultural Economics Emeritus, Australian National University, Canberra ACT 0200, Australia
peter.warr@anu.edu.au

Abstract

Changes in the global food economy involve both supply-side and demand-side forces. This paper focuses on two potentially important demand-side shifters: urbanization and ageing. An analytical problem in the literature on this subject has been separating the effects of these shifters from the effects of income growth, which has been correlated with them. The evidence suggests that urbanization raises the demand for energy-dense foods that are more easily prepared than traditional foods such as staple grains. It does not seem to increase total intake of calories per person, but to substitute one source of calories for another, with more consumption per person of animal products, including meat and dairy products, more consumption of vegetable oils and wheat products, and less consumption of traditional staples, including most grains, other than processed products made from them, and pulses. In nutritional terms, urbanization leads to more consumption of animal and vegetable fats and less consumption of complex carbohydrates and fiber. The effects of ageing of the population are less well studied. They seem to be qualitatively similar to, though smaller than, the effects of urbanization: less consumption of staple grains and more consumption of wheat products, meat, fish and fruit.

Keywords: Food demand, structural shifters, urbanization, ageing, staple foods.

1. Introduction

Most discussions of the global food economy rightly focus on supply and the factors driving changes in aggregate food availability. But actual changes in food consumption depend on the interaction between demand and supply, both of which are changing over time. Changes in food demand are potentially important for food consumption outcomes, as well as changes in supply. The standard tool for understanding food demand and changes in it is the economic theory of demand, which explains changes in consumption per person, both at the aggregate level and the household level, in terms of changes in incomes, food prices and the prices of other goods, recently supplemented by factors that drive demand from sources other than final food consumption, such as use in production of fuels. Total demand depends on these determinants of demand per capita and population. But this analytical apparatus may miss important changes in the demand for food.

Changes in the global economy suggest the possibility of important structural shifters in the relationship between food demand and the standard explanatory variables — income and prices. This paper explores the evidence on two such possible demand shifters: urbanization and the ageing of the population. Both of these potential shifters are known to be relevant for the supply of food, but they have also been mentioned as possible shifters in demand. This paper focuses on the literature dealing with their relevance, if any, for the demand for food.

The issue is important for our understanding of the world food economy, including projections of the quantities and prices of food that may be available in the future. These projections typically distinguish between supply and demand forces and the sources of structural shifts in both. If structural shifters are important for the demand for food, projections should take these variables explicitly into account.

Section 2 provides an overview of recent changes in global food consumption. The next two sections review the available literature on the impact on food demand of urbanization and human ageing, respectively. The final section concludes and discusses the biases that may arise in demand estimation and demand projections if these shifters are not considered explicitly.

2. Changes in Global Food Consumption

Over the last few decades, global per capita food consumption has increased substantially. Between 1970 and 2005, per capita caloric intake from all sources increased by 17%. The proportional increase was largest in the developing countries, where per capita caloric intake increased by 27% (2,143–2,722 calories per person per day), whereas in the developed countries the increase was smaller, at 9%, though starting from a higher level (3,136–3,418).[1] In the developing countries, undernutrition has declined as a proportion of the total population, but remains a serious problem (Warr, 2014). In the developed countries, over-consumption with resulting obesity and associated health problems, including diabetes, is a major concern, as it is increasingly in many developing countries. Beneath these increased mean levels of caloric intake lie important issues of the distribution across individuals of consumption, the consistency over time of food intake, the changing composition of caloric intake, between carbohydrates, fats and protein, the intake of nutrients other than calories, and the commodity composition of food consumption. In all these respects, the experience of individual countries varies widely.

India and China, which together account for about one third of the global population, have both experienced large increases in aggregate per capita caloric intake. In 1970, per capita consumption was about 2,000 calories per person per day in both countries. By 2005 this had increased

[1] *Source*: Data in this and the following five paragraphs are from FAOSTAT. Available at: http://www.fao.org/faostat/en/#home.

by 50% in China (to 3,000) and by 25% in India (to 2,500). The increase was negligible in Sub-Saharan Africa (SSA), taken together, with several countries experiencing declines in per capita consumption. In the countries of the former Soviet Union, per capita food consumption declined following their independence in the early 1990s, but levels of consumption recovered in the 2000s. In Latin America, food consumption rose, but at a lower rate than in Asia.

Associated with these increases in aggregate caloric intake was a change in the composition of the global diet towards more energy dense foods, especially vegetable oils and dairy/meat products. The share of vegetable oils in global caloric intake increased 67% over the three and a half decades to reach 11% of total caloric intake in 2005. Improvements in transportation and storage capabilities facilitated these changes. In contrast, consumption of some traditional foods declined, including pulses and root crops. The share of meat in total caloric intake increased by 80% to 8% of total caloric consumption. Figure 1 summarizes the data on this issue.

Figure 2 distinguishes between developed and developing countries in this overall story. It compares the changes in composition of the diets of developed and developing countries from 1970 to 2005. In the developed countries, the share of cereals in total consumption remained relatively constant, at around 40% of total caloric intake, but meat consumption increased by 30%, reaching 12% of total intake. Fruit consumption increased even more rapidly, but reached only 4% of total intake by 2005. The shares of animal fats and sugar declined, by 80% and 10%, respectively. In the case of animal fats this presumably reflects health warnings about links to cardiovascular disease. Nevertheless, fat consumption from all sources increased due to the substitution of vegetable oils for animal fats. In the case of sugar, the reason was the increased consumption of sugar substitutes such as high fructose corn syrup and artificial sweeteners.

Developing countries represent around 70% of the global population and that population is growing at double the rate of the developed countries. Accordingly, these countries dominate global food demand and its prospects. Grains continue to be the largest source of total caloric intake in the developing countries, but the increase in total calories derived from this source was only 8%, compared with a 27% increase in total caloric

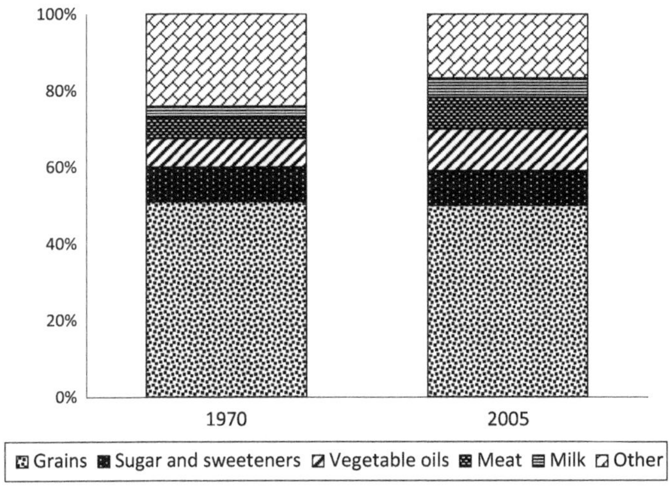

Figure 1. Global diet composition, 1970 and 2005.

Source: Author's calculations, based on Shapouri and Rosen (2007) using data from FAOSTAT.

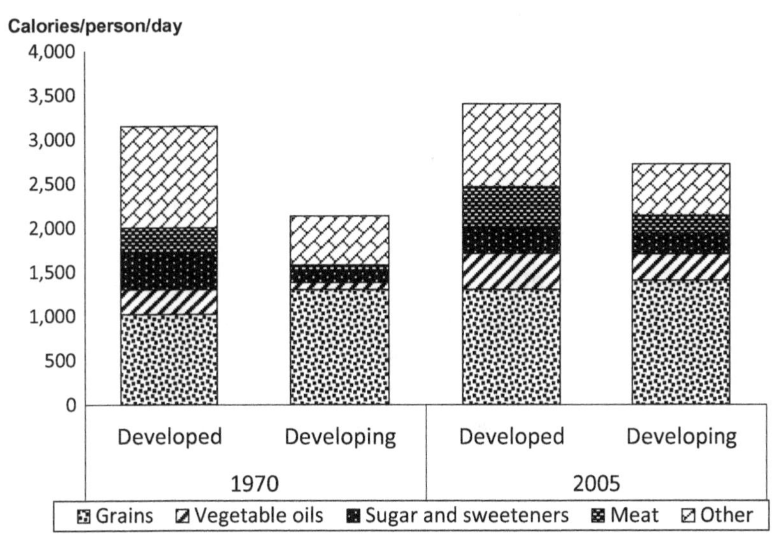

Figure 2. Developed and developing countries diet composition, 1970 and 2005.

Source: Author's calculations, based on Shapouri and Rosen (2007) using data from FAOSTAT.

intake. The per capita consumption of higher valued food items, including meat, eggs and vegetable oils roughly tripled and consumption of sugar increased by two thirds. The story is rather different in the least developed countries (incomes below US$500). Per capita consumption increased by 10% (2,000–2,200). Consumption of vegetable oils increased by 28%, followed by sugar, eggs, meat and milk. But consumption of vegetables, fruits and pulses all declined.

In summary, the developing countries' diets have become more like those of the developed countries, a process described by Popkin (2004) as "the nutrition transition". Popkin, Adair and Ng (2012) point out that dietary changes that took up to two centuries in the developed countries are occurring in just a few decades in today's developing countries, and that although total caloric intake continues to increase in the developing countries, this is not necessarily taking the form of more nutritious foods.

Changes in incomes and prices clearly played a major role in these demand shifts. Over this 35-year period, developed country incomes doubled and developing country incomes almost tripled, except that in the least developed countries income growth was much slower. Despite short-term volatility, the relative prices of staple foods and beef have declined to well below their 1970 levels (Shapouri and Rosen, 2007).[2] The well-known OECD-FAO projections of food demand and supply (Alexandratos and Bruinsma, 2012) predict relatively flat demand for staple foods for the period ending in 2025, and relatively stable real prices on average, with the qualification that livestock product prices are expected to rise relative to crop prices. These projections are based on the demand-side factors mentioned in the introduction. But other demand-side factors, not considered in these projections, may also be important. Urbanization and ageing of the population have been suggested as additional drivers of food demand, among other factors (Huang and Bouis, 1996). We turn now to the evidence on these potential demand shifters.

[2] Shapouri and Rosen's data relate to the period prior to the food price shocks of 2007–2008, during which staple food prices soared, but since those shocks staple food prices have again declined to be well below 1970 levels.

3. Urbanization

Urbanization refers to the shift of much of the population from a rural existence, centred on farming, to urban life, centred on non-agricultural occupations. Increasing rates of urbanization are a well-documented reality and the process seems inexorable. Figure 3 summarizes World Bank data comparing levels of urbanization in the years 1970 and 2015. In 2015, 54% of the world's population lived in urban areas, compared with 37% in 1970. The proportional increase was especially high in the East Asia and Pacific region and when countries are classified by income per capita, the increase was highest in the upper middle-income countries, where the proportion of the population living in urban areas doubled.

Since everyone eats, the urbanization process implies a decline in the ratio of the number of producers of food to consumers of it. Many studies have speculated that urbanization has been a driver of changes in global food prices. For example, in a report responding to the

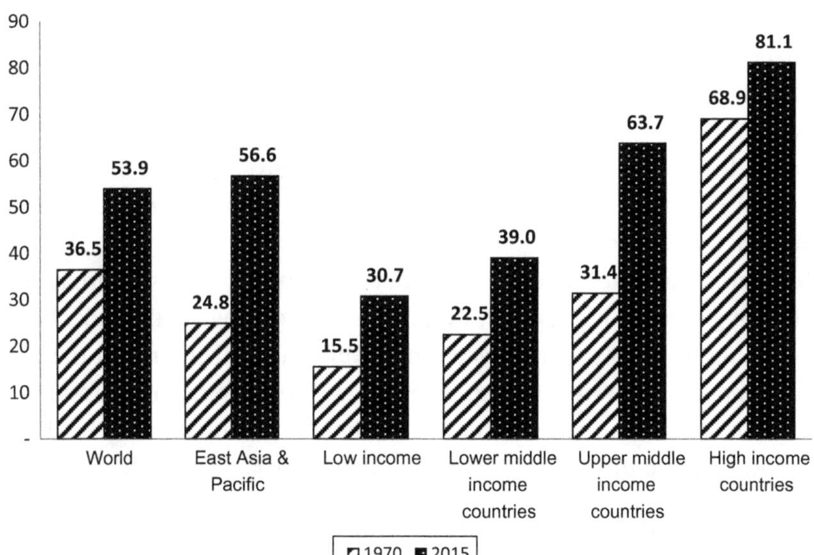

Figure 3. Share of population living in urban areas, 1970 and 2015 (%).

Source: Author's calculations, using data from World Bank, *World Development Indicators*.

2007–2008 increases in food prices, an UNCTAD study lists the causes of higher prices as

> "... population growth, urbanization and rapid economic development ... amplified by recent droughts, slow supply response, the fall in the dollar, high energy prices and ... increased demand for biofuels." (UNCTAD 2008)

Urbanization is identified as a driver of food prices in this and similar statements, though the mechanics of this relationship are unspecified. Many studies suggest that the effect that urbanization may have on food prices operates through supply-side forces, reducing supply by diminishing the availability of agricultural land and possibly the supply of labour for on-farm work. Demand-side influences have also been suggested, pointing to the different patterns of average consumption of rural and urban households, generally implying that urbanization increases the total demand for food. This discussion relates mainly to the developing countries, where rates of rural to urban migration can be very high. In most developed countries, the rural share of the population is already so low that further urbanization is no longer a potential driver of food demand.

Unfortunately, most studies claiming that urbanization affects the demand for food do not distinguish between urbanization itself and the higher average incomes that normally accompany it. The link between urbanization and incomes takes two forms. First, on average, the richer the country, the higher the rate of urbanization: in a cross-section of countries, the level of urbanization is correlated with national income per person; and over time, as income increases in a particular country, the level of urbanization tends to increase. Second, the average incomes of urban residents are generally higher than those of the remaining rural residents.

Failing to distinguish between the level of urbanization and the level of income could be misleading. Suppose we compare average food consumption between urban and rural households, finding them to be different, and attribute the difference to the effect of urbanization. In fact, many studies do just that. But what if income differences between urban and rural households explained the observed difference in the demand for food? Urbanization would in fact be playing no role in driving demand and there would be no need to allow for the degree of urbanization in studies of the demand for food, separately from the level of income.

Regmi and Dyck (2001) recognize the analytic distinction between the effects of urbanization, on the one hand, and income, on the other. They argue that for households of a given level of income, urbanization affects food demand through its effect on caloric requirements, food availability and female labour status. The evidence these authors provide is primarily based on qualitative speculation, rather than econometric analysis. Other authors emphasize the possible effects of changing preferences, the availability of refrigeration and the impact of supermarkets, but these claims too are generally based on casual theorizing rather than quantitative analysis. The empirical question that remains is whether, controlling for income, urbanization affects the demand for food, and if so, in what way.

3.1. *Urbanization and the Total Demand for Food*

It is important to distinguish between the impact that urbanization may have on the total demand for food from its possible effect on the composition of that demand. In an important study, Stage *et al.* (2010) examine the relationship between total food expenditures and overall expenditures in China and India using household survey data. In the case of China, using data for 2005, this relationship appears to be identical for rural and urban areas. These data are reproduced in Figure 4. Data for India show a similar story. Comparing rural and urban households with similar incomes, the total demand for food is very similar. Studies on Vietnam (Hoang *et al.*, 2008) and Tanzania (Mafuru and Marsh, 2003) use similar methods to this and reach similar conclusions.

The evidence presented by these authors seemingly indicates that at the same level of income, urban and rural households have almost identical expenditures on food; urbanization itself has negligible impact on total food demand per person. People migrating from rural to urban areas typically do so in the hope of higher incomes. If they are successful in this, by attaining higher incomes, their food consumption increases, just as it does for higher-income rural households who do not move. If rural to urban migrants are unsuccessful in raising their incomes, their total food consumption does not rise. The move from rural to urban areas may

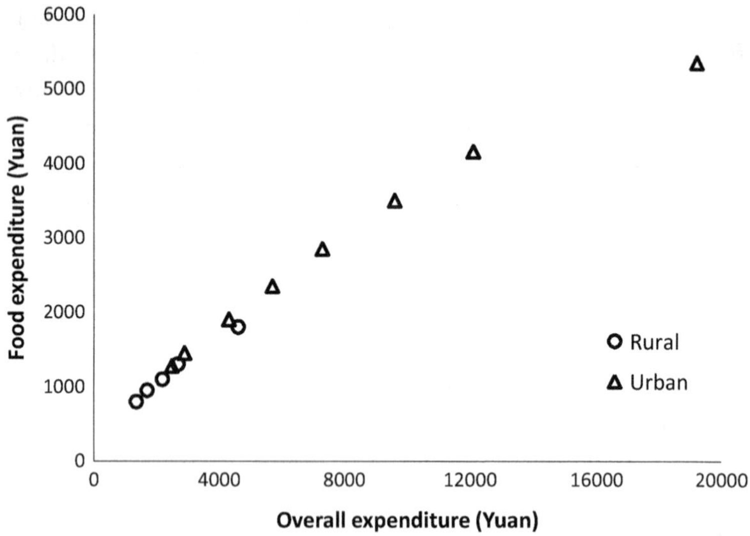

Figure 4. China: Average annual expenditure on food and overall expenditures, rural and urban areas (2005).

Source: Based on Stage *et al.* (2008) using data from National Bureau of Statistics of China (2006), *China Statistical Yearbook 2006*, China Statistics Press, Beijing.

in many cases be the vehicle for raising incomes, but any other source of increased income would have had a similar effect if the household had not migrated to an urban area. The argument of Stage *et al.* is therefore that it is income growth, not urbanization as such that is responsible for the increased total food intake. Urbanization and increased per capita demand for food may be correlated, but the relationship is not causal. If these authors are right, projections of total demand for food do not need to take explicit account of the level of urbanization, provided they account properly for income.

On closer inspection, the evidence provided by Stage *et al.* is open to question. First, referring to Figure 4, only five rural observations and eight urban observations are shown. The range of rural income observations is so narrow that comparison of rural and urban households at similar levels of income is possible only over the bottom one quarter of the range of urban incomes shown in their diagram.[3] The reason is that only group data, averages of large numbers of household observations, are presented. The number of observations shown for the India part of the study is larger, but again only a small number of group average observations, based on state level data, are presented. In both cases, the original survey-based data sets contain thousands of individual household level observations, covering a wider range of incomes than that captured by a small number of group averages.

The appropriate way to test the hypothesis that food expenditures are the same in urban and rural areas at the same levels of income would be to access the original household level observations. The dependent variable would be household food expenditure per person. Independent variables would include household income and control variables not intrinsic to urbanization but which could influence the relationship between food expenditures and incomes at the household level. These control variables would include, among others, educational attainment, number of children, and whether the household has access to electricity. The test of the hypothesis would then be whether a shifter dummy variable for urban or rural residence was statistically significant.

There is a further possible concern. The research strategy of comparing food expenditures of rural and urban households at the same levels of income makes sense only if urbanization and income levels are independently determined. What if income growth was itself (at least partly) caused by urbanization? If it was, the Stage *et al.* analysis would become invalid because urbanization would then cause higher levels of food demand through its effect on income. Economic geographers often claim that cities are inherently highly productive, because they offer

[3] Stage *et al.* (2005, p. 203) describe these observations as referring to "various income quintiles and deciles in rural and urban areas". It is not clear from this why there are five rural observations and eight urban observations. Were some observations omitted? The source indicates that the data are obtained from the published *China Statistical Yearbook 2006*, which of course can provide only group data and not household level observations. The India data they present are similarly based on average group data obtained from a published report of the National Sample Survey Organization.

economies of scale and minimize transactions and transport costs, so that urbanization itself raises incomes. Bloom *et al.* (2008) test this proposition empirically. They note that the proportion of a country's population living in urban areas is highly correlated with its average level of income. In their statistical analysis, using a cross-section of 180 countries, Bloom *et al.* ask whether income levels are Granger-caused by the level of urbanization, meaning that the level of urbanization is a statistically significant predictor of the subsequent growth of income. They conclude that it is not. Their findings support the notion that the level of urbanization is an indicator, rather than a cause, of economic development. The Stage *et al.* analysis thus seemingly survives this possible objection.

It may be true that, as Stage *et al.* claim, urbanization as such does not significantly affect total per capita consumption of food, but it may affect long-term total demand for food through a less obvious channel. Demographers have demonstrated that urbanization reduces the rate of population growth (Mace, 2008). The mechanism seems to be that urbanization lowers fertility because child rearing is more costly in urban than in rural areas. First, the opportunity cost of the mother's time is higher. Second, the availability of grandparents to care for children may be absent. As an illustration of this phenomenon, Mace points to historically high rates of infanticide and child abandonment in urban areas, reflecting these cost differences in raising children between urban and rural areas. For most urban women, not having so many children, and investing in child quality instead of child numbers, is obviously a preferable solution. But this line of thought has opposite implications from the presumption, cited above, that urbanization raises the demand for food. By lowering population growth in the long term, urbanization may actually reduce the total demand for food, even if it does not affect total food demand per person.

The evidence is thin and far from conclusive, but based on the available studies, if the level of urbanization does affect the total demand for food, that effect seems to be small. Even the sign of any such effect is uncertain. However, Stage *et al.* identify an important qualification to this conclusion. Because urban households have greater access to commercial supplies of food and are heavily dependent on them, rather than their own production, urban households are more likely than rural households to hoard food if they expect future price increases. This was indeed a feature of the urban food panics that resulted from the 2007–2008 food price shock and apparently accentuated the magnitude of the temporary food price increases that occurred then. In several countries, urban stocks of food, available in the commercial markets, disappeared. The potential implication is that urbanization may increase the volatility of total food demand, even if it does not significantly influence its long-term mean level. However, this possibility awaits formal statistical testing.

3.1.1. *Urbanization and the composition of food demand*

After reviewing the available evidence, Regmi and Dyck (2001) conclude that the effect of urbanization is primarily on the composition of food demand, rather than total food consumption. They emphasize the greater availability of food in urban areas and the greater scope for choice. Urban consumers are less constrained than rural residents by the foods that happen to be produced in their own locality.[4] Urban residents may be more exposed to dietary and other influences coming from other cultures. The evidence suggests that urban consumers have moved in the direction of a "global urban diet", including the consumption of many Western-style foods, and away from the traditional diets prevalent in rural areas, a phenomenon described earlier, in the context of OECD countries, by Blandford (1984).[5]

Stage *et al.* (2007) dispute these conclusions. Having argued that urbanization does not affect the total demand for food, these authors go on to argue that urbanization does not affect the composition of food demand,

[4] For example, Huang and Rozelle (1998) find that in China the rural demand for foodstuffs is restricted by the incompleted development of markets, especially markets for meat. Wu (1999) reports that in the 1990s rural residents in China still produced on average half of their own food.

[5] Casual observation suggests that this same global convergence among urban people is also true in other aspects of urban life, including dress, musical tastes and work patterns.

either, once allowance is made for income differences between urban and rural households. But the evidence they present is thin and the literature on this point does not support them. In reviewing this literature it must be emphasized that not all studies arguing that urbanization alters the composition of food demand distinguish properly between the effects of urbanization and rising incomes. This is particularly true of the nutrition literature, such as Popkin (1999), Mendez and Popkin (2004) and Ruel *et al.* (1980, 1999, 2017). This literature tends to assume that when the food consumption of rural and urban populations are found to differ, the difference must be due to urbanization itself. Stage *et al.* are right to point out the analytical problem with this form of evidence, but they do not seem to be right in claiming that urbanization has no effect independently of income. Studies that distinguish between urbanization and income are not numerous, but they do suggest that urbanization has an effect independent of income.

In an early study, Huang and David (1993) use cross-country data for Asian countries from 1960 to 1988 in which they distinguish clearly between differences in urbanization and differences in incomes. They show that in higher income Asian countries, urbanization led to a movement away from the local staple, rice, and coarse grains and towards more processed wheat products, based on imported wheat. In lower income countries, demand for cereal grains either increased or remained the same with urbanization. That is, the effect that urbanization has on food demand depends on the level of income of the country.

Huang and Bouis (1996, 2001) estimate demand functions for food in Taiwan, using household survey data for 1981 and 1991, taking explicit account of prices, incomes and structural shifters, including urbanization. The effect of urbanization is both statistically significant and large. They report that the move to urban areas has negative effects on the demand for rice (–23%) and positive effects on the demand for wheat products (+19%), meat (+5%), fish (+10%) and fruit (+38%).

Shapouri and Rosen (2007) summarize data from various countries showing that at the same level of income, those countries with greater urban population shares consume diets with more fat (both vegetable and animal). This corresponds to a greater share of processed foods in urban food consumption, a trend also reflected in the larger share of processed foods, rather than staple foods, in international agricultural trade than in total consumption. The highest rate of growth of processed food imports is found in the developing countries.

Seto and Ramankutty (2016) summarize data indicating that "With few exceptions, highly urbanized countries consume more animal protein — in the form of pork, poultry, beef and dairy products — than the world average" (p. 943) and that both higher incomes and higher degrees of urbanization contribute to this outcome. In nutritional terms, these changes imply a shift from complex carbohydrates, such as those found in grains, vegetables and fruits, towards animal proteins, refined fats, refined sugars, alcohols and oils (Tilman and Clark, 2014).

These trends have obvious implications for international trade in food. Opening to international trade makes it possible for urban consumers to move away from traditional diets, dominated by the foods that happen to be produced in their particular region, in that particular season. Rural residents do not have the same flexibility, although the penetration of commercial food markets into rural areas is changing this situation by making greater choice available to rural people (Reardon *et al.*, 2004, 2009), just as it has already for urban people. This analysis implies that as commercial food markets extend their reach into rural areas, the differences between the composition of urban and rural food demand may diminish. Urbanization may become a less important determinant of dietary composition, even at the same level of income, because the choices available to rural residents may become more like those found in urban areas.

What drives these differences between the composition of urban and rural food demand? The greater choice of foods available in urban areas through commercial channels, discussed above, is clearly a major factor. But urban areas also offer a much greater range of economic opportunities in general than rural areas. This applies particularly to women. The increased opportunity cost of women's time when they move from rural to urban locations raises the demand for "fast food" options (Shapouri and Rosen, 2007). Senauer *et al.* (1986) demonstrate the role of the higher opportunity cost of women's time in driving the demand for bread among urban households in Sri Lanka, and Kennedy and Reardon (1994) report similar findings among quasi-urban residents in Kenya.

3.2. *Ageing*

It is well known that as a country becomes richer, birth rates decline, mortality rates fall and life expectancy increases. The age distribution of the population first shifts such that surviving young people form a higher proportion of the population and eventually, as they age and live longer than their parents, older people form a larger proportion. Figure 5 summarizes data on the changing age distribution of the world population over the period 1970–2015. These demographic changes are more rapid in Asia than for the world as a whole and more rapid for less developed than more developed countries.

Several Asian societies have now reached the ageing component of this demographic transition. Older people are less physically active and require less food energy than the young. If food consumption adjusted correspondingly to this physiological reality, obesity among the middle-aged and older segments of the population would not be a problem. The facts indicate otherwise. Accordingly, it is not clear that older people really consume less food than the young, even though they may "need" less food and consuming less may be better for their health. How does the ageing of the population really affect global food demand?

Unfortunately, the evidence is very thin indeed. The available studies are primarily concerned with nutrition. Their focus is normative — on judging whether observed changes in diet are in line with healthy outcomes, or not — rather than with positive analysis of how ageing actually affects the demand for food. The evidence is that older people do indeed consume fewer calories than the young. Wakimoto and Block (2001) summarize a large number of epidemiological studies in the United States using cohort and cross-section data. Between ages 20 and 80, mean caloric intake declines by 1,000 to 1,200 calories per day in men and by 600 to 800 calories per day in women. The authors attribute these declines to a combination of reduced activity and reduced muscle mass. Intake of other nutrients, including protein and micronutrients, also declines, but the authors conclude that it not yet possible to assess whether these declining intakes of non-calorie nutrients constitute a health threat. In contrast, Tucker and Buranapin (2001) state that although requirements for energy decline with age, requirements for

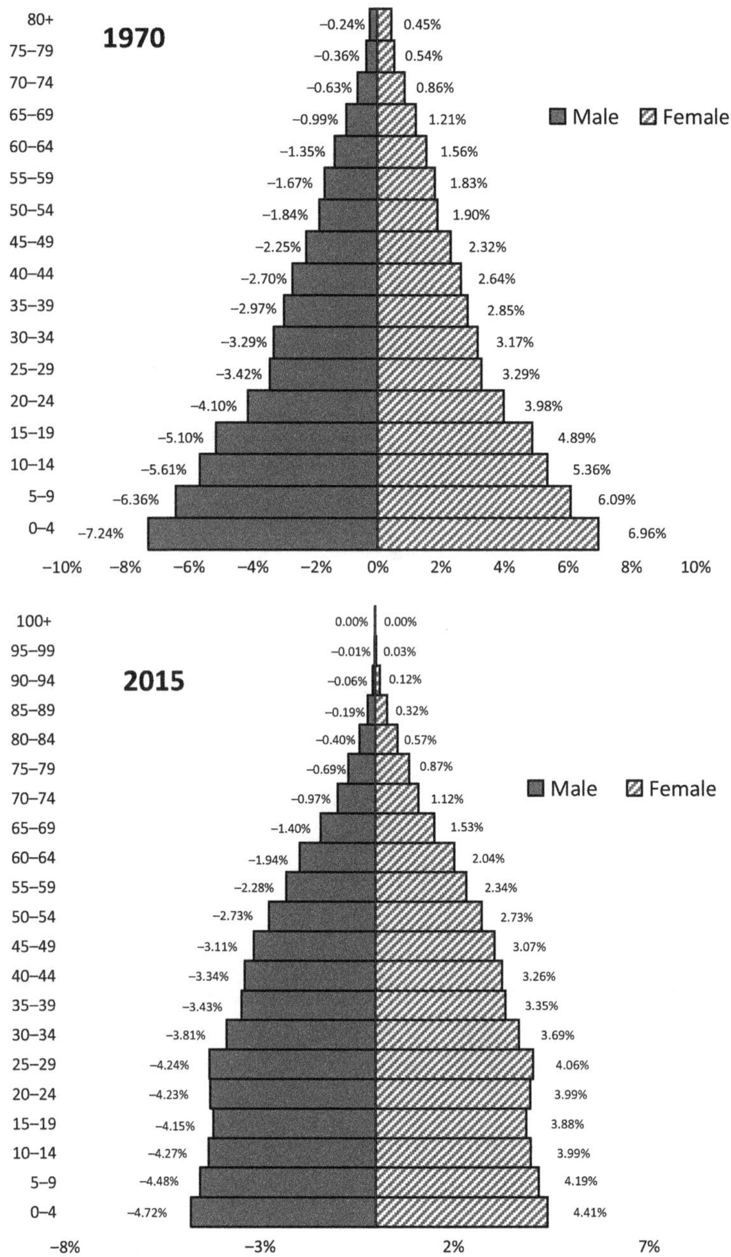

Figure 5. Population Pyramid for the World, 1970 and 2015.

Source: Author's calculations using data from www.populationpyramid.net.

micronutrients increase. According to these authors, the decline in micronutrient intakes with age is indeed a health problem. They argue that as people age, they should substitute fruit and vegetables for foods high in fat and refined grains, and are highly critical of the "fast food" culture. They are probably right, but this sheds no light on the actual demand for food as people age.

Huang and Bouis (1996, 2001) is a rare example of a demand study that estimates the effect that population ageing has on commodity demand, controlling for income, price and level of urbanization. Using household survey data for Taiwan, as described above, the authors find that changes in age composition affect food consumption in two ways. First, older people demand fewer calories, but second, generational differences in tastes mean that they are less likely than the young to adapt to more modern diets, which are more energy dense and higher in animal protein and fat than traditional diets. Extrapolating from these results, the higher the proportion of older people in the population, the lower will be the total demand for calories per person. But the effect of other variables, including higher incomes, urbanization, and changing tastes coming from other sources, will be muted by the fact that older people are more likely than the young to stick with their traditional diets.

The estimated pattern of ageing effects is that people over 50 years reduce their demand for rice and increase demand for wheat products, meat, fish and fruit, roughly mirroring the effects of urbanization, discussed above. But the estimated effects of ageing are very small compared with the effects of urbanization. For example, the estimated reduction in demand for rice as people move into the over-50 age group is 0.3%, compared with the 23% reduction in demand arising from urbanization, described above. The increased demand for wheat products resulting from the same degree of ageing, was 1.3%, compared with 19% from urbanization.

4. Conclusions

The evidence reviewed in this chapter indicates that urbanization raises the demand for energy-dense foods that take less time to prepare than traditional foods, and reduces the demand for hard-to-prepare staples. It does not seem to increase total intake of calories per person, but its effect is mainly to substitute one source of calories for another. In commodity terms, urbanization leads to more consumption per person of animal products, including meat and dairy products, more consumption of vegetable oils and wheat products and less consumption of traditional staples, including most grains, other than processed products made from them, and pulses. In nutritional terms, urbanization leads to more consumption of animal and vegetable fats and less consumption of complex carbohydrates and fibre.

The effects of ageing of the population are not well studied, but seem to be qualitatively similar to the effects to urbanization — less consumption of staple grains and more consumption of wheat products, meat, fish and fruit. But these demand effects are apparently much smaller than the effects of urbanization.

Recognition of the importance of these structural shifters is important for projections of food demand. The process of urbanization seems inexorable and irreversible. The rate at which it happens is positively correlated with income, but the relationship between these two variables is not and cannot be constant. In early stages of development, rates of urbanization may be very high, as in China over the past three decades. But eventually, as the population becomes highly urbanized, as in Japan, Korea and Taiwan today, the rate of urbanization must necessarily decline, because the rural population has become small, and this must happen regardless of the rate of income growth.

If time-series based demand estimation does not control for the rate of urbanization, the effect of urbanization will partly be attributed to income, depending on the degree to which these two variables are correlated over the estimation period. Income elasticities of demand will be overestimated, for those commodities whose demand is enhanced by urbanization and underestimated for commodities whose demand declines with urbanization. In projections of food demand, this would not necessarily be a problem if the two variables, income and urbanization, could be relied upon to move together in the future, in a regular manner. But this is not and cannot be the reality.

In countries at advanced levels of urbanization, such as Japan and Korea, future rates of urbanization must be lower than past rates. When projections of food demand are based on statistical demand studies that do not distinguish the impact of urbanization independently of income, the effects of slowing urbanization will be missed. For products whose demand rises with urbanization, including wheat products, meat, dairy products and vegetable oils, the projected increase in their demand as incomes rise will be over-stated, because the statistically-estimated income elasticities of demand also capture the contribution of past high rates of urbanization. The greater the projected rate of income growth, the greater the degree of overestimation. For products whose demand declines with urbanization, including staple grains and vegetables, the absolute decline in their demand will similarly be overestimated.

References

Alexandratos, N. and J. Bruinsma (2012) "World Agriculture Towards 2030/2050: The 2012 Revision", ESA Working paper No. 12-03, FAO, Rome. Available at: http://www.fao.org/docrep/016/ap106e/ap106e.pdf.

Blandford, D. (1984) "Changes in Food Consumption Patterns in the OECD Area", *European Review of Agricultural Economics*, Vol. 11, pp. 43–65.

Bloom, D. E., Canning, D. and G. Fink (2008) "Urbanization and the Wealth of Nations", *Science*, Vol. 319, pp. 772–775.

Hoang, X. T., Dinh, T. T. P., Nguyen, T. H. and C. Tacoli (2008) "Urbanization and Rural Development in Viet Nam's Mekong Delta: Livelihood Transformations in Three Fruit-Growing Settlements, Rural–Urban Interactions and Livelihood Strategies Series", Working Paper 14, IIED, London. Available at: http://pubs.iied.org/pdfs/10555IIED.pdf.

Huang, J. and C. C. David (1993) "Demand for Cereal Grains in Asia: The Effect of Urbanization", *Agricultural Economics*, Vol. 8, pp. 107–124.

Huang J. and H. Bouis (1996) "Structural Changes in the Demand for Food in Asia", Discussion Paper 11. Washington, DC: International Food Policy Research Institute.

Huang J. and H. Bouis (2001) "Structural Changes in the Demand for Food in Asia: Empirical Evidence from Taiwan", *Agricultural Economics*, Vol. 26, pp. 57–69.

Huang, J. and S. Rozelle (1998) "Market Development and Food Demand in Rural China", *China Economic Review*, Vol. 9, pp. 25–45.

Kennedy, E. and T. Reardon (1994) "Shift to Non-traditional Grains in the Diets of East and West Africa: Role of Women's Opportunity Cost of Time", *Food Policy*, Vol. 1, pp. 45–56.

Mace, R. (2008) "Reproducing in Cities", *Science*, Vol. 319, pp. 764–766.

Mafuru, J. M. and T. L. Marsh (2003) "An Analysis of Household Food Expenditure Systems in Tanzania, Kansas State University", Unpublished manuscript. Available at: http://ageconsearch.umn.edu/bitstream/36007/1/sp03ma02.pdf.

Mendez, M. and B. M. Popkin (2004) "Globalization, Urbanization and Nutritional Change in the Developing World", *Journal of Agricultural Development Economics*, Vol. 1, pp. 220–241.

Popkin, B. M. (1999) "Urbanization, Lifestyle Changes and the Nutrition Transition", *World Development*, Vol. 27, pp. 1905–1916.

Reardon, T., Timmer, C. P. and J. Berdegué (2004) "The Rapid Rise of Supermarkets in Developing Countries: Induced Organizational, Institutional, and Technological Change in Agrifood Systems", *Journal of Agricultural and Development Economics*, Vol. 1, pp. 168–183. Available at: http://www.fao.org/docrep/Article/ejade/ae226e/ae226e00.htm.

Regmi, A. and J. Dyck (2001) "Effects of Urbanization on Global Food Demand", in *Changing Structure of Global Food Consumption and Trade*, ed. A. Regmi, Agriculture and Trade Report WRS-01–1. Washington, DC: Market and Trade Economics Division, Economic Research Service, US Department of Agriculture. Available at: https://www.ers.usda.gov/webdocs/publications/wrs011/14974_wrs011e_1_.pdf?v=42262.

Ruel, M. T., Garrett, J., Morris, S., Maxwell, D., Oshaug, A., Engle, P., Menon, P., Slack, A. and L. J. Haddad (1980) "Urban Challenges to Nutrition Security: A Review of Food Security, Health and Care in the Cities", Food Consumption and Nutrition Division Discussion Paper 51. Washington DC: International Food Policy Research Institute.

Ruel, M. T., Haddad, L. J. and J. L. Garrett (1999) "Some Urban Facts of Life: Implications for Research and Policy", *World Development*, Vol. 27, pp. 1917–1938.

Ruel, M. T., Garrett, J., Yosef, S. and M. Olivier (2017) "Urbanization, Food Security and Nutrition", in *Nutrition and Health in a Developing World*, eds. S. de Pee, D. Taren and M. W. Bloem, 3rd edn. Springer, Heidelberg, pp. 705–735.

Senauer, B., Sahn, D. and H. Alderman (1986) "The Effect of the Value of Time on Food Consumption Patterns in Developing Countries: Evidence from Sri Lanka", *American Journal of Agricultural Economics*, Vol. 68, pp. 920–927.

Seto, K. C. and N. Ramankutty (2016). "Hidden Linkages between Urbanization and Food Systems", *Science*, Vol. 352, pp. 943–945.

Shapouri, S. and S. Rosen (2007) "Global Diet Composition: Factors behind the Changes and Implications of the New Trends", *Food Security Assessment*, [Internet], pp. 28–37. Available at: http://162.79.45.209/media/205655/gfa19b_1_.pdf.

Stage, J., Stage, J. and G. McGranahan (2010) "Is Urbanization Contributing to Higher Food Prices?" *Environment and Urbanization*, Vol. 22, pp. 199–215.

Tilman, D. and M. Clark (2014) "Global Diets Link Environmental Sustainability and Human Health", *Nature*, Vol. 515, pp. 518–522.

Tucker, K. L. and S. Buranapin (2001) "Nutrition and Aging in Developing Countries", *Journal of Nutrition*, Vol. 45, pp. 2417S–2423S.

Wakimoto, P. and G. Block (2001) "Dietary Intake, Dietary Patterns, and Changes with Age: An Epidemiological Perspective", *Journals of Gerontology*, Vol. 56A, pp. 65–80.

Warr, P. (2014) "Food Insecurity and its Determinants", *Australian Journal of Agricultural and Resource Economics*, Vol. 58, pp. 519–537.

Wu, Y. (1999) *China's Consumer Revolution: The Emerging Patterns of Wealth and Expenditure*. Massachusetts, USA: Edward Elgar.

Chapter 4

Conflict, Climate Change and Food Security in South Asia

Simrit Kaur*,‡ and Harpreet Kaur†,§

**Respectively Professor of Economics and Public Policy,
Faculty of Management Studies,
(Presently, Principal, Shri Ram College of Commerce),
University of Delhi, India
†Assistant Professor, Sri Guru Gobind Singh
College of Commerce, University of Delhi, India
‡kaur.simrit@gmail.com
§har_preetkaur@hotmail.com*

Abstract

Densely populated South Asia faces the challenge of reducing hunger and food insecurity while combating vulnerability to climate change, natural disasters and conflicts. Home to about 36 per cent of the undernourished people in the world, the region (along with Middle East and North Africa and Sub-Saharan Africa) accounted for 84 percent of violent terrorist attacks and 95 percent of related fatalities in the world. Higher instances of temperature extremes and altered rainfall patterns accompanied with sea level rise are affecting livelihoods and pushing migration both at national and sub-national levels. In this context, the study examines conflicts (through dummies considering combinations of conflict/no conflict in the present and preceding years) and climate change (as captured by rainfall and temperature over the period 1901 to 2014) as correlates of food security using fixed-effects panel data regression analysis over the period 1991 to 2014. Our econometric findings indicate that both conflicts and climate change worsen the already precarious food security situation in South Asia. In fact, the impact is even greater when prolonged conflicts are considered. Analyzing conflict–climate interactions, food insecurity appears to further worsen with temperatures deviating from their pre-structural break averages, when considered along with prolonged armed conflicts. The study concludes by recommending policies addressing food insecurity, *conflicts, and climate change adaptation and mitigation.*

Keywords: Climate change, conflict, food security, structural breaks, panel data, South Asia.

1. Introduction

Sustainable Development Goals (SDGs), the successors of the Millennium Development Goals (MDGs), have ensured a renewed commitment to end hunger and global poverty by 2030. Specifically, the second SDG calls for measures "to end hunger, achieve food security and improved nutrition, and promote sustainable agriculture" (von Grember *et al.*, 2016). Taking stock of the current situation, the Global Hunger Index (GHI) Report, 2016 states that world hunger even today remains at a "serious" or "alarming" level for 50 countries in the World (out of the 118 studied in the Report). Despite achieving the largest absolute improvements since 2000, South Asia continues to experience high levels of hunger,[1] with its GHI at 29%.[2] The region faces the challenge of reducing hunger and food insecurity, while at the same time combating challenges in the form of limits to agricultural growth and productivity, uncertain crude oil prices, food price volatility, biofuel developments and enhanced vulnerability to climate change, natural disasters and conflicts.

Armed conflict disrupts food systems, destroys livelihoods, displaces people and leaves those who do not flee both terrified and unsure when

[1] South Asia's GHI is second only to Sub-Saharan Africa.

[2] This is higher than the average for developing countries which is at 21.3%.

they will eat their next meal (von Grember *et al*., 2015). About 172 million people in the World today have been affected by conflict. Those affected include not only refugees but also populations who do not flee their homes — and who tend to fare even worse than those displaced (CRED, 2013).[3] There are also people, who are victims of violence in "peaceful" countries — victims of violent crime, gang violence, brutality by state enforcement bodies, etc. — who account for the vast majority of violence globally (Geneva Declaration, 2011). Of the estimated 780,000 people who died worldwide from violence and its immediate effects each year between 2004 and 2009, 66% were killed in non-conflict settings (mainly due to crimes), 27% died from hunger and disease due to conflict, and 7% died as a direct consequence of war (von Grember *et al*., 2015).

Global warming and climate change is yet another threat being faced by agricultural production systems. The World Meteorological Organization (WMO) estimates the recent five year period, 2011–2015, as the warmest five-year period until now. The world experienced several extreme weather events, such as heat waves, primarily a result of the ongoing climate change (WMO, 2015). The IPCC's Fifth Assessment Report (AR5) on Climate Change, Working Group (WG) I, also states that the earth has been successively warmer in the last three decades compared to any preceding decade since 1850 (IPCC, 2013). The combined land and ocean surface temperature (averaged globally) has risen by about 0.85°C since 1880. Over the period 1901–2010, global mean sea level rose by 0.19 m, an increase not experienced in the last two millennia. Regarding future projections, the report states global mean surface temperature is projected to rise by 0.4–2.6°C by 2050. Further, intense precipitation events would occur more frequently, and contrasts in precipitation between wet and dry regions and between wet and dry seasons are also expected to increase. Global mean sea level will also continue to rise with increased warming and acidification of oceans (IPCC, 2013).

Massive disruptions to food systems caused by climate-related disasters and destruction and displacement of armed conflict take a severe toll on food security. With this background, the present study discusses the food security situation in South Asia in Section 2. This is followed by an

[3]CRED, Centre for Research on the Epidemiology of Disasters.

analysis of civil conflicts in the region in Section 3. Section 4 discusses the climate change trends being experienced in the region. A synoptic overview of empirical literature on conflict, climate change and food security is presented in Section 5. Data, empirical methodology and the results of our econometric exercise are presented in Section 6. Finally, Section 7 concludes from a broad policy perspective.

2. Food Security in South Asia

Food security as a concept is complex and has evolved over time, moving away from a strong focus on food availability to a multifaceted approach that also takes into account food accessibility, food utilization and food stability. According to FAO (1996), "food security exists when all people, at all times, have physical and economic access to sufficient, safe and nutritious food that meets their dietary needs and food preferences for an active and healthy life". The four characteristics on which food security is based are food availability, accessibility, utilization and vulnerability/stability.[4]

2.1. *Food Security Situation in South Asia*

South Asia is home to about 36% of the undernourished people in the world.[5] Within South Asia, the number of malnourished people in India stands at a staggering figure of 194.6 million or about 70% of the undernourished people in South Asia (FAO, 2015). Pakistan, Bangladesh, Afghanistan, Sri Lanka and Nepal have about 15%, 9%, 3%, 2% and 1% of the undernourished people. In Figure 1(a), we plot the depth of food deficit,

[4] *Food Availability* is concerned with domestic food production, food stocks, food aid and imports. *Food Accessibility* focuses on purchasing powers, poverty levels, inter and intra household inequalities, and existence of appropriate infrastructure facilities. *Food Utilization* focuses on factors such as the availability of clean water and adequate sanitation. *Food Stability* concentrates on the time dimension of food security. It accounts for vulnerability to external conditions such as natural disasters, conflicts, political instability, unemployment, rising food prices and volatility that impact food security status.

[5] According to the FAO, Food security Indicators database, 792.5 million people (or just over one in 10) in the world are undernourished.

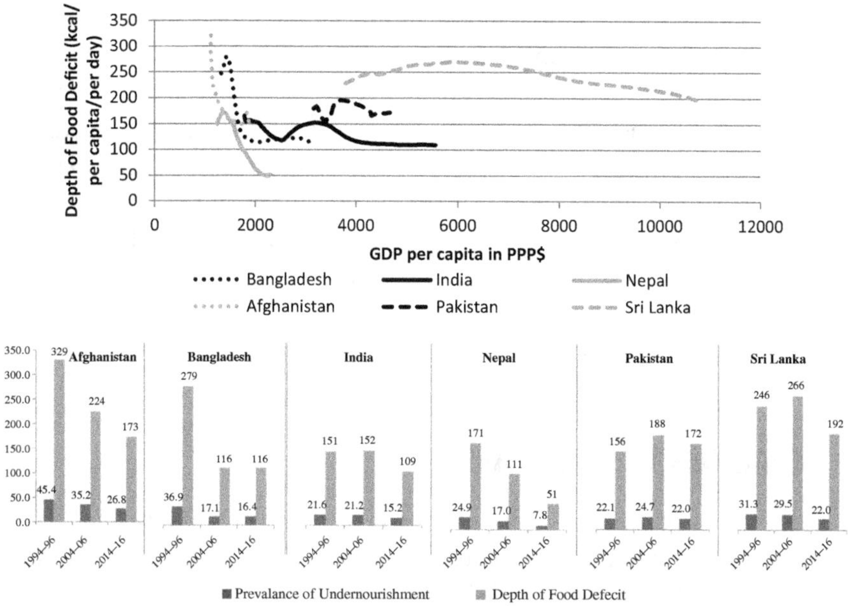

Figure 1. Depth of food deficit and prevalence of undernourishment.

Note: For the bottom panel, the vertical axis measures the Prevalence of Undernourishment (in percentage) and the Depth of Food Deficit (in kcal/per capita/day).
Source: Based on data from FAO-Food Security Indicators (2016).

undernourishment and GDP per capita (in PPP US$) for six South Asian countries. Pertinent observations based on Figure 1 are as follows:

- Increases in real per capita incomes between 1990 and 2015 have resulted in a decrease in the depth of food deficit.
- With respect to intra-regional differences, the decline in the depth of food deficit is sharper in Afghanistan, Bangladesh and Nepal as compared to that in India, Pakistan and Sri Lanka. It also shows that the decline in the depth of food deficit is greater at lower levels of income. It also illustrates that within South Asia, Bangladesh has seen the steepest decline in its depth of food deficit, despite only a marginal increase in its per capita GDP. On the other hand, Sri Lanka has experienced the largest increase in its per capita GDP, with a not-so-large decline in its depth of food deficit.

- The bottom panel of the figure shows that with respect to prevalence of undernourishment, Nepal has experienced the steepest decline from 24.9% in 1994–1996 to 7.8% in 2014–2016. Afghanistan has also made tremendous progress followed by Bangladesh, India and Sri Lanka. For Pakistan, the percentage of undernourished population fell only marginally from 22.1 to 22.0 over the period 1994–1996 to 2014–2016.
- Also, presently, the depth of the food deficit in terms of kilocalories per capita per day is highest in Sri Lanka, followed by Afghanistan, Pakistan, Bangladesh, India and Nepal (192, 173, 172, 116, 109 and 51 kcal/caput/day, respectively).

3. Conflicts in South Asia

South Asia is one of the most violent places on earth (Ghazi and Iyer, 2010). According to the Global Terrorism Index Report, 2016, South Asia along with Middle East and North Africa and Sub-Saharan Africa accounts for 84% of violent terrorist attacks and 95% of related fatalities in the world. The region has also witnessed considerable increases in conflict. In 2015, there were 4,566 incidents of conflict in the region, up from only 12 reported in 1980. Further, these conflicts led to about 8,280 fatalities, rising from 40 fatalities reported in 1980 (Global Terrorism Database -GTD, START, 2017).[6]

Within South Asia, Afghanistan is the most volatile and unstable country (South Asia Terrorism Portal).[7] It struggles with internal conflict and Islamic terrorism.[8] Pakistan and Bangladesh too have experienced violence on account of Islamic radicals. India has experienced insurgency and terror-

[6]According to the GTD, information on "terrorism" incidents and causalities are based on the following definition of terrorism; covering acts of intentional violence perpetrated by subnational non-state actors. Further, the acts must satisfy two of the following three criteria: they must be aimed at attaining a specific political, economic, religious or social goal; there must be evidence of an intention to coerce, intimidate or convey some message to a larger audience than the immediate victims and/or the actions must be outside the context of legitimate warfare activities.

[7]http://www.satp.org/satporgtp/southasia/index.html

[8]https://www.insightonconflict.org/conflicts/afghanistan/conflict-profile/

ism-related events in Jammu & Kashmir, Maoist violence in central parts of the country and insurgencies across the north eastern parts based on ethnic and minority issues. Nepal has also experienced violence on account of Maoist insurgents and the present protests against the constitution by the Madhesis. Sri Lanka faces violent ethnic separatist conflict, primarily involving the Sri Lankan Tamils and the larger Sinhalese population.

Figure 2 shows the time trend of incidents and resulting fatalities for the South Asian region from 1972 to 2015. Analysis of Figure 2 reveals following trends:

(i) From 1970 to 1983 (Phase I), conflicts in the region stagnated at low levels. Thereafter, in Phase II, they gradually increased and reached a peak in 1989, only to fall to very low levels by 1993.

(ii) The period 1993–1995 experienced a sharp rise in conflicts. In fact, the number of conflicts reached a relatively high peak in 1995, before falling until 1998 (Phase III).

(iii) Increases were witnessed again till 2001 with a minute drop in 2002 (Phase IV). Thereafter, in Phase V (from 2003 to 2014), the region witnessed a steady and steep increase in number of conflicts, as well as the related casualties.

(iv) The casualties resulting from these conflicts have also shown a similar pattern. The number of fatalities resulting from violent conflicts

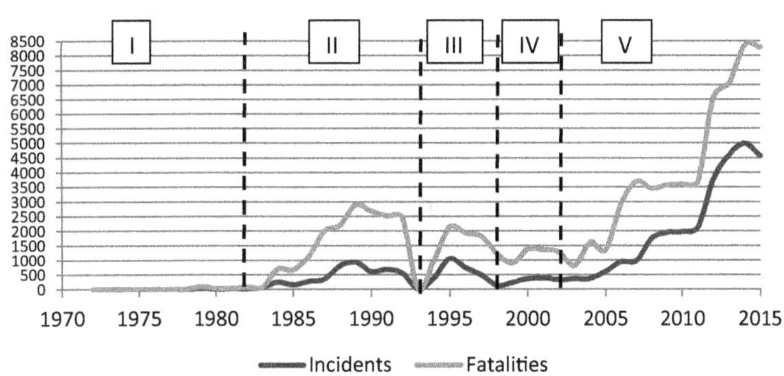

Figure 2. Number of conflicts and fatalities in South Asia (1972–2015).

Source: Authors representation based on Global Terrorism Database — GTD, START (2017).

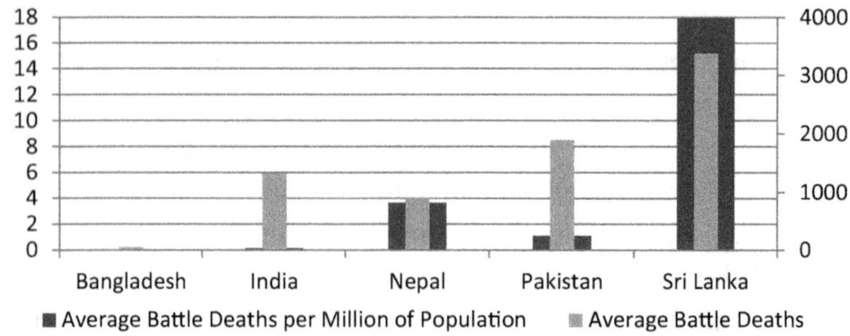

Figure 3. Average battle deaths in South Asia (1990–2014).

Source: Authors representation based on data from PRIO/Uppsala armed conflict dataset, Allansson *et al.* (2017).

> crossed 500 in 1984, and 1,000 per annum in 1989. Throughout the post-2000 period, the number of casualties in the region did not fall below 800 per year. The largest number of casualties of 8,356 was witnessed in 2014.

Based on the PRIO/Uppsala armed conflict dataset, Allansson, Melander and Themnér (2017),[9] Figure 3 provides the country-wise distribution of conflicts and battle deaths over the period 1990–2014. Sri Lanka experienced the largest number of battle deaths during the said period both in terms of the absolute numbers (3373) as well as in terms of population per million (17.9). It was followed by Nepal, Pakistan and India if fatalities per million of population are considered. However, in absolute numbers Pakistan and India witnessed higher battle deaths at 1894 and 1313, respectively, compared to Nepal's 901. Bangladesh experienced the least battle deaths both in absolute and relative terms.

In Figure 4, the spatial location of conflicts is also analyzed. In the first period from 1981 to 1990, the largest number of conflicts occurred in

[9]According to the Uppsala Conflict Data Program, UCDP, a conflict is a contested incompatibility that concerns government, territory or both, in which the use of armed force between two parties, of which at least one is the government of a state, results in at least 25 battle-related deaths.

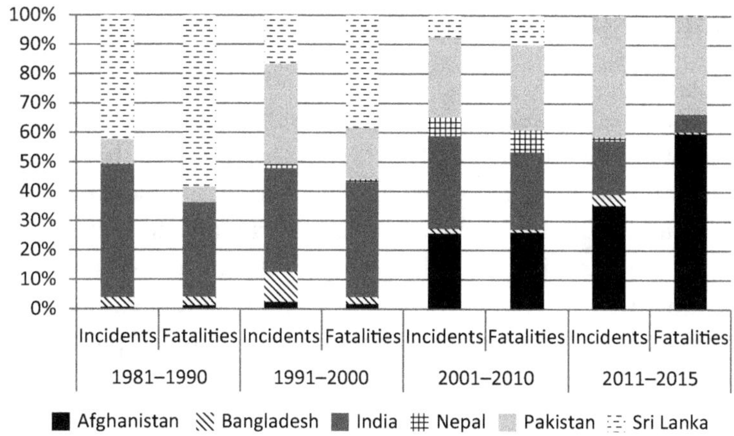

Figure 4. Cumulative number of conflicts and fatalities in South Asia.

Source: Authors representation based on Global Terrorism Database — GTD, START (2017).

India followed by Sri Lanka (1,567 and 1,460, respectively) comprising 45.3% and 42.3% of the total incidents in the region. In the following decade, India continued to experience the largest number of conflicts. However, Pakistan overtook Sri Lanka, having witnessed 1,566 armed conflicts compared to Sri Lanka's 768. Nepal and Bangladesh had the lowest number of conflict events comprising 0.26% and 3.33% of the total incidents in the region. In the decade 2001–2010, Afghanistan experienced an increase in conflicts, which was more than 20 times compared to the previous decade. It became the third most conflict-prone country in the region accounting for more than 25% of the total incidents. In the latest five-year period, conflicts in Pakistan and Afghanistan have been the highest, accounting for over three fourths of the conflicts. Sri Lanka is the only country in the region to have witnessed a steady decline in the cumulative number of conflicts over the periods considered.

With respect to fatalities in the region, Afghanistan and Pakistan together accounted for more than 90% in the latest five-year period. The absolute number of fatalities in Afghanistan has gone up by more than 135 times from 150 in 1981–1990 to 20,359 in 2011–2015. Once again, Sri Lanka is the only country in the region to have witnessed a steady decline in the fatalities over this period.

4. South Asia: Climate Change Trends

According to WGI's Report (IPCC, 2013), warming has occurred across most of South Asia. There have also been higher instances of temperature extremes with the numbers of cold days and nights likely to have decreased and the numbers of warm days and nights increased. Altered rainfall patterns with lower average seasonal rainfall and greater variability over the decades, increased frequency of deficit monsoons and heavy precipitation events have also been observed in the region. Sea level rise is also a serious risk, potentially affecting livelihoods and pushing migration both at national and sub-national levels.

4.1. *Annual Average Temperature*

South Asia has been experiencing an increase in *annual average temperatures* at the country level (Hijioka *et al.*, 2014). The annual average temperature graphs for select south Asian countries, as represented in Figures 5 and 6, shows that while Nepal is the coldest country in the region, Sri Lanka is the hottest, with their respective average temperatures being 8.3°C and 26.9°C. Over the period, Bangladesh, India and Pakistan have had average temperatures of 25°C, 23.7°C and 20.22°C. Further,

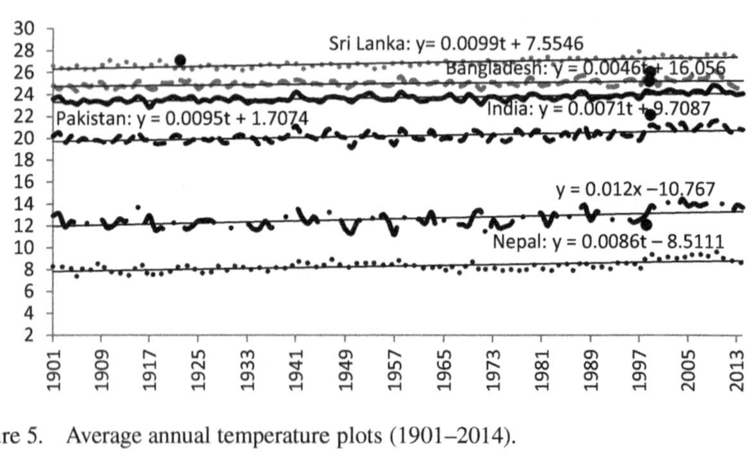

Figure 5. Average annual temperature plots (1901–2014).

Source: Authors computation based on data from CRU TS3.23 (Harris and Jones, 2015).

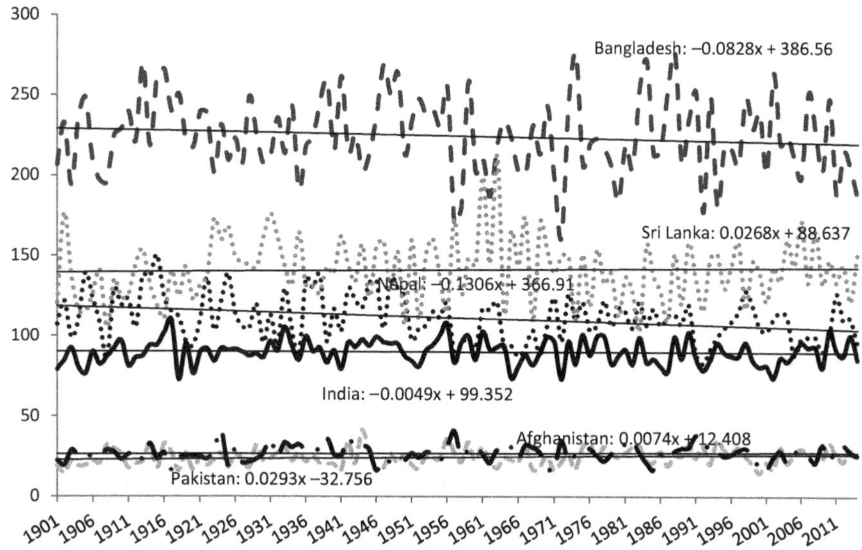

Figure 6. Average annual precipitation plots (1901–2014).

Source: Authors computation based on data from CRU TS3.23 (Harris and Jones, 2015).

Pakistan followed by Nepal and Sri Lanka has exhibited the largest volatility in terms of average annual temperatures.[10]

It is interesting to note that all South Asian countries have experienced an increase in average temperatures over the study period. The average temperatures have been growing at an average annual trend rate[11] of between 0.01°C and 0.03°C over the period 1981–2014. Average temperatures in Sri Lanka and Pakistan have experienced the highest absolute increases of 0.8°C and 0.6°C between 1901 and 2014. The annual *average maximum and minimum temperatures* have also been increasing significantly.[12]

---

[10]Over the period of 1901–2014, the standard deviation of average annual temperatures was 0.74 for Afghanistan, followed by 0.51 for Pakistan, 0.48 for Nepal and 0.4 for Sri Lanka. India and Bangladesh exhibited lower standard deviations of 0.34 and 0.33, respectively.

[11]Significant at 1%.

[12]The average maximum temperatures in these countries have been growing at an average annual trend rate of between 0.005°C (Bangladesh) and 0.01°C (Sri Lanka) over the period 1901–2014. The average minimum temperatures have also been significantly increasing with an average annual trend rate of 0.004°C (Bangladesh) and 0.014°C (Afghanistan).

4.2. *Average Annual Precipitation in South Asian Countries*

The average annual precipitation plots over the period 1901–2014 along with their linear trend lines for the five south Asian countries are given in Figure 6. Two salient observations based on Figure 6 are: first, Bangladesh, Nepal and India show a declining trend in average precipitation levels over the period 1901–2014. However, for the same period, Afghanistan Pakistan and Sri Lanka show an increasing trend. Second, the regression estimates show that while the trends for Nepal and Pakistan are significant,[13] for the other four countries they are non-significant.

4.3. *Structural Breaks in Temperature and Precipitation Trends in South Asia*

Since countries in the region may have experienced changes in climate trends at different points of time, respective structural breaks for both temperature and rainfall have been identified and explored in the present study. Structural breaks are points in time at which the statistical patterns of a time series change (Andrews, 1993; Bai and Perron, 2003). Identification of such break points enables better understanding of the behaviour of time series. Using the Bai (1997) and Bai and Perron (1998, 2003) estimation procedure, these break points are identified. Based on the estimates of a single structural break, we report the pre- and post-structural break point averages for both precipitation and temperatures, in Table 1.

Some important observations based on Table 1 are as follows:

(i) For average precipitation, only Afghanistan, Nepal and India appear to have witnessed significant breaks in their trends, occurring at 1946, 1951 and 1965, respectively. Interestingly, the average precipitation has decreased for all the three countries as reflected by the averages of the post-break years. However, while the volatility in this context has increased for India, the same has decreased for Afghanistan and Nepal.

---

[13] Significant at 1% and 10%, respectively.

Table 1. Bai–Perron structural breaks and statistics.

Country	Average precipitation (mm)			Average maximum temperature (°C)			Average minimum temperature (°C)		
	Bai-Perron structural break	Pre-break	Post-break	Bai-Perron structural break	Pre-break	Post-break	Bai-Perron structural break	Pre-break	Post-break
Afghanistan	1946**	27.07	26.91	1998***	19.61	20.84	1977***	5.19	6.32
		(5.09)	(4.95)		(0.66)	(0.4)		(0.54)	(0.62)
Bangladesh	1957	229.7	219.33	1967**	29.48	29.67	1943**	20.44	20.54
		(20.59)	(26.78)		(0.32)	(0.37)		(0.28)	(0.39)
India	1965**	90.93	88.48	1998**	29.56	30.15	1933**	17.57	17.2
		(7.495)	(7.91)		(0.27)	(0.23)		(0.23)	(0.37)
Nepal	1951*	117.33	106.43	1971**	14.81	15.01	1959**	1.591	1.99
		(15.62)	(11.33)		(0.41)	(0.55)		(0.38)	(0.62)
Pakistan	1998	24.541	24.35	1998**	27.06	27.92	1949**	12.99	13.53
		(5.58)	(5.02)		(0.41)	(0.332)		(0.38)	(0.58)
Sri Lanka	1974	143.07	137.42	1987**	26.63	26.90	1922**	22.94	23.25
		(21.19)	(16.61)		(0.29)	(0.189)		(0.26)	(0.39)

Notes: ***, ** and * denote significance at a 1%, 5% and 10%, respectively. Results generated by E-views 9.
The figures in parenthesis are the corresponding standard deviations.
Source: Authors computation based on data from CRU TS3.23 (Harris and Jones, 2015).

(ii) Taking into account average maximum temperatures, the structural breaks experienced by all the six countries are significant. Bangladesh was the first to experience a structural break in 1967, followed by Nepal in 1971. Sri Lanka experienced the same in 1987. Afghanistan, India and Pakistan experienced a structural break in the context of average maximum temperatures in the year 1998. While the average maximum temperatures have increased in the post-break years for all the six countries, the volatility has been higher only for Bangladesh and Nepal in the post-break years. For Afghanistan, India, Pakistan and Sri Lanka, the volatility has been lower.

(iii) Regarding average minimum temperatures, the structural breaks once again remain significant and, interestingly, occur prior to those of average maximum temperatures. Sri Lanka experienced a break as early as 1922, followed by India and Bangladesh in 1933 and 1943, respectively. Pakistan experienced it in 1949, and Nepal in 1959. Afghanistan experienced a structural break much later in 1977. Interestingly, India is the only country for which average minimum temperatures are lower in the post-break years. The volatility with respect to average minimum temperatures has been higher for all the six countries in the post-break period.

5. Literature Review

5.1. *Conflict and Food Security*

While there is no consensus in the literature regarding the key drivers of conflict across countries, often explanations fall under either the "Greed" or the "Grievance" hypothesis (Collier and Hoeffler, 2004).[14] Food insecurity can also trigger, fuel or sustain conflict in many different ways. Sudden food price rises, competition for limited food production resources

[14]According to the "Greed" hypothesis, it is the economic opportunity and the ability to finance armed rebellion that is the key driver of conflict. The "Grievance" hypothesis on the other hand attributes conflict to the grievances of certain groups of population that are marginalized on the basis of religion, ethnicity, caste, etc. These grievances are generally political in nature, and conflict on this basis mostly occurs in societies where political means to seek redress are limited.

and inequities affecting food security can exacerbate grievances and thereby promote conflict. Violent conflicts, in turn, create food insecurity, malnutrition and — in some instances — famine. Thus, food insecurity can perpetuate conflict, although its effects depend on the context, with the strongest links evident in states that already have fragile markets and weak political institutions (Collier *et al.*, 2003). Jeanty and Hitzhusen (2006) apply instrumental variable panel data techniques to estimate the adverse effect of civil wars and conflicts on food security in developing countries. Adams (2013), after making appropriate methodological adjustments to account for endogeneity, applies the negative binomial regression model to predict the event of conflict due to food insecurity. Wischnath and Buhaug (2014) also investigate how year-on-year fluctuations in food production affect the severity of ongoing armed conflicts in states of India. Their findings suggest that harvest loss is robustly associated with increased levels of political violence.

Several other studies have examined the link between food prices and conflict. However, the results remain largely ambiguous (Berazneva and Lee, 2013; Smith, 2014; Bellemare, 2015). For instance, in a study by Bellemare (2015), the impact of food prices on food-related political unrest using monthly data (January 1990 to January 2011) at the international level has been analyzed. Using natural disasters as instruments for food prices, they find that while increase in food prices increase political unrest, increase in food price volatility on the other hand decreases political unrest. Chen (2015) studies the relationship of commodity prices and the onsets of conflict events in Sudan. Using Structure Vector Auto-Regression (SVAR) and Linear Non-Gaussian Acyclic Model (LiNGAM), he concludes that wheat price is a cause of conflict events in Sudan. The study, however, does not find any causal link going from conflict to commodity prices. McGuirk and Burke (2016) use a panel grid dataset to study if exogenous shocks to world food prices cause civil conflict in Africa. Results based on a panel fixed-effects model show that higher prices lead to fewer civil conflict battles in areas (cells) that produce food and more civil conflict battles in cells that consume food. They thus conclude that negative income shocks cause civil conflict, as rising prices increase income for producers and decrease income for consumers in real terms.

5.2. *Climate Change and Food Security*

Climate change is projected to have a significant adverse impact on agricultural production and thereby food security in South Asia (Nelson *et al.*, 2009; Müller *et al.*, 2010; Knox *et al.*, 2012). According to Nelson *et al.* (2009), South Asia is expected to experience a decline in the yield of wheat (with no CO_2 fertilization) of about 43.7–48.8% compared to 29.2% and 33.5% for all developing countries taken together. Similarly, for millets, the region is expected to face productivity declines between 9.5% and 19% compared to declines of between 6.9% and 7.5% for Sub-Saharan Africa. According to Müller *et al.* (2010), South Asia is likely to experience average declines in crop yield at a rate of 16.4%[15] compared to 7.6% for Sub-Saharan Africa and 6.5% for the World as a whole. Knox *et al.* (2012) also conclude that average yield declines for all crops in the region would be about 7.7%. Further, maize and sorghum are two crops that are expected to experience the most significant variations. The average yield decline for maize is expected to be 17.6%, while that of sorghum is 10.8%. Several other studies (notably ADB, 2013; IPCC, 2014; Kelkar and Bhadwal, 2007; Lee *et al.*, 2012) have also projected a similar decline in agricultural productivity in South Asia due to climate change. Country-specific studies have also highlighted the impact of climate change on crop yields (for instance Karim *et al.*, 1996; Sarker *et al.*, 2012 for Bangladesh; Mall and Agarwal, 2002; Kumar and Sharma, 2013 for India; Malla, 2008 for Nepal; Hussain and Mudassar, 2006; Mahmood *et al.*, 2012 for Pakistan; Seo *et al.*, 2005 for Sri Lanka).

5.3. *Conflict, Climate and Food Security*

Few studies have also analysed the critical link between conflict, climate and food insecurity. However, often the dependent variable is conflict. Malik (2011) empirically examines the association between food insecurity, landlessness, unemployment and human under-development on violent conflicts across districts in Pakistan with data on the number of violent attacks in each district in 2009, as collected by Pakistan Institute of Policy Studies (PIPS, 2009). The study uses a linear probability model.

[15]Percentage change in 2046–2055 relative to 1996–2005 on current (2000) crop land considering no CO_2 fertilization.

The dependent variable is defined on the basis of presence/absence of violent attacks in a particular district. Results indicate that in addition to the provincial-level fixed characteristics, landlessness and food insecurity are positively and robustly associated with the probability of violent attacks across districts in Pakistan. Crost *et al.* (2015) use province-level data from the Philippines for the period 2001–2009 to study the relationship between rainfall and agricultural production to explore the connection between rainfall and civil conflict. They study the differential impact of dry and wet season rainfall on rice and corn production along with the effect of (lagged) rainfall on conflict variables (incidents/casualties). They find that lagged rainfall affects the number of violent incidents initiated by insurgents but not the number of incidents initiated by government forces. Buhaug *et al.* (2015) investigate the empirical association between climate variability, food production and political violence across Sub-Saharan Africa. Their analysis reveals that agricultural output and violent conflict appear to be weakly and inconsistently connected.

Given the limited research initiated in understanding the links between conflict, climate and food security, the current study attempts to study these crucial links for six South Asian countries. The panel study attempts to draw conclusions in terms of the impacts of *conflict* and *climate change* on food security in the region.

6. Econometric Analysis: Methodology, Data Sources and Results

In this section, we undertake an econometric analysis to study the impact of conflict and climate change on food security in South Asia. Specifically, the impact of armed conflict and climate change as proxied by rainfall and temperature, and food security indicators captured by Dietary Energy Supply Adequacy (DES_{Adq}), Prevalence of Undernourishment (POU_N) and Depth of Food Deficit ($\text{Food Deficit}_{Depth}$) is undertaken. The period of the study is 1991–2014.

Based on literature, there seems to be endogeneity between conflict and food insecurity, as armed conflict could be both a cause as well as a consequence of food insecurity. To address this problem econometrically, use of Instrumental Variables (IV) regression analysis (2SLS) is suggested instead of Ordinary Least Squares (OLS), as OLS is likely to give inconsistent results (Woolridge, 2009). We too began our analysis using 2SLS regressions. However, based on our econometric results, despite using a set of several instruments, the technique had to be rejected in favour of OLS. The details of the same are hereby provided.

6.1. *Rationale for Rejecting IV Estimation and Accepting OLS*

Based on a review of literature pertaining to determinants of conflicts (Collier, 2000; Collier and Hoeffler, 2004; Jeanty and Hitzhusen, 2006), data was collected on variables that impact household's *grievance* and *greed*, motivating them to become anti-nationals. Factors impacting grievance were proxied by variables such as unemployment, school enrolment (especially for males) and availability of domestic credit provided by financial institutions. Variables such as rents received on natural resources and corruption[16] were included to represent motivation in joining anti-state organizations for *greed*.

Typically, in a regression of X on Y:

$$Y = \beta_0 + \beta_1 X + \mu,$$

if X is endogenous, IV regression analysis involves selecting an appropriate instrument Z (or a combination of instruments) such that $\text{cov}(Z, X) \neq 0$ and $\text{cov}(Z, \mu) = 0$. Hence, the application of IV regression analysis requires certain prerequisites that need to be met. However, in our case the perquisites pertaining to (i) endogeneity of armed conflict, (ii) a value of F statistic greater than 10 in the first stage regression and (iii) appropriate instruments that are relevant and not weak did not hold simultaneously.[17]

A select sample of our results, using several instruments (either independently or in combination with more instruments), is appended as Annexure Table A.1. In general, the set of control variables included (though varying across model specifications) have been irrigation, arable

[16]For instance, corruption is expected to promote prevalence of black money that may be disbursed to youth in large quantities, motivating greed.

[17]Refer to Table A.1.

land (hectares per person), road density, GDP per capita in constant US dollars, food aid, food imports as a proportion of total merchandise imports, political stability index, inflation and variants of climate variables. Our findings clearly indicate that using an IV technique may not be appropriate. Under such circumstances, Woolridge (2009, p. 514) states that when instruments are weak, i.e. when the correlation between Z and X is low, "*the IV estimator can have a large asymptotic bias even if Z and μ are only moderately correlated*". In such circumstances, it is advisable to use OLS regression instead of IV. Therefore, henceforth our preferred model specification is OLS.

6.2. *OLS: Methodology and Results*

Given that nearly all combinations of instruments that we used were estimated to be weak, the fixed effects panel data regression analysis was adopted to study conflicts and climate change as correlates of food security in six South Asian Countries (Afghanistan, Pakistan, India, Bangladesh, Sri Lanka and Nepal). Specifically, the following econometric equations have been estimated:

$$\begin{aligned} Y_{jit} = {} & \alpha_0 + \beta_1 Irr_{it} + \beta_2 Land_{it} + \beta_3 AC_{D_{1it}} + \beta_4 AC_{D_{2it}} + \beta_5 AC_{D_{3it}} + \beta_6 CVT_{jit} \\ & + \beta_7 CVP_{jit} + \beta_8 Urb_{pop\,Gr_{it}} + \beta_9 Inflation_{it} + \beta_{10} GDP_{pc\,Gr_{it}} \\ & + \beta_{11} Road_{Den_{it}} + \beta_{12} PSI_{it} + \beta_{13} AC_{D_{1it}} * CVT_{jit} + \beta_{14} AC_{D_{2it}} * CVT_{jit} \\ & + \beta_{15} AC_{D_{3it}} * CVT_{jit} + \mu_{it}, \end{aligned} \quad (1)$$

where Y_j represents Food Security. It is captured in the following three forms:

- Dietary Energy Supply Adequacy (DES_{Adq}),
- Prevalence of Undernourishment (POU_N), and
- Depth of Food Deficit (Food $Deficit_{Depth}$).

(i) **DES_{Adq}:** Dietary Energy Supply Adequacy is a country's average supply of calories for food consumption normalized by the average dietary energy requirement estimated for its population to provide an index of adequacy of the food supply in terms of calories.

(ii) **POU_N:** Prevalence of Undernourishment is the probability that a randomly selected individual from the population consumes an amount of calories that is insufficient to cover her/his energy requirement for an active and healthy life.

(iii) **Food $Deficit_{Depth}$:** Depth of Food Deficit is the average intensity of food deprivation of the undernourished. It is estimated as the difference between the average dietary energy requirement and the average dietary energy consumption of the undernourished population (food-deprived), multiplied by the number of undernourished to provide an estimate of the total food deficit in the country. This is then normalized by the total population.

Armed Conflict (AC). To analyze the impact of conflict, our preferred specification has been to capture it as dummy variable that takes a specific value depending on whether the current year is "with" or "without" a conflict, along with distribution of conflicts in previous 2 years. We expect that while households may have coping mechanisms to deal with food insecurity pertaining to conflict in the short run, say a year, such mechanisms may fail over longer time periods. As such, three Conflict Dummies were created, representing various combinations of conflict/no conflict in the present and preceding years.

Specifically,

(i) AC_{D1} represents the dummy when armed conflict takes place in the current year, coupled with no conflict in the preceding t–1 period. However, period t–2 could be with or without conflict. Thus, it encompasses observations pertaining to C_t,NC_{t-1},NC_{t-2} as well as C_t,NC_{t-1},C_{t-2} (where C represents conflict and NC represents no conflict). In our sample, there were a total of eight observations (5 + 3, respectively) in this category.

(ii) AC_{D2} represents the dummy when armed conflict takes place in the current year, as well as in the immediate preceding period only. That is, it represents armed conflict in the current year, coupled with conflict in the preceding t–1 period but no conflict in period t–2 (C_t,C_{t-1},NC_{t-2}). In our sample, there were a total of five observations in this category.

(iii) AC_{D3} represents the dummy for armed conflict when armed conflict takes place in the current year, as well as in the preceding two periods (C_t,C_{t-1},C_{t-2}).

(iv) The base category represents no conflict in the current period. This may include combinations of conflict/no conflict in previous years. In our sample, majority of observations in this category (39 out of 54) represent *no conflict* in all the 3 years (NC_t,NC_{t-1},NC_{t-2}).

Irr represents area equipped for irrigation as a percentage of agricultural area.

Land is arable land measured as hectares per person.

CVT_j represents variants of Climate Variable related to Temperature. The specific variants of CVT_j included in the regression analysis are deviations of average maximum and minimum temperatures from their respective averages during the *pre-structural break point* years.

CVP_j represents deviations of average annual precipitations from average annual precipitation during the *pre-structural break point* years.

$Urb_{Pop\ Gr}$ represents growth rate of urban population.

Inflation is the inflation rate based on GDP deflator.

$GDP_{pc\ Gr}$ is the per capita GDP growth rate.

$Road_{Den}$ is a measure of physical infrastructure. It is the kilometre of road per 100 km^2 of land area.

PSI represents political stability index, and is expected impact food security favourably.

*AC*CVT*, the last three terms represent interactions between conflict and climate variables. For instance, the impact on food security is expected to be larger when the combined effect of armed conflict and increased temperature deviations are considered. Specifically,

(i) $AC_{D1}*CVT_j$ is the interaction between armed conflict in the current period and deviations of temperature variables from their pre-structural break averages.

(ii) $AC_{D2}*CVT_j$ is the interaction between armed conflict in the current and immediate preceding period and deviations of temperature variables from their pre-structural break averages.

(iii) $AC_{D3}*CVT_j$ is the interaction between armed conflict in the current and immediate preceding two periods and deviations of temperature variables from their pre-structural break averages.

Data for the dependent variables, viz., Dietary Energy Supply Adequacy (DES_{Adq}), Prevalence of Undernourishment (POU_N) and Depth of Food Deficit ($Food\ Deficit_{Depth}$), are from FAO's Suite of Food Security Indicators, 2016. The armed conflict data is from the PRIO/Uppsala armed conflict dataset, Allansson, Melander, and Themnér (2017). The climate data has been collected for the period 1901–2014 from Climatic Research Unit (CRU), University of East Anglia; CRU TS3.23 (Harris and Jones, 2015). The long period climate data is used to measure deviations. Deviations are estimated with respect to estimated structural breakpoint years. For most of the other variables, data is primarily sourced from Food and Agricultural Organisation (FAO) and World Development Indicators (WDI). Data related to infrastructure (road density per square km) as well as political stability[18] are from FAO. Data for irrigation (area equipped for irrigation as a percentage of agricultural area) has been calculated from FAOSTAT database (by dividing area equipped for irrigation by agricultural area).[19] Data on arable land (hectares per person), urban population growth rate, inflation[20] and GDP per capita growth rate are sourced from WDI (2016).

6.3. *Empirical Results*

The econometric results of the impact of armed conflict and climate change on DES_{Adq}, POU_N and $Food\ Deficit_{Depth}$ are reported in Tables 2 and 3. In Table 2, the estimated coefficients of armed conflict and climate change on DES_{Adq} are reported. In Table 3, the results of regression analysis considering the impact of armed conflict and climate change on POU_N and $Food\ Deficit_{Depth}$ are presented. In both the tables, climate variations are considered in terms of deviations of temperature (maximum and minimum) and precipitation from their pre-structural break averages.

---

[18] Produced by: Brookings Institution (Daniel Kaufmann); World Bank Development Research Group (Aart Kraay); and World Bank Institute (Massimo Mastruzzi). The original source of data is www.govindicators.org.

[19] http://www.fao.org/faostat/en/#data/RL

[20] Based on GDP deflator.

Table 2. Impact of armed conflict and climate change on DES_{Adq}.

	DES_{Adq}					
	(1)	(2)	(3)	(4)	(5)	(6)
Irr	0.396**	0.385***	0.381***	0.349	0.373***	0.368***
	(0.125)	(0.058)	(0.079)	(0.173)	(0.082)	(0.077)
Land	−15.624	5.415	5.006	49.586	0.863	−5.360
	(7.793)	(6.415)	(26.203)	(34.266)	(27.860)	(21.068)
AC_{D1}	−1.967	−1.814*	−1.397	−0.793	−0.479	1.958
	(1.559)	(0.880)	(0.911)	(0.440)	(1.098)	(1.652)
AC_{D2}	−1.228	−1.911	−1.341	0.964	−1.788	−3.727
	(2.024)	(1.591)	(1.456)	(0.993)	(1.614)	(2.791)
AC_{D3}	−3.720**	−3.310*	−3.175*	0.131	−3.255*	−0.702
	(1.227)	(1.562)	(1.506)	(1.614)	(1.541)	(1.681)
$CVT_{Min\ Dev\ (Brk\ Pt)}$		8.436**	6.677**	7.260**	6.748**	8.609***
		(2.194)	(2.239)	(1.981)	(2.156)	(1.542)
$CVT_{Max\ Dev\ (Brk\ Pt)}$		−7.075**	−5.991**	−5.522**	−6.080***	−6.659***
		(1.836)	(1.627)	(2.108)	(1.406)	(1.210)
$CVP_{Dev\ (Brk\ Pt)}$		0.015	0.015	0.021	0.014	0.008
		(0.015)	(0.013)	(0.015)	(0.013)	(0.010)
$Urban\ Pop_{Gr}$		−1.836**	−2.332***	−2.164**	−2.296**	−2.200***
		(0.623)	(0.564)	(0.673)	(0.576)	(0.482)
$Inflation_{GDP\ Deflator}$			0.034	0.024	0.032	0.045
			(0.074)	(0.057)	(0.077)	(0.085)
$GDP_{pc\ Gr}$			−0.044	0.042	−0.042	−0.052
			(0.080)	(0.094)	(0.080)	(0.076)
$Road_{Den}$				0.031		
				(0.042)		
PSI				0.912		
				(1.281)		
$AC_{D2} * CVT_{Max}$					1.457	
					(1.766)	
$AC_{D1} * CVT_{Max}$					−1.999	
					(2.003)	
$AC_{D3} * CVT_{Min}$						−2.884*
						(1.248)
$AC_{D2} * CVT_{Min}$						2.792
						(2.464)

(Continued)

Table 2. (*Continued*)

	DES_{Adq}					
	(1)	**(2)**	**(3)**	**(4)**	**(5)**	**(6)**
$AC_{D1} * CVT_{Min}$						−4.084
						(2.129)
Constant	96.579***	96.567***	98.899***	87.624***	99.664***	99.159***
N	138	138	126	92	126	126
Groups	6	6	6	6	6	6
R^2 Within	0.277	0.569	0.601	0.445	0.606	0.623
R^2 Between	0.375	0.346	0.162	0.082	0.167	0.202
R^2 Overall	0.295	0.379	0.166	0.224	0.169	0.188
Rho	0.755	0.804	0.854	0.882	0.853	0.863

Note: Robust Standard errors in parentheses $*p < 0.10$, $**p < 0.05$ and $***p < 0.01$.

Table 3. Impact of armed conflict and climate change on POU_N and $Food\ Deficit_{Depth}$.

	POU_N			$Food\ Deficit_{Depth}$		
	(1a)	**(2a)**	**(3a)**	**(1b)**	**(2b)**	**(3b)**
Irr	−0.566**	−0.606*	−0.548**	−5.227*	−5.575	−5.037**
	(0.188)	(0.266)	(0.196)	(2.092)	(3.219)	(1.783)
Land	52.747	−7.852	60.510	342.470	−259.953	389.754
	(64.514)	(51.499)	(66.242)	(765.607)	(659.888)	(818.803)
AC_{D1}	1.289	1.395***	−0.516	17.935**	20.887**	−7.073
	(0.810)	(0.305)	(1.722)	(6.794)	(5.676)	(21.464)
AC_{D2}	1.534	0.665	1.836	16.213*	14.020	60.792*
	(1.030)	(0.725)	(1.333)	(7.973)	(7.139)	(29.592)
AC_{D3}	2.848**	0.787	3.005**	22.596*	6.262	25.873**
	(0.945)	(0.871)	(0.959)	(10.864)	(7.699)	(8.997)
$CVT_{Min\ Dev\ (Brk\ Pt)}$	−6.184**	−6.480*	−6.206**	−35.022	−20.997	−35.153
	(2.371)	(2.590)	(2.198)	(30.479)	(32.754)	(27.766)
$CVT_{Max\ Dev\ (Brk\ Pt)}$	6.110**	6.005*	6.024**	41.263	28.709	40.105
	(2.210)	(2.744)	(1.891)	(26.215)	(32.524)	(21.391)
$CVP_{Dev\ (Brk\ Pt)}$	0.009	−0.006	0.010	0.241**	0.150	0.250**
	(0.014)	(0.004)	(0.016)	(0.088)	(0.076)	(0.081)
$Urban\ Pop_{Gr}$	1.450**	1.583**	1.385**	8.740*	8.001	7.605
	(0.412)	(0.610)	(0.408)	(3.625)	(6.300)	(7.666)

(*Continued*)

Table 3. (*Continued*)

	POU_N			$Food\ Deficit_{Depth}$		
	(1a)	**(2a)**	**(3a)**	**(1b)**	**(2b)**	**(3b)**
$Inflation_{GDP\ Deflator}$	0.003	0.048	0.010	0.473	0.839	0.540
	(0.088)	(0.073)	(0.089)	(0.699)	(0.622)	(0.683)
$GDP_{pc\ Gr}$	–0.054	–0.084	–0.061	–0.742	–1.418	–0.882
	(0.093)	(0.110)	(0.091)	(0.878)	(1.067)	(0.851)
$Road_{Den}$		–0.031			–0.169	
		(0.039)			(0.319)	
Political Stability Index						1.934
						(17.341)
$AC_{D2} * CVT_{Max}$			–1.039			30.661*
			(2.270)			(15.193)
$AC_{D1} * CVT_{Max}$			3.891			48.927
			(2.707)			(34.462)
$AC_{D2} * CVT_{Min}$						–66.680
						(37.030)
$AC_{D1} * CVT_{Min}$						–1.655
						(23.482)
Constant	31.825*	45.763**	30.380	275.936	397.846	268.567
N	126	92	126	121	88	121
Groups	6	6	6	6	6	6
R^2 Within	0.669	0.531	0.678	0.568	0.379	0.584
R^2 Between	0.243	0.138	0.239	0.078	0.071	0.076
R^2 Overall	0.182	0.151	0.179	0.093	0.135	0.094
Rho	0.935	0.925	0.938	0.940	0.928	0.939

Note: Robust Standard errors in parentheses $*p < 0.10$, $**p < 0.05$ and $***p < 0.01$.

In general, irrespective of the model, specification irrigation (*Irr*) has been estimated to have a positive impact on DES_{Adq} (Table 2). This reinstates the significance of promoting irrigation for not only food production but food security as well. Correspondingly, irrigation in general has a significant negative impact on both "prevalence of food security" and "depth of food deficit" (POU_N and $Food\ Deficit_{Depth}$), thereby once again reinforcing the need for promoting irrigation across economies of South Asia. The results are reported in Table 3.

Land surprisingly is not significant in any of the specifications in both the tables. Thus, it does not appear to be important in combating food insecurity in the region.

The coefficients for dummies related to AC remain negative when their impact on dietary energy supply is analyzed. This implies that relative to the reference category of no conflict in the current period, prevalence of conflict impedes food security. Further, in general, the coefficients are greater in magnitude and also significant when conflicts in the present year are accompanied by conflicts in two preceding years as well. This implies that persistence of conflict over time adversely impacts households to effectively adopt conflict *coping* and *mitigating* strategies. Additionally, as shown in Table 3, similar patterns emerge when impacts are considered on "prevalence of undernourishment" and "depth of food deficit". In general, the coefficients are positive, implying that conflicts worsen food insecurity. The coefficients pertaining to AC_{D3} are significant as well, implying that prolonged armed conflicts aggravate food insecurity in these economies.

Considering the climate variable CVT_j, our analysis reveals that deviations in both types of temperature (maximum and minimum) impacts food security significantly, when measured by DES_{Adq}. However, the impacts are different (refer to Table 2). While increase in deviations of minimum temperature from their respective pre-structural break averages impacts dietary energy supply favourably, increases in deviations of maximum temperature from their respective pre-structural break averages impacts the same adversely. With respect to impact on "prevalence of undernourishment", largely a similar picture emerges. While increase in deviations of minimum temperature lowers food insecurity, increases in deviations of maximum temperature aggravate food insecurity. Further, changes in temperature deviations have been estimated to have a non-significant impact on "depth of food deficit".

With respect to precipitation, our results indicate that deviations in rainfall from their respective pre-structural break averages aggravate the problem of depth of food deficit significantly. However, rather interestingly, the same does not impact DES_{Adq} and POU_N significantly (Table 3).

Urban Pop_{Gr} in general has a significant negative impact on food security. Our estimates indicate that DES_{Adq} falls significantly with a rise in urban population growth (Table 3). Similarly, POU_N and *Food* $Deficit_{Depth}$ also rises significantly with growth in urban population.

Variables such as Inflation and GDP_{pcGr} have been estimated to have a non-significant impact on food security (DES_{Adq}, POU_N and *Food* $Deficit_{Depth}$). Infrastructure too as measured by $Road_{Den}$ has a non-significant impact. Rather surprisingly, political stability (*PSI*) too does not impact indicators of food security significantly. However, inclusion of "Roads" and "PSI" as control variables make armed conflict non-significant (model specification (4) in Table 2).

We also interacted climate variables with conflict dummies to study the differential interaction impacts. Few interesting results emerge. For instance, analysis of Table 3 reveals that when minimum temperature deviations are considered along with prolonged armed conflict, the interaction term AC_{D3} * CVT_{Min} is negative and significant. This implies that while on its own, minimum temperature deviations from their pre-structural break averages increase DES_{Adq}, the favourable impact lowers when we consider it along with prolonged armed conflicts. Similarly, as shown in Table 3, *Food* $Deficit_{Depth}$ increases significantly when the combined impact of average maximum temperature deviations and two year continuous armed conflicts is considered (Model 3a). Our results also reveal that the differential impact of maximum temperature deviations from their pre-structural break averages on DES_{Adq} and POU_N are non-significant.

7. Conclusion and Policy Implications

South Asia is one of the most densely populated regions in the world with large proportions of people living in abysmal poverty. These poor and vulnerable populations are increasingly facing threats of climate change and rise in armed conflicts. Our econometric findings indicate that both conflicts and climate change worsen the already precarious food security situation in South Asia. It is thus imperative that policies addressing *food insecurity, conflicts*, *climate change, adaptation* and *mitigation* be adopted.

Despite having made substantial efforts to ensure food availability for the poor, South Asian countries still face the key challenges of improving food and nutritional security as well as reducing poverty (IFPRI, 2015). In order to break the vicious cycle of deprivation, while economic growth is essential, evidence suggests that this happens at a modest rate. Thus targeted interventions, say, in the form of direct investments in nutrition are desirable (Alderman, 2005). Sen's concept of development as freedom (Sen, 2000) also justifies state actions to secure and expand the freedom of individuals. Studies by Kaur (2007, 2008) also corroborate Sen's view. Her findings indicate that while higher economic freedom (as measured by the Frazer's Institute's economic freedom index) promotes growth, it does not necessarily expand *larger freedoms*, as measured by freedom from want and deprivation. However, according to the World Bank Report on Social Safety Nets, 2015, the coverage gap of social safety net programs in South Asia is rather acute, with only one-fifth of the poorest 20% having access to social safety nets (World Bank, 2015). In recognition of this fact, many countries have enshrined the right to adequate food in their national constitutions. However, several studies, such as by Jha *et al.* (2011, 2013, 2014), Gaiha (2014), Kaur (2014) and Svedberg (2012), critically analyze the effectiveness of food interventionist policies.[21]

It is well documented that increasing public investments in agricultural research and development, rural infrastructure and education can help sustain long-term growth in agricultural production (Fan *et al.*, 2008). The importance of these factors is reinforced in view of *climate change* experienced globally, including in economies of South Asia. However, agriculture investments have not only been traditionally low in South Asia, but have remained stagnant as well. For instance, agricultural capital stock per worker in most countries of South Asia did not show any increase over the 20 year period from 1987 to 2007

[21] Some other studies that critically analyze targeted food subsidy programmes are: Bhattacharya and Rana (2008), Jha and Srinivasan (2001), Jha *et al.* (1999, 2013), Kochar (2005), Khera (2008, 2011), Kumar (2010), Svedberg (2012) and Planning Commission (2008).

(FAO, 2012). Further, public spending per worker in agriculture for South Asia was only US$79 (Constant 2005 PPP) in 2005–2007, much lower than the US$677 which the high income countries spent. An important way to assess whether government expenditure on agriculture reflects the economic importance of the sector is the Agricultural Orientation Index (AOI).[22] For South Asia, the AOI was only 0.27 in 2005–2007, a value lower than all regions of the world (except Sub-Saharan Africa).[23]

With respect to *climate mitigation policies* in agriculture, the State of Food and Agriculture (SOFA) Report, 2016 states that "rapid transformations of food and farming systems" are essential to cope with a warmer world (IPCC, 2014). Promotion of land-based mitigation policies involving agriculture, forestry and other land uses (AFOLU) sector are important, and include both supply and demand side mitigation measures. *Supply-side* policies related to land management include improved crop varieties, crop rotation, perennial cropping systems and adoption of agricultural biotechnology. Improved water availability in cropland including water harvesting and application also remains important. Improved management of carbon and nitrogen in agriculture is equally important (FAO-SOFA, 2016). Adoption of *demand-side* mitigation policies include cutting down on food losses experienced in the supply chain as well as inducing changes in human diets towards less "emission intensive products".[24] Further, addressing supply chain losses is also essential and includes adoption of measures integrating marketing and value chain aspects into existing extension systems as well as building linkages between farmers and other agencies to support the bargaining position of

---

[22]It is the share of agriculture in total government expenditure divided by the share of agriculture in total GDP.

[23]The AOI for East Asia and the Pacific was the highest at 0.59, followed by that of Latin America and the Caribbean (0.38).

[24]To substantiate, a comparison of three meals served in Sweden with similar energy and protein content based on (1) soy, wheat, carrots and apples; (2) pork, potatoes, green beans and oranges and (3) beef, rice, cooked frozen vegetables and tropical fruits revealed GHG emissions of 0.42 kg CO_2 eq for the first option, 1.3 kg CO_2 eq for the second and 4.7 kg CO_2 eq for the third, i.e. a factor of >10 difference (AFOLU, 2014, p. 39).

farmers (ADB, 2013). It is also important to address the system of cross subsidies on fertilizers, water and electricity prevalent in the region. These subsidies encourage the abuse of resources with a detrimental impact on environment.

With reference to conflicts, greed and grievance are its primary causes. Grievances in terms of high inequalities, absence or lack of political freedom and rights as well as religious and ethnic fractionalizations cause conflicts (Collier and Hoeffler, 2004). In addition, lack of economic opportunities resulting from low levels of education, high population growth, poverty, low GDP growth rates and greater competition over natural resources also encourages conflicts. For instance, Collier (2000) reports that a 10% increase in the number of youth in secondary education cuts the risk of conflict by 4%. Similarly, a cut in population growth rate and an increase in economic growth by one percentage point lower the risk of conflict by 2.5% and 1% points, respectively. Needless to say, economies of South Asia need to address these issues to mitigate occurrence of armed conflicts.

To conclude, South Asia faces the challenge of reducing hunger and food insecurity while at the same time combating challenges in the form of enhanced vulnerability to climate change, natural disasters and conflicts. Appropriate policies need to be adopted on an urgent basis; else the existing fragile food security situations will only worsen.

Appendix

Table A.1. Instrumental variables regression test statistics.

	Endogenity test	**Kleibergen–Paap Wald rk F statistic (weak identification test)**	**Kleibergen–Paap rk LM statistic (underidentification test)**	**Hansen J statistic (overidentification test of all instruments)**
Null Hypothesis	*The specified endogenous regressors can actually be treated as exogenous.*	*Equation is weakly identified.*	*The equation is underidentified.*	*The instruments are valid instruments.*
		Single Instruments		
Trade (% GDP)	8.186***	5.74	4.613**	
Trade (% GDP)	8.137***	5.73	4.659**	
Trade (% GDP)	10.112***	5.1	4.310**	
Trade (% GDP)	10.25***	5.36	4.480**	
Trade (% GDP)	8.96***	5.13	4.586**	
$GER_{Males\ Sec}$	30.62***	0.86	0.81	
Unemployment (% of Total Labour Force)	10.97***	1.64	1.301	
Domestic Credit provided by the financial sector (% of GDP)	43.93***	12.02	9.673***	

(Continued)

Table A.1. (*Continued*)

	Endogenity test	**Kleibergen–Paap Wald rk F statistic (weak identification test)**	**Kleibergen–Paap rk LM statistic (underidentification test)**	**Hansen J statistic (overidentification test of all instruments)**
Combination of Instruments				
$GER_{Males\ Sec}$ & Unemployment (% of Total Labour Force)	12.236***	8.11	6.522**	2.83*
Trade (% GDP), Domestic Credit provided by the financial sector (% of GDP) and Urban Population Growth Rate	5.446**	7.85	14.42***	39.74***
Trade (% GDP), Domestic Credit provided by the financial sector (% of GDP) and Urban Population Density	5.332**	7.61	15.04**	39.72***
Trade (% GDP) and Domestic Credit provided by the financial sector (% of GDP)	6.259**	7.88	8.32**	16.30***

Notes: Different combinations of the following variables — *Irr*, *Land*, $Road_{Den}$ and GDP_{pc} — *in constant US Dollars*, *food imports as a proportion of total merchandise imports*, the *PSI* and *food aid per million population* along with different variants of the climate variables. CVT_j *and CVP* were used as control variables.

References

Adams, C. S. (2013) *Bread and Riots: Assessing the Effect of Food Security on Political Stability*. Georgetown University.

ADB (2013) *Food Security in Asia and the Pacific*. Mandaluyong City, Philippines: Asian Development Bank. Retrieved from http://reliefweb.int/sites/reliefweb.int/files/resources/food-security-asia-pacific.pdf.

Alderman, H. (2005) "Linkages Between Poverty Reduction Strategies and Child Nutrition: An Asian Perspective", *Economic and Political Weekly*, 4837–4842.

Allansson, M., Melander, E. and L. Themnér (2017) "Organized Violence, 1989–2016", *Journal of Peace Research*, Vol. 54, No. 4, pp. 574–587.

Bai, J. (1997) "Estimation of a Change Point in Multiple Regression Models", *The Review of Economics and Statistics*, Vol. 79, No. 4, pp. 551–563.

Bai, J. and P. Perron (1998) "Estimating and Testing Linear Models with Multiple Structural Changes", *Econometrica*, 47–78.

Bai, J. and P. Perron (2003) "Computation and Analysis of Multiple Structural Change Models", *Journal of Applied Econometrics*, Vol. 18, No. 1, pp. 1–22.

Bellemare, M. F. (2015) "Rising Food Prices, Food Price Volatility, and Social Unrest", *American Journal of Agricultural Economics*, Vol. 97, No. 1, pp. 1–21.

Berazneva, J. and D. R. Lee (2013) "Explaining the African Food Riots of 2007–2008: An Empirical Analysis", *Food Policy*, Vol. 39, pp. 28–39.

Bhattacharyya, D. and K. Rana (2008) "Politics of PDS Anger in West Bengal", *Economic and Political Weekly*, pp. 63–69.

Buhaug, H., Benjaminsen, T. A., Sjaastad, E. and O. M. Theisen (2015) "Climate Variability, Food Production Shocks, and Violent Conflict in Sub-Saharan Africa", *Environmental Research Letters*, Vol. 10, No. 12, p. 125015.

Chen, J., Kibriya, S., Bessler, D. and E. Price (2015) A Causal Exploration of Conflict Events and Commodity Prices of Sudan.

Collier, P. (2000) *Economic Causes of Civil Conflict and Their Implications for Policy* (pp. 1–23) Washington, DC: World Bank.

Collier, P. and A. Hoeffler (2004) "Greed and Grievance in Civil War", *Oxford Economic Papers*, Vol. 56, No. 4, pp. 563–595.

Collier, P., Elliott, L., Hegre, H., Hoeffler, A., Reynal-Querol, M. and N. Sambanis (2003) *Breaking the Conflict Trap: Civil War and Development Policy*. Washington, DC: World Bank.

CRED (2013) *People Affected by Conflict 2013: Humanitarian Needs in Numbers*. Louvain, Belgium.

Crost, B., Duquennois, C., Felter, J. and D. I. Rees (2015) *Climate Change, Agricultural Production and Civil Conflict: Evidence from the Philippines* (IZA Discussion Paper No. 8965). Retrieved from: http://legacy.iza.org/en/webcontent/publications/papers/viewAbstract?dp_id=8965.

Fan, S., Gulati, A. and S. Thorat (2008) "Investment, Subsidies, and Pro-Poor Growth in Rural India", *Agricultural Economics*, Vol. 39, No. 2, pp. 163–170.

FAO (1996) *Rome Declaration on World Food Security and World Food Summit Plan of Action*. World Food Summit 13–17 November, 1996, Rome, Italy: Food and Agriculture Organization.

FAO (2012) *2012 The State of Food and Agriculture: Investing in Agriculture for a Better Future*. Rome, Italy: Food and Agriculture Organization.

FAO (2015) *Regional Overview of Food Insecurity, Asia and the Pacific: Towards a Food Secure Asia and Pacific*. Bangkok, Thailand: Food and Agriculture Organization.

FAO-Food Security Indicators (2016) Retrieved from www.fao.org/economic/ess/ess-fs/ess-fadata/en/.

FAO-SOFA (2016) *2016 The State of Food and Agriculture: Climate Change, Agriculture and Food Security*. Rome, Italy: Food and Agriculture Organization. Retrieved from http://www.fao.org/3/a-i6030e.pdf.

FAOSTAT (2016) Retrieved from http://www.fao.org/faostat/en/#data.

Gaiha, R., Jha, R., Kulkarni, V. S. and N. Kaicker (2015) "Diets, Nutrition, and Poverty", In *The Oxford Handbook of Food, Politics, and Society* (Publication no. 10.1093/oxfordhb/9780195397772.013.029).

Ghani, E. and L. Iyer (2010) *Conflict and Development: Lessons from South Asia* (No. 10157). The World Bank.

Harris, I. and P. D. Jones (2015) CRU TS3.23: Climatic Research Unit (CRU) Time-Series (TS) Version 3.23 of High Resolution Gridded Data of Month-by-month Variation in Climate (January 1901–December 2014). Centre for Environmental Data Analysis. http://dx.doi.org/10.5285/4c7fdfa6-f176-4c58-acee-683d5e9d2ed5.

Hijioka, Y., Lin, E., Pereira, J. J., Corlett, R. T., Cui, X., Insarov, G. and A. Surjan (2014) Chapter 24: Asia. *Working Group II Contribution to the IPCC Fifth Assessment Report Climate Change*, 1858–1925.

Hussain, S. S. and M. Mudasser (2007) "Prospects for Wheat Production Under Changing Climate in Mountain Areas of Pakistan — An Econometric Analysis", *Agricultural Systems*, Vol. 94, No. 2, pp. 494–501.

IFPRI (2015) *2014–2015 Global Food Policy Report*. Washington, DC: International Food Policy Research Institute.

IPCC (2013) "Climate Change 2013: The Physical Science Basis", In Stocker, T. F., Qin, D., Plattner, G. K., Tignor, M., Allen, S. K., Boschung, J., Nauels, A., Xia, Y., Bex, V. and Midgley, P. M. (eds.), *Contribution of Working Group I to the Fifth Assessment Report of the Intergovernmental Panel on Climate Change*. Cambridge, United Kingdom and New York, NY, USA: Cambridge University Press.

IPCC (2014) "Climate Change 2014: Impacts, Adaptation, and Vulnerability", Part A: Global and sectoral aspects. In Field, C. B., Barros, V. R., Dokken, D. J., Mach, K. J. , Mastrandrea, M. D., Bilir, T. E., Chatterjee, M., Ebi, K. L. , Estrada, Y. O., Genova, R. C., Girma, B., Kissel, E. S., Levy, A. N., MacCracken, S., Mastrandrea, P. R. and White, L. L. (eds.), *Contribution of Working Group II to the Fifth Assessment Report of the Intergovernmental Panel on Climate Change*. Cambridge, United Kingdom and New York, NY, USA: Cambridge University Press.

Jeanty, P. W. and F. Hitzhusen (2006, July) "Analyzing the Effects of Conflicts on Food Security in Developing Countries: An Instrumental Variable Panel Data Approach", *Conference Paper at the American Agricultural Economics Association Annual Meeting 2006*.

Jha, S. and P. V. Srinivasan (2001) "Taking the PDS to the Poor: Directions for Further Reform", *Economic and Political Weekly*, 3779–3786.

Jha, R., Bhattacharyya, S. and R. Gaiha (2011) "Social Safety Nets and Nutrient Deprivation: An Analysis of the National Rural Employment Guarantee Program and the Public Distribution System in India", *Journal of Asian Economics*, Vol. 22, No. 2, pp. 189–201.

Jha, R., Gaiha, R., Pandey, M. K. and N. Kaicker (2013) "Food Subsidy, Income Transfer and the Poor: A Comparative Analysis of the Public Distribution System in India's States", *Journal of Policy Modeling*, Vol. 35, No. 6, pp. 887–908.

Jha, R., Kaur, S., Gaiha, R. and M. K. Pandey (2014) "National Rural Employment Guarantee Scheme and Targeted Public Distribution Scheme in Rajasthan and Madhya Pradesh: Complements or Substitutes?", *Journal of Asian and African Studies*, Vol. 4, No. 2, pp. 164–186. http://jas.sagepub.com/content/early/2013/05/01/0021909613479312.full.pdf+html.

Jha, R., Murthy, K. B., Nagarajan, H. K. and A. K. Seth (1999) "Real Consumption Levels and Public Distribution System in India", *Economic and Political Weekly*, 919–927.

Karim, Z., Hussain, S. G. and M. Ahmed (1996) "Assessing Impacts of Climatic Variations on Foodgrain Production in Bangladesh", In *Climate Change*

Vulnerability and Adaptation in Asia and the Pacific (pp. 53–62). Netherlands: Springer.

Kaur, S. (2007) "Economic Freedom, Inequality and Poverty: Re-Examining the Role of Government", *The Indian Economic Journal*, Vol. 55, No. 2, pp. 96–118.

Kaur, S. (2008) "Economic Freedom, Larger Freedoms and State Intervention", In *Forum on Public Policy: A Journal of the Oxford Round Table*. Forum on Public Policy. Accessible online at: http://forumonpublicpolicy.com/archivespring08/kaur.pdf.

Kaur, S. (2014) "Food Entitlements, Subsidies and Right to Food: A South Asian Perspective", In Jha, R., Gaiha, R. and Deolalikar, A. B. (eds.), *Handbook on Food: Demand, Supply, Sustainability and Security*. Edward Elgar Publishing.

Kelkar, U. and S. Bhadwal (2007) "South Asian Regional Study on Climate Change Impacts and Adaptation: Implications for Human Development" *Human Development Report Office, Occasional Paper*, United Nations Development Programme.

Khera, R. (2008) "Access to the Targeted Public Distribution System: A Case Study in Rajasthan", *Economic and Political Weekly*, 51–56.

Knox, J., Hess, T., Daccache, A. and T. Wheeler (2012) "Climate Change Impacts on Crop Productivity in Africa and South Asia", *Environmental Research Letters*, Vol. 7, No. 3, p. 034032.

Kochar, A. (2005) "Can Targeted Food Programs Improve Nutrition? An Empirical Analysis of India's Public Distribution System", *Economic Development and Cultural Change*, Vol. 54, No. 1, pp. 203–235.

Kumar, P. (2010) Targeted Public Distribution System Performance and Inefficiencies. New Delhi: Academic Foundation.

Lee, J., Nadolnyak, D. A. and V. M. Hartarska (2012) "Impact of Climate Change on Agricultural Production in Asian Countries: Evidence from Panel Study", *Southern Agricultural Economics Association*: Birmingham, AL.

Mahmood, N., Ahmad, B., Hassan, S. and K. Bakhsh (2012) "Impact of Temperature and Precipitation on Rice Productivity in Rice-Wheat Cropping System of Punjab Province", *The Journal of Animal and Plant Sciences*, Vol. 22, No. 4, pp. 993–997.

Malik, S. M. (2011) *An Empirical Investigation of the Relationship Between Food Insecurity, Landlessness, and Violent Conflict in Pakistan*. Working Papers and Research Reports.

Mall, R. K. and P. K. Aggarwal (2002) "Climate Change and Rice Yields in Diverse Agro-Environments of India Evaluation of Impact Assessment Models", *Climatic Change*, Vol. 52, No. 3, pp. 315–330.

Malla, G. (2009) "Climate Change and Its Impact on Nepalese Agriculture", *Journal of Agriculture and Environment*, Vol. 9, pp. 62–71.

McGuirk, E. F. and M. Burke (2016) "Economic Shocks and Varieties of Conflict: Global Prices, Real Income and Local Violence in Africa (October 21, 2016)". Available at: SSRN: https://ssrn.com/abstract=2776263 or http://dx.doi.org/10.2139/ssrn.2776263.

Müller, C., Bondeau, A., Popp, A., Waha, K. and M. Fadar (2010) "Climate Change Impacts on Agricultural Yields", Background Note for the World Development Report 2010. *Development and Climate Change. Potsdam Institute for Climate Impact Research (PIK).* Washington, DC: World Bank.

National Consortium for the Study of Terrorism and Responses to Terrorism (START) (2017) Global Terrorism Database [Data file]. Retrieved from https://www.start.umd.edu/gtd.

Nelson, G. C., Rosegrant, M. W., Koo, J., Robertson, R., Sulser, T., Zhu, T., Ringler, C., Msangi, S., Palazzo, A., Batka, M., Magalhaes, M., Valmonte-Santos, R., Ewing, M. and D. R. Lee (2009) *Climate Change Impact on Agriculture and Costs of Adaptation* (Vol. 21). Washington, DC: International Food Policy Research Institute.

Planning Commission (2008) *Eleventh Five-Year Plan*. New Delhi.

Sarker, M. A. R., Alam, K. and J. Gow (2012) "Exploring the Relationship Between Climate Change and Rice Yield in Bangladesh: An Analysis of Time Series Data", *Agricultural Systems*, Vol. 112, pp. 11–16.

Sen, A. (2001) *Development as Freedom*. Oxford University Press.

Seo, S. N. N., Mendelsohn, R. and M. Munasinghe (2005) "Climate Change and Agriculture in Sri Lanka: A Ricardian Valuation", *Environment and Development Economics*, Vol. 10, No. 05, pp. 581–596.

Smith, P., Bustamante, M., Ahammad, H., Clark, H., Dong, H., Elsiddig, E. A., Haberl, H., Harper, R., House, J., Jafari, M., Masera, O., Mbow, C., Ravindranath, N. H., Rice, C. W., Robledo Abad, C., Romanovskaya, A., Sperling, F., and F. Tubiello (2014) "Agriculture, Forestry and Other Land Use (AFOLU)", In: Edenhofer, O., Pichs-Madruga, R., Sokona, Y., Farahani, E., Kadner, S., Seyboth, K., Adler, A., Baum, I., Brunner, S., Eickemeier, P., Kriemann, B., Savolainen, J., Schlömer, S., von Stechow, C., Zwickel, T. and J. C. Minx (eds.), *Climate Change 2014: Mitigation of Climate Change. Contribution of Working Group III to the Fifth Assessment Report of the Intergovernmental Panel on Climate Change*. Cambridge, United Kingdom and New York, NY, USA: Cambridge University Press.

Smith, T. G. (2014) "Feeding Unrest: Disentangling the Causal Relationship Between Food Price Shocks and Sociopolitical Conflict in Urban Africa", *Journal of Peace Research*, Vol. 51, No. 6, pp. 679–695.

South Asia Terrorism Portal (http://www.satp.org/).

Stiglitz, J. E. (2012) *The Price of Inequality: How Today's Divided Society Endangers Our Future*, Stiglitz, J. E.: W. W. Norton & Company.

Svedberg, P. (2012) "Reforming or Replacing the Public Distribution System with Cash Transfers?" *Economic and Political Weekly*, Vol. 27, No. 7, pp. 53–62.

von Grember *et al.* (2015) *2015 Global Hunger Index: Armed Conflict and the Challenge of Hunger*. Bonn Washington, DC and Dublin: Welthungerhilfe, International Food Policy Research Institute, and Concern Worldwide. http://dx.doi.org/10.2499/9780896292260.

von Grember *et al.* (2016) *2016 Global Hunger Index: Getting to Zero Hunger*. Bonn Washington, DC and Dublin: Welthungerhilfe, International Food Policy Research Institute, and Concern Worldwide. http://dx.doi.org/10.2499/9780896292260.

Wischnath, G. and H. Buhaug (2014) "Rice or Riots: On Food Production and Conflict Severity Across India", *Political Geography*, Vol. 43, pp. 6–15.

WMO (2015) WMO Statement on the Status of the Global Climate in 2014. Retrieved from https://public.wmo.int/en/media/press-release/wmo-2015-likely-be-warmest-record-2011-2015-warmest-five-year-period.

Wooldridge, J. M. (2009) *Introductory Econometrics: A Modern Approach* (4th edn.). India: South-Western Cengage Learning.

World Bank (2015) *The State of Social Safety Nets 2015*. Washington, DC: World Bank. doi:10.1596/978-1-4648-0543-1.

World Development Indicators (2016) http://data.worldbank.org/data-catalog/world-development-indicators.

Part II
Food Security in China and India

Chapter 5

The Chinese Dual Malnutrition: Facts, Challenges and Perspectives

Jing You* and Zekun Du

School of Agricultural Economics and Rural Development Renmin University of China, 59 Zhongguancun Street, Beijing 100872, China
**jing.you@ruc.edu.cn*

Abstract

China has achieved huge success in alleviating nutrient deprivation over the past four decades. The prevalence of child undernutrition in terms of stunting, underweight and infant mortality has dropped well below the world average. This chapter reviews China's successful experiences in improving health and nutrition, and points out the challenge of overnutrition in terms of child overweight and obesity. Income growth increases diet adequacy, while the westernized dietary transition during fast urbanization, preferences towards meat and oil, and the traditional social norm highlighting a fat body shape for children give rise to overnutrition. Children of rural or migrant families have higher prevalence of overnutrition than that of their urban counterparts. It is worth addressing dual malnutrition — remaining nutrient deprived as well as overweight and obesity — if China aims to realize its national blueprint "Healthy China 2030".

Keywords: Malnutrition, overweight, obesity, China.

1. Introduction

China has made great efforts in improving population health since the 1990s. Per capita expenditure on health has risen dramatically from US$21 in 1995 to US$419.7 in 2014. The government's total expenditure on health accounted for 3.53% and 5.55% of GDP in 1995 and 2014, respectively. The government first raised the aim of setting up free child vaccination in 1990, made child vaccination free in 2004, and expanded child vaccine to 12 varieties in 2008. Agricultural production has also achieved great success over the past decade. Grain yields have increased every year for more than a decade, from 452.6367 million tons in 2001 to 621.4392 million tons in 2015, equivalent to 355.89 kg and 453.2 kg per capita, respectively.[1]

More support to health and agricultural success have entailed China to achieve many of the United Nations' Millennium Development Goals (MDGs). The number of people with malnutrition between 2012 and 2014 dropped by 138.1 million compared to that between 1990 and 1992, and the proportion of the population with malnutrition to the entire population dropped from 23.9% between 1990 and 1992 to 10.6% between 2012 and 2014, down by 55.6%.[2]

According to the United Nations Population Division and the World Population Prospects, life expectancy at birth has increased from 43 years old in 1960 to 1976 in 2015, surpassing the world average of 71.676. The

[1]Data come from *China Statistical Yearbooks* published annually by the National Bureau of Statistics of China (NBS).

[2]Data come from (UNDP) China Office. Available at: http://www.cn.undp.org/content/china/en/home/post-2015/mdgoverview/overview/mdg1/ [accessed June 13, 2017].

State Council further sets up the life expectancy at 79 by 2030 in their flagship national plan "Healthy China 2030" released in October 2016. Infant mortality rates have dropped from 84.1‰ in 1970 to 9.2‰ in 2015, well below the world average of 31.7. Access to improved water source has risen from 67% in 1990 to 96% in 2015, which included mainly rural households whose access rate increased from 47 to 93%. 64% (87%) of rural (urban) households had access to improved sanitation facilities in 2015 as opposed to 40% (68%) in 1990. Registering a decrease of prevalence of underweight from 19.1% in 1990 to 3.6% in 2010, China has achieved the MDG 1, i.e. halving the prevalence of underweight between 1990 and 2015 (MFA, 2015).

The present chapter reviews China's remarkable success in fighting against child malnutrition and highlights an emerging burden — overnutrition in terms of overweight and obesity. Section 2 reviews the dietary transition in China over the past three decades underlying the changes in nutritional status. Sections 3 and 4 discuss under- and overnutrition for children, respectively. In each of these two sections, we will begin by showing the facts over the past decades mainly based on official surveys and then, challenges in the present and prospects ahead in terms of policy intervention and actions. Section 5 concludes.

2. Overview of Chinese Dietary Transition

Chinese diets have been undergoing dramatic changes from traditionally low-fat and high-fibre diets to a westernized lifestyle being characterized by high-fat, high energy density and low dietary fibre (Su *et al.*, 2015). The official nutrition survey, China National Nutrition Survey (CNNS) in Table 1, shows that the total energy intake decreases as income grows. As found by You *et al.* (2016), this is also documented in China Health and Nutrition Survey (CHNS) between 1989 and 2009, a panel household data set that covers seven to nine provinces from coastal to inland China and has been designed and implemented by the Carolina Population Center at the University of North Carolina at Chapel Hill in collaboration with the National Institute for Nutrition and Health (NINH, former National Institute of Nutrition and Food Safety) at the Chinese Center for Disease

Control (CDC) and Prevention.[3] Despite remarkable success in tackling child undernutrition to be discussed in the next section, the overall decreasing energy intake and persistently low energy intake in poor rural areas (e.g. Gansu and Inner Mongolia in You *et al.*, 2017) impose huge challenges in eliminating persistent and remaining nutrition poverty in the future.

A prominent feature in Chinese dietary transition is excessive fat intake when realizing better economic well-being. As shown in Table 1, the proportion of fat has been doubled over the period 1982–2012 and accounted for one third of daily total energy intake. This excessive increase in fat seems to concentrate in rural population. In the meanwhile, however, for both urban and rural populations, the proportion of protein has only climbed by one percentage point!

The strong tendency of fat intake is accompanied by rapid spread of fast food restaurants all over China (Xue *et al.*, 2016). Given that dietary changes are one of the important determinants of obesity epidemic, one essential task facing the government is to establish a reasonable dietary regime, following the principles of a "balanced diet", to help people form healthy eating habits (Ji *et al.*, 2013) and to encourage the young generation to appreciate and adopt traditional ingredients and recipes (Ji and Cheng, 2009).

Looking into micronutrient intake in Table 2, the most dramatic increases in retinol equivalent took place in the 1980s, while the intake of many micronutrients decreased, such as vitamins B1, A and C, nicotinic acid, potassium, phosphorus, sodium, calcium, iron, zinc and selenium. Children bear the brunt of shortage of crucial micronutrients, leading to iron and zinc deficiency.

Compared with malnutrition measured by weight or height, nutrition deficiency is less noticeable to both the government and the public. In the traditional Chinese culture, people view plumpness as a signal of high economic well-being, bright prosperity and good health; whereas thinness is viewed as poverty, bad luck, and illness (Watson, 2000). As a result, Chinese parents may tend to spoil their children by feeding them more

---

[3] See the project website for more details: http://www.cpc.unc.edu/projects/china/ [accessed June 15, 2017].

Table 1. Energy intake and its components (kcal per person per day, 1982–2012).

	Average				Urban				Rural			
Energy intake	**1982**	**1992**	**2002**	**2012**	**1982**	**1992**	**2002**	**2012**	**1982**	**1992**	**2002**	**2012**
Total energy	2473.3	2310.3	2234.2	2180.3	1285.9	2361.7	2118.7	2060.2	2581.6	2283.5	2279.1	2295.4
	(100%)	(100%)	(100%)	(100%)	(100%)	(100%)	(100%)	(100%)	(100%)	(100%)	(100%)	(100%)
Macronutrient												
Protein	266.8	272	263.6	258	267.2	300.4	276.0	261.6	266.4	257.2	258.4	254.4
	(10.79%)	(11.77%)	(11.80%)	(11.83%)	(20.78%)	(12.72%)	(13.03%)	(12.70%)	(10.32%)	(11.26%)	(11.34%)	(11.08%)
Fat	432.9	524.7	685.8	719.1	614.7	699.3	769.5	754.2	356.4	434.7	654.3	685.8
	(17.50%)	(22.71%)	(30.70%)	(32.98%)	(47.80%)	(29.61%)	(36.32%)	(36.61%)	(13.80%)	(19.04%)	(28.71%)	(29.88%)
Carbohydrate	1773.6	1513.6	1284.8	1203.2	404.0	1362.0	1073.2	1044.4	1958.8	1591.6	1366.4	1355.2
	(71.71%)	(65.52%)	(57.50%)	(55.19%)	(31.42%)	(57.67%)	(50.65%)	(50.69%)	(75.88%)	(69.70%)	(59.95%)	(59.04%)

Note: The calories are calculated according to the following conversion: 1 g protein = 4 kcal; 1 g fat = 9 kcal; 1 g carbohydrate = 4 kcal.

Source: Authors' calculation and compilation of aggregated data from two official surveys — the China National Nutrition Survey (CNNS) from 1982 to 2002, and The China Household Nutrition and Health Surveillance (CHNHS) in 2012. These aggregated data are available in the *China Health and Family Planning Statistical Yearbooks* published annually by the National Health and Family Planning Commission (NHFPC) since 2003.

food with high calories, which may result in a greater consumption of high-fat diets by children (Yang, 2007) but with less attention to micronutrient intake or its structure.

3. Child Undernutrition

3.1. *Undernutrition for Children Under 5 or 7 Years of Age*

China has established the registration system for pregnant women and the health management system for infants and children. The death rate of pregnant women dropped sharply from 80 per 100 thousand in 1990 to 20.1 per 100 thousand in 2015, with narrowing urban–rural ratio, from 1:2.2 in 1991 to 1:1.1 in 2013 (MFA, 2015). As shown in Figure 1, more

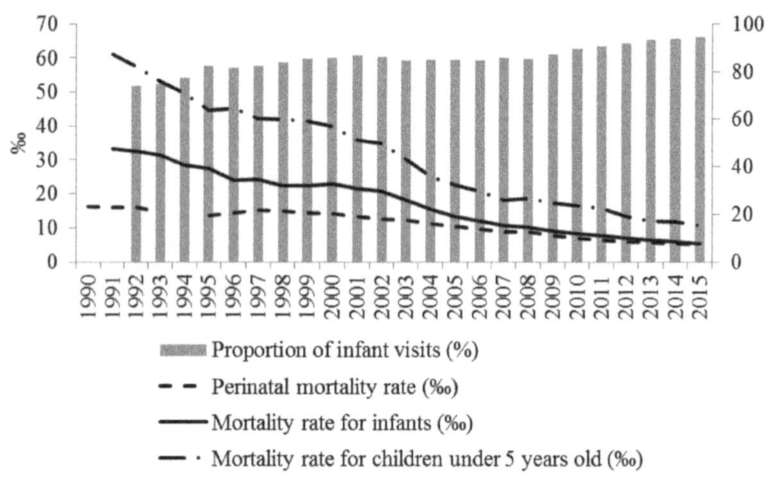

Figure 1. Health care and mortality (1990–2015).

Notes: Infants are defined as those who are aged between 0 and 27 days. The proportion of infant visits is calculated as the ratio of infants who are visited for at least once over the total number of infants survived. The perinatal mortality rate is calculated as number of stillbirths and deaths in the first week of life per 1,000 total births that completed 28 weeks of gestation or were weighted at least 1 kg at birth.

Source: Authors' compilation of data *from China Health and Family Planning Statistical Yearbooks* published annually by the National Health and Family Planning Commission (NHFPC) since 2003.

than three quarters of infants are visited by community health centres at least once within the first month of birth; and this proportion approached 100% at the end of 2015. During the visit, the community health centre checks the living conditions, family environment, infant's health and anthropometrics and gives advice and instructions on infant feeding. The perinatal mortality rate has declined continuously from 16‰ in 1990 to 5‰ in 2015. The mortality rates for both infants and children under 5 years of age declined, from 33.1‰ in 1991 to 5.4‰ in 2015 for the former and from 61 to 10.7‰ for the latter at the same time. The proportional reduction is also similar between two groups — 83.7% for the former and 82.5% for the latter. The Chinese government seems to put same efforts in increasing survival of young children. As shown in Figure 3, the coverage rates of health monitoring system and health care for children under 3 and 7 years of age increased in parallel with that of infants shown in Figure 1.

Benefiting from the nearly unitary monitoring system for child health, China has successfully addressed child underweight and outpaced other countries. The official data suggest that the rate of underweight among children under 5 years of age was 1.5% in 2015 (Figure 2), a 78.3% decrease from 6.9% in 1992, while the world average rate of underweight for children under 5 years of age was 16% and only registered a 36% proportionate decrease between 1990 and 2011 (UNICEF, 2012). The infant underweight saw a quick drop between 1991 and 1992, and then became stable around 2.5%.

Survey data reaffirm success in improving child health in official statistics. Figures 3 and 4 compiled empirical results for children under 5 years old based on different data sets. The prevalence of child underweight in Figure 3 was about 8% in 1993, which was 3 percentage points higher than the official estimate of 5.1% in Figure 2. The difference shrank in the following survey years and both pointed to about 2% after the 2000s. The overall downward trend of child underweight retains, while the temporary increase of prevalence between 2004 and 2006 for the whole sample population lacks robustness given decreasing underweight in other studies and in its rural and urban subsamples.

Wasting remained at a lower prevalence compared with underweight and stunting and decreased from 3% to 1%, but there was a sharp rise in

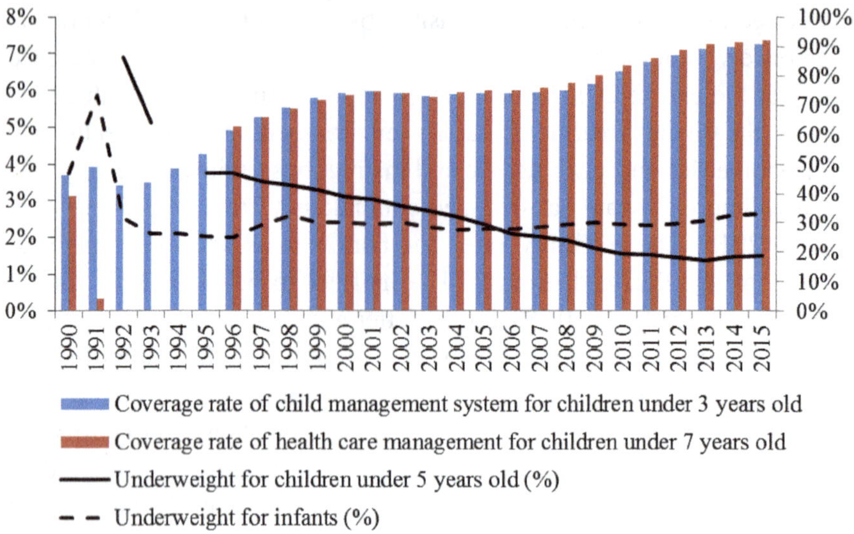

Figure 2. Health care and underweight (1990–2015).

Notes: Child management system for children under 3 years of age is to monitor growth and development. Health care management for children under 7 years of age is to monitor anthropometrics. Underweight for children under 5 years is defined as that of the WHO, i.e. lower weight than the 2 standard deviations of the median weight among children in each age. The median weight is adopted by the WHO's standard. Underweight is defined as weight at birth being lower than 2.5 kg. The infant underweight rate is the proportion of underweight infants in all infants survived.

Source: Authors' compilation of data from *China Health and Family Planning Statistical Yearbooks* published annually by the National Health and Family Planning Commission (NHFPC) since 2003.

2006 up to 8% ascribed to measurement or reporting errors rather than an implication of undernutrition (Piernas *et al.*, 2015; Yu *et al.*, 2016).

Despite overall reduction in child undernutrition, there is heterogeneity in age and gender. Stunting and underweight are age-specific. Among children under 5 years old, incidence of stunting and underweight peaks during 24–47 months and 48–59 months, respectively; whereas the lowest incidence occurs during 0–6 months (Yu *et al.*, 2011; Zhang *et al.*, 2011a). An assessment of child nutrition in Xiamen (in Fujian province) shows that wasting occurs mainly among children aged 3–4 years (Chen *et al.*, 2016). The risk of wasting of children under 5 years of age in rural areas halves after 6 months and remains at low prevalence (Zhang *et al.*, 2011a; Yu *et al.*, 2011).

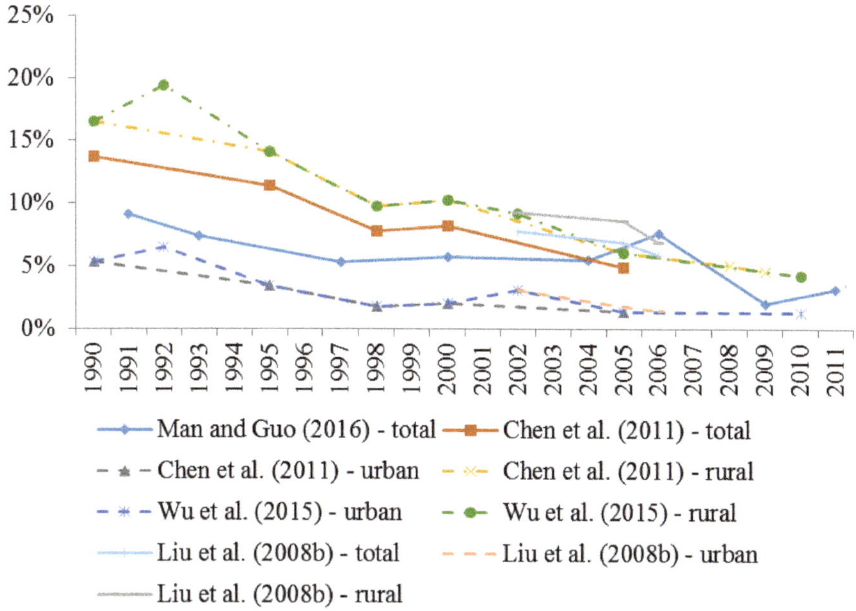

Figure 3. Prevalence of underweight for children under 5 years of age (1989–2011).

Notes: Man and Guo (2016) use the CHNS in 1991, 1993, 1995, 1997, 2000, 2004, 2006, 2009 and 2011. Chen *et al.* (2011) use the National Food and Nutrition Surveillance System in 1990, 1995, 2000, 2005, 2008 and 2009. Wu *et al.* (2015) use the National Food and Nutrition Surveillance System and the CNNS between 1990 and 2010. Liu *et al.* (2008b) use the CNNS in 2002, the National Food and Nutrition Surveillance System in 2005 and the Survey of Children and Women Development Indicators in 2006. This last nation-wide survey was to collect information on children and women development indicators set up by the State Council in 2001 for the period 2001–2010. All surveys, except the CHNS, are officially sampled and conducted by different government sectors.
Source: Authors' compilation of estimates in the literature.

Nutritional status between genders remains inconclusive. Adopting the 2000 National Center for Health Statistics (NCHS) Growth Charts to the rural sample of the CHNS, Ren *et al.* (2014) find that the probability of being mildly stunted, e.g. *z*-score ranging between −2 and −1, is 5 percentage points higher for girls aged from 6 months to 10 years than for boys in the same cohort. This is later demonstrated again by Zhang *et al.* (2016), whose research shows that girls under 5 years of age in rural areas suffered from a higher risk of undernutrition than boys. On the contrary, in Yu *et al.* (2011), boys under 5 years of age are

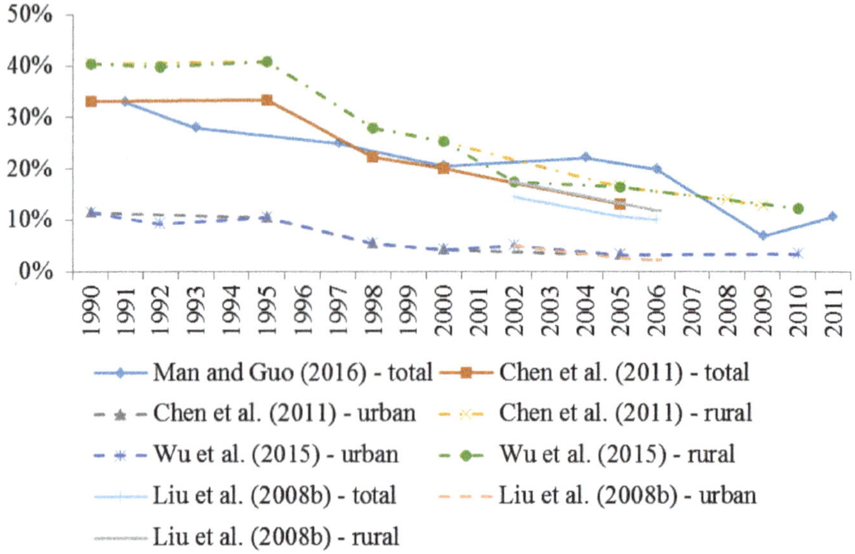

Figure 4. Prevalence of stunting for children under 5 years of age (1990–2011).

Note: See Figure 3.

Source: See Figure 3.

more vulnerable than girls in terms of stunting, while underweight and wasting did not vary significantly. Neutral results were reported by Liu *et al.* (2013) based on the CHNS from 1989 to 2006. They find that girls are slightly more stunting than boys, but this difference is not significant.

3.2. *Undernutrition for Children Older than 5 and 7 Years of Age*

Different from the unitary monitoring system for infants and children under 5 years of age, there are no annual official data on malnutrition or health monitoring system on the annual basis for this cohort. The Chinese government implements national nutrition surveys and student surveys for the purpose of tracking dynamics of health and physique. We thus resort to these official surveys, together with other nation-wide surveys conducted by research institutes, in this section.

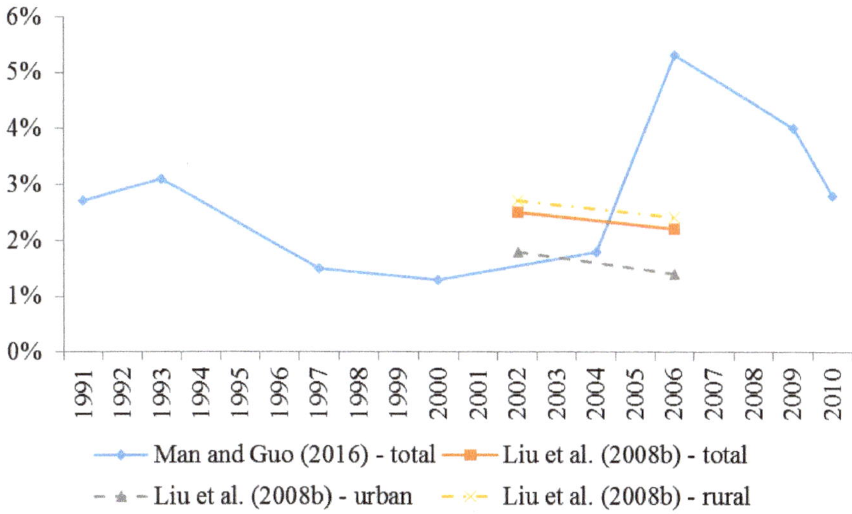

Figure 5. Prevalence of wasting for children under 5 years of age (1990–2010).

Note: See Figure 3. Measured by height-for-age (stunting) and weight-for-height (wasting) in the CHNS, Figures 4 and 5 also illustrate downward trends of child undernutrition. Although stunting was substantially more prevalent than underweight and wasting at the beginning of 1990s, it followed a faster decline for more than two decades, from about 33% to 10% in around 2010 (NHFPC, 2012), and further to 8.1% in 2013 (Yu *et al.*, 2016).

Source: See Figure 3.

A downward trend can be found again in official surveys. In the China National Nutrition Survey (CNNS), which is the official nation-wide survey conducted in 1959, 1982, 1992 and 2002, 10.6% of children aged 12–18 years were underweight in 1982 (i.e. BMI<18.5 according to International Obesity Task Force (IOTF) standard) and this proportion grew to 13.1% in 1992 (Du *et al.*, 2014). A downward trend of undernutrition has turned up since the early 1990s. In the CHNS, the prevalence of underweight (BMI-for-age <5th percentile based on the 2000 NCHS Growth Charts) for children aged 6–17.9 years declined from 14.8% in 1991 to 9.4% in 2004 with an annual proportionate reduction of 2.8%, while the prevalence of stunting (height-for-age <5th percentile based on the 2000 NCHS Growth Charts) showed a larger and quicker reduction, from 37.2% to 16.0%, over the same period with an annual speed of 4.4% (Dearth-Wesley *et al.*, 2008). In the 2002 CNNS (also known as the China

National Nutrition and Health Survey, CNNHS), Chang and Wang (2016) summarize that 6.3% and 13.4% children aged 6–17 years were stunted and wasted, respectively, based on the new national standard (i.e. the screening standard for malnutrition of school-age children and adolescents, WS/T 456-2014, issued by the NHFPC in June 2014 and implemented from December 2014). Applying this 2014 criteria to the Chinese National Survey on Student Constitution and Health (CNSSCH) led by the Ministry of Education and conducted in roughly every 5-year time since 1979, Dong *et al.* (2016) find that 15.4% of students aged 7–12 years in 2005 suffered from malnutrition to different extents, comprising 2% of stunting, 7.3% of mild wasting and 6.1% of severe wasting. These proportions only marginally declined to 1.2%, 6.3% and 5.4%, respectively, for stunting, mild wasting and severe wasting in 2010. The CNNHS in 2012 suggests that 2.8% of children aged 6–17 years in 2012 were stunting and 9% were wasted, registering 25% and 14% of reduction, respectively, from 2002 (Chang and Wang, 2016). The average height increased by 2.3 cm for boys and 1.8 cm for girls between 2002 and 2012 (*ibid*).

There is, however, heterogeneity in the estimates of undernutrition, especially in age–specific undernutrition. Based on the IOTF standard, 14.5% of boys aged 6–11 years in 2004 were underweight (Seo and Niu, 2014). This proportion increased to 17.6% in 2006 and continued to rise to 20.1% in 2009. Similarly, 19.4%, 24.7% and 23.6% of girls of the same age were underweight in 2004, 2006 and 2009, respectively. The downward trend of underweight was driven by boys aged 12–18 years — the prevalence decreased gradually from 18.6% in 2004 to 17.9% in 2006 and further down to 14.2% in 2009, while the prevalence of girls of same age remained at 20.4%, 20.5% and 20.7% in 2004, 2006 and 2009, respectively.

Figure 6 compares the prevalence of stunting and wasting by gender and by urban–rural divide for children aged 7–18 years in the 2010 CNSSCH. Wasting is more prevalent than stunting and is the main nutrition problem for older children. The prevalence of stunting remained stable when children grew up and the gender disparity was trivial. By contrast, wasting conveys another and more complicated story. In both rural and urban subsample, boys were more likely to be wasted when they grew up, while girls suffered from less wasting until about 18 years old.

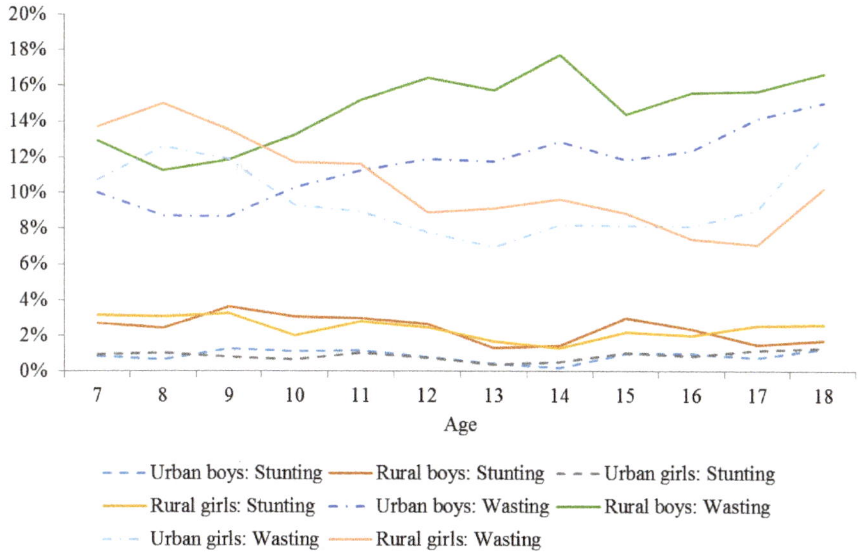

Figure 6. Child growth and development (aged 7–18 years in 2010).

Notes: The standard of undernutrition is the WS/T 456 released by the NHFPC in 2014. Stunting and wasting are defined as falling into age-specific ranges of (low) height and (low) BMI, respectively.
Source: Authors' compilation of aggregated data from the CNSSCH in 2010.

When children were below about 11–12 years old, wasting was more prevalent among girls than among boys in both urban and rural subgroups, but when beyond 11–12 years old, boys were more likely to be wasting than girls.

Comparing the estimates of underweight for children aged 7–18 years and those for children aged below 5 years, the prevalence seems to be higher for the former than for the latter.

3.3. *Challenges*

3.3.1. *Persistent but narrowing urban–rural disparity*

Rural children are more likely to be stunted and underweight than their urban counterparts. As shown in Figure 4, despite a larger reduction of stunting for rural children aged below 5 years than for their urban counterparts, 12.1% (3.4%) of the former were stunted (underweight) in 2010 as opposed to 3.4% (1.3%) of the latter (Wu *et al.*, 2015). Similar result were found by Zong and Li (2014). In 2013, the prevalence of stunting, underweight and wasting in rural population were 11.2%, 3.1% and 1.4%, respectively, while in urban, they were 4.3%, 1.5% and 1.3%, respectively (Yu *et al.*, 2016).

Among children aged above 7 years, the CHNS 2004–2009 showed consistently better nutrition status for urban than for rural children. The prevalence of underweight varies between 9.4% and 21.7% among urban children, while it was between 15.8% and 25.8% among rural ones (Seo and Niu, 2014). The only exception is girls aged 12–18 years, among whom rural prevalence of underweight (9.4%) was lower than that of the urban (15.8%). When gender differences are also taken into account, as shown in Figure 6, rural girls were more likely to be wasted than urban ones until 16 years old, while rural boys were worse off than urban ones in terms of the prevalence of undernutrition at all ages before adulthood.[4]

In the meanwhile, the urban–rural gap in nutrition narrowed. The gap in terms of the ratio of prevalence of stunting (underweight) between urban and rural children was 5.3 (4.6) in 2006 (Liu *et al.*, 2008b), which shrank to about 2 (3) in around 2013 (Chang and Wang, 2016). Nevertheless, this by no means indicates that undernutrition is less of a problem or can be neglected in rural areas. Rural children, especially those in poorer rural areas, have long lagged behind their urban counterparts. The CNSSCH shows that nutritional status of children under 5 years of age in poor rural areas did not improve between 1998 and 2000, but rather worsened. Specifically, there had still been 12.3% and 21% of rural children under 5 years of age who were underweight and stunted, respectively, by the end of 2005, twice as many as the rural average (Chang *et al.*, 2006). The CDC set up the Monitoring Information System for Children under 6 Years in Poor Areas in 2005

[4]Nevertheless, the CNSSCH in 2005 and 2010 do not reveal average gender differences between boys and girls at all ages between 7 and 11 years (see Dong *et al.*, 2016, Table 2). Both genders suggest significant decreases in underweight and stunting with equivalent magnitude. Gender differences are nested in the urban–rural disparity.

and expanded it in later years to cover 100 poor counties out of 27 provinces that were designated by the State Council. The data in 2009 show that 15.9% of children under 5 years old in poor rural areas were stunted; 7.8% and 3.7% were underweight and wasted, respectively (Yu *et al.*, 2011). Comparing them with the national average prevalence of underweight in Figure 1 (2.4% in 2009), children in poor rural areas are 3.25 (=7.8%/2.4%) times likely to suffer from undernutrition as if they had been average children.

3.3.2. *Regional disparity*

The Chinese remarkable improvement in child nutrition is not distributed evenly across areas. Geographic disparity persists and is even broadened over time. Compared with low rates of stunting (4.9%) and underweight (3.5%) in the eastern region in 2005, the western region exhibited the highest prevalence at 13.9% and 7.8%, respectively, and the central region lies in between — 11.8% and 7%, respectively (Liu *et al.*, 2008b). In 2011, 14.3% of eastern children under 5 years of age suffered from any form of undernutrition (namely, stunting, underweight and wasting), while the proportion in the central and western regions were 27.5% and 41.4%, respectively (Man and Guo, 2016). This underlines the east–west ratio of 2.9.

More specifically, compared with northeastern provinces such as Liaoning and Heilongjiang and coastal provinces like Jiangsu, children in the central provinces, such as Henan, Hubei and Hunan, were associated with higher probabilities of stunting, while children in western provinces such as Guangxi and Guizhou were worse in all health and nutritional outcomes (Liu *et al.*, 2013). Based on the new national nutrition standard (i.e. WS/T456-2014)[5] and the CNSSCH sampling students aged 7–12 years in 2010, malnutrition concentrates in western provinces such as Guizhou and Yunnan suffered from persistent child malnutrition. Tibetan

[5]The criteria are age-specific upper and lower thresholds of BMI, and are higher than those of the WHO. Consequently, the prevalence of child malnutrition is higher under the Chinese national criteria than under WHO's. For the estimates under WHO's standards in 2007, see Ji (2009) over the period 1985–2005.

students suffered severer malnutrition: the prevalence of mild wasting (severe wasting) increased dramatically from 4.5% (2.5%) in 2005 to 10.1% (9.2%) in 2010. It seems that improvement in child nutrition is driven by eastern provinces, nevertheless, even within provinces suggesting low (<10%) or moderate (10–20%) prevalence, a few provinces witnessed increasing malnutrition. For example, Jiangsu, an eastern province, had the prevalence of mild wasting (severe wasting) at 3.8% (2.4%) in 2005, but 4.2% (3.6%) in 2010. Severe wasting even gets worse by 1.1 to 2.3 percentage points in the Northeast, such as Heilongjiang, Jilin and Liaoning provinces.

Even within the same region, provincial disparities are prominent. A study in six western provinces in 2009 (Sichuan, Guangxi, Guizhou, Gansu, Xinjiang and Inner Mongolia) reveals substantial variations across provinces (Zhang *et al.*, 2011b). Guangxi ranked first in stunting (26.2%) and underweight (15.9%), while Inner Mongolia (5.6%) and Xinjiang (2.5%) witnessed the lowest prevalence in two dimensions, respectively.

3.3.3. *Migrant children and left-behind children*

China has witnessed perhaps the largest internal (rural-to-urban) migration all over the world. The NBS documents 292 million internal migrants in 2016, accounting for of one fifth of China's total population. The average age of migrants was 29.3 in 2015 and the size of family in migration was 2.61 persons (NHFPC, 2016). According to the most recent Census at the end of 2010, there were more than 61 million left-behind children (aged under 18 years) in China, accounting for around 21.88% of total Chinese children. A typical social problem brought about by such a large size of migrants is how to arrange parenting, for both left-behind children who stay at home villages with local household registration but lack family care and migrant children who move with parents to cities but without local household registration (linking to local social welfare). Existing studies have not achieved consensus on health or nutritional well-being of children in different parenting patterns.

A typical concern with children living away from parents is their low health and nutrition status due to lack of parental care. Indeed a strand of literature has confirmed this, yet with heterogeneity in results. In addition to higher risk of mental health (Shi *et al.*, 2016), children aged under 5 years in 2009 with migrant mothers were 48.3% (54%) more likely to be stunted (underweight) than those with non-migrant mothers (NHFPC, 2012). Using the CHNS, de Brauw and Mu (2011) find that the negative association between child underweight and migrating family members was driven by older children aged 8–14 years. On the contrary, Chen (2012) and Mo *et al.* (2016) find that parental migration brings significantly negative impact on nutrition and health conditions for children under 6 years of age. Xiao *et al.* (2015) warn that early childhood is critical for children's growth in later life and being left behind during early childhood, as compared with living with parents, could lead to slower growth rates of height and weight. Mothers play a vital role in making sure children are normally nourished. In the CHNS, rural children having their mother as the caregiver generally have 20% lower incidence of illness or chronic diseases (Li *et al.*, 2015). The prevalence of stunting was the lowest (14.9%) among children being cared for by their mother, followed by grandparents (18.4%) and by fathers (21.8%) (Ban *et al.*, 2015). In another survey in Shandong province in 2013, grandparental care yields the highest prevalence of wasting (5.3%), compared with being left-behind (4%) and maternal care (3.9%) (Mo *et al.*, 2016).

One reason underlying positive association between parental (especially maternal) care and child nutrition is attributed to intra-household allocation: with men at home, women allocate more household economic resources on food and other inputs into child nutrition and health (Ning and Cheng, 2013). Another reason is that migrating parents result in less time spent preparing and buying food and this in turn causes lower quality and smaller amounts of food consumed by left-behind children (de Brauw and Mu, 2011). An interesting perspective to explain the "not-so-good" role of grandparental care on child nutrition is from intergenerational beliefs about a healthy diet. Using self-collected data in a central and agricultural province (Henan) from 2013 to 2014, Zhang *et al.* (2015) document different beliefs across generations. The grandparent generation who experienced the Great Famine in the late 1950s was concerned about not having enough food and tended to emphasize the importance of starchy foods for children's growth, while the parental generation was concerned about food safety and paid more attention to protein-source foods including meat, eggs and milk. As such, left-behind children cared for by grandparents would be at higher risk of malnutrition. It is also alarming that parents in their study tended to offer children high-energy food, which was viewed as a sign of economic status, rather than as part of a balanced diet. This carries potential risk of overnutrition, which will be explored in Section 4.

In contrast to a negative view on left-behind children's nutrition, a comprehensive data set covering 141 thousand rural children out of 10 provinces over the period 2009 and 2013 show that left-behind children outperform their rural counterparts living with parents in nutrition, health and education, because out-migration is self-selected (or afforded) by richer rural families (Zhou *et al.*, 2015). Correcting this endogeneity, Mu and de Brauw (2015) find no significant impact of parental migration on child height, but find positive impact on weight, which is likely to be a result of improved access to tap water in migrant households.

Further, migrant children confront similar or even higher risk of undernutrition. Based on the CHNS from 2006 to 2009, Lu *et al.* (2016) compare left-behind and migrant children in many dimensions of well-being. 6.85% of rural non-left-behind children were underweight, as opposed to 5.74% of migrant children and 3.25% of left-behind children. 6.67% of migrant children smoked, followed by 2% of left-behind children and 1.79% of rural non-left-behind children.

Local city life does not necessarily benefit migrant children's health and nutrition given institutional barriers like *Hukou* (household registration) which is linked to local social welfare schemes, while migrants have to stick to their *Hukou* at home villages. Using the CHNS between 1993 and 2009, Liu *et al.* (2015) calculate the child nutritional indicators based on their *Hukou* status. Children with urban *Hukou* had 0.25 higher height z-scores and 0.15 higher weight z-scores than children with rural *Hukou*, and the difference between them based on *Hukou* was larger than the difference in height and weight (0.23 and 0.09, respectively) by urban vs. rural residence. Controlling for place of residence, children with urban *Hukou* still had 0.18 higher height z-scores and 0.17 higher weight z-scores than children with rural *Hukou*. Although the authors also document declining the *Hukou*-induced nutritional gap after 2000, migrant children are still as vulnerable as those being left-behind in rural areas, and perhaps require different policy intervention given their residency and family living arrangements.

3.3.4. *Nutrient deficiency*

As shown previously in Table 2, key micronutrient intake declines over time, especially in rural population. Indeed, an alarming phenomenon among rural children is nutrient deficiency, leading to anaemia and future to low cognitive skills and worse educational outcomes. This is detrimental to the child's life-long achievements.

The prevalence of nutrient deficiency is higher than that of stunting or underweight. The anaemia rate was 24.9% among 4,000 rural students in Grades 4 and 5 in 2009 out of 10 poor counties in Ningxia and Qinghai provinces (Luo *et al.*, 2011). In an adjacent and poor province, Gansu, the rate was 10.4% for 2,000 primary school children over the period 2000 and 2004 (You, 2013).

3.3.5. *Dynamics of undernutrition over time*

The survey estimates in Figures 3–5 show reversionary trends in child undernutrition after the late 2000s. In Wu and Qi's (2016) investigation, poor provinces like Guangxi exhibit such reversal in underweight among children under 18 years of age. This corresponds to an official report revealing the doubled size of stunted children under 12 months in poor rural areas after the financial crisis in 2008 (NHFPC, 2012). Dong *et al.* (2016) warn that rich provinces having been characterized by low malnutrition are at higher risk of regressing than poor provinces. Seo and Niu (2014) find that among boys aged 6–11 years, the proportions of underweight were almost doubled for three subpopulations — those who lived in low-income families, who lived in urban areas, and, interestingly, who watched TV or did homework for more than 2 hours a day.

When dynamics of nutrient intake is taken into account, we would have reasons to be concerned with not only the "new entries" of undernutrition but also those who "returned" due to various reasons. This calls for longer-term monitoring and management of child nutrition, which is

Table 2. Nutrient intake (per person per day, 1982–2012).

Nutrient	Average				Urban				Rural			
	1982	1992	2002	2012	1982	1992	2002	2012	1982	1992	2002	2012
Macronutrient												
Protein (g)	66.7	68.0	65.9	64.5	66.8	75.1	69.0	65.4	66.6	64.3	64.6	63.6
Fat (g)	48.1	58.3	76.2	79.9	68.3	77.7	85.5	83.8	39.6	48.3	72.7	76.2
Carbohydrate (g)	443.4	378.4	321.2	300.8	101.0	340.5	268.3	261.1	489.7	397.9	341.6	338.8
Dietary fibre (g)	8.1	13.3	12.0	10.8	6.8	11.6	11.1	10.8	8.7	14.1	12.4	10.9
Micronutrient												
Retinol equivalent (mcg)	119.0	476.0	469.2	443.5	147.3	605.5	547.2	514.5	107.8	409.0	439.1	375.4
Thiamine (Vitamin B1, mg)	2.5	1.2	1.0	0.9	2.1	1.1	1.0	0.9	2.6	1.2	1.0	1.0
Riboflavin (Vitamin B2, mg)	0.9	0.8	0.8	0.8	0.8	0.9	0.9	0.8	0.9	0.7	0.7	0.7
Vitamin A (mg)	253				346				108			
Vitamin E (mg)			35.6	35.9			37.3	37.5			35.0	34.3
Vitamin C (mg)	122.0	100.2			109.0	95.6			143.0	102.6		
Carotenes (mg)	3.5	4.8			2.6	6.1			4.5	4.1		
Nicotinic acid (mg)	17.0	15.7			17.0	16.9			18.0	15.0		
Potassium (mg)			1700.1	1616.9			1722.4	1660.7			1691.5	1574.3
Phosphorus (mg)	1623.2	1057.8	978.8		1574.0	1077.4	973.2		1644.0	1047.6	981.0	
Sodium (mg)			6268.2	5702.7			6007.7	5858.8			6368.8	5554.6
Calcium (mg)	694.5	405.4	388.8	366.1	563.0	457.9	438.6	412.4	750.0	378.2	369.6	321.4
Iron (mg)	37.3	23.4	23.2	21.5	34.2	25.5	23.7	21.9	38.6	22.4	23.1	21.2
Zinc (mg)			11.3	10.7			11.5	10.6			11.2	10.8
Selenium (mg)			39.9	44.6			46.5	47.0			37.4	42.2

Source: Authors' calculation and compilation of aggregated data from two official surveys — the China National Nutrition Survey (CNNS) from 1982 to 2002, and The China Household Nutrition and Health Surveillance (CHNHS) in 2012. These aggregated data are available in the *China Health and Family Planning Statistical Yearbooks* published annually by the National Health and Family Planning Commission (NHFPC) since 2003.

beyond the current system stopping at age 7. Older children (aged 7–18 years) need gender-specific advice on nutrition. This could be particularly useful for girls given that preference of thinness in adolescence might tempt them to go on diet and lose weight.

3.4. *Perspectives*

On realizing the MDGs in nutrition, the Chinese government has proposed ambitious goals in the next 5-year plan. The State Council issued the National Scheme of Child Development (2011–2020) in 2011, listing 33 measurable indicators for monitoring purposes, and further issued the National Scheme of Food and Nutrition (2014–2020) in 2014, inserting more targets for adults and the elderly and emphasizing nutrition interventions. In particular, for children under 5 years of age, the Scheme aims to reduce the prevalence of stunting to 7% and underweight to 5% and reduce the prevalence of anaemia to 12% by 2020. While these latter two had been achieved by 2015 (1.49% for underweight and 4.79% for anaemia),[6] far ahead of the schedule, the goal of reducing stunting has not been reached yet with only 2 more years to go.

That having been said, China's progress in fighting against stunting seems to be still on track. The WHO targets to reduce the number of stunted children under 5 years of age by 40% by 2025 (Onis *et al.*, 2013). Given China's prevalence of stunting of 9.9% in 2010, China has to make it decline to 5.9% by 2025 should China choose to step in line with the WHO. In a national child nutrition survey implemented by the NHFPC in every decade, China's prevalence of stunting was 12.1% in 2010 and reduced to 11.3% in 2013 according to the rural child survey led by the Chinese Maternal and Child Health Association.[7] The annual "speed" of reduction is just equivalent to the WHO's. Nevertheless, heterogeneity creates problems again. As discussed in previous subsections, urban–rural

---

[6] Data derived from the NBS. Available at: http://www.stats.gov.cn/tjsj/zxfb/201611/t20161103_1423705.html [in Chinese, accessed June 17, 2017].

[7] Data derived from internal memo. Public news summarizing some statistics can be found at: http://money.163.com/16/0608/18/BP2C15KK00253B0H.html [accessed June 17, 2017, in Chinese].

and provincial disparities create "lagged-behind" populations. The prevalence of child stunting was even as high as 19.5% in poor areas in 2013 in the aforementioned official surveys.

Given that rural, especially poor rural population, are most attacked by undernutrition, the government has initiated poverty-alleviation programs in order to take advantages of the income effects to eliminate undernutrition. Nevertheless, as found by You *et al.* (2016) in the CHNS between 1989 and 2009, higher income does not necessarily push nutrient intake in China, especially in rural areas where the absolute and relative levels of food prices, their volatility and the households' physical activities and preferences can confound the income effects on nutrient intake. Another ambitious program, the Nutrition Improvement Program for Rural Students in Compulsory Education was launched by the Ministry of Education in 2012. It covered 26 million students in 669 counties out of 22 provinces, accounting for about 30% of students in central and western China (Zhang *et al.*, 2016). The Program encourages schools to use catering chains serviced by food enterprises according to the nutrient criteria. Using rural data in Shaanxi province (poor western areas), Luo *et al.* (2009) find facilities of student dormitories and canteens are under-equipped and the services are of low quality, resulting in even lower height-for-age *z*-scores for boarding students than that for non-boarding ones.

At the same time, programs targeting maternal health and health behavior are put onto the agenda. Aiming to raise the breastfeeding rate among infants under 6 months up to 50% by 2020, the National Center for Women and Children's Health at the CDC initiated a breastfeeding campaign — "10 m^2 of Mother Love" in collaboration with the UNICEF in 2013.[8] It facilitates breastfeeding in public places and at work by helping constructing/setting up breastfeeding rooms. In the newly revised Advertisement Law in 2014, companies are prohibited to advertise infant formula, beverage and food claiming its function as full or partial replacement of breastfeeding.[9]

[8]The project website is http://10m2.unicef.cn/ [accessed June 17, 2017].

[9]The official news from the government webpage can be found at http://www.npc.gov.cn/npc/xinwen/lfgz/flca/2014-08/31/content_1876199.htm [accessed in June 17, 2017, in Chinese].

To tackle nutrient deficiency, the government initiated "one egg per day" project, first in Ningxia province in 2009, aiming to supplement rural children's daily nutrient intake. However, Kleiman-Weiner *et al.* (2013) evaluate the project and with little effects, but find chewable vitamins increase blood haemoglobin concentration. At the individual level, education in terms of informing parents of their children's anaemia, face-to-face education sessions and distributing health education materials does not seem to be effective (Luo *et al.*, 2012a), while a simple daily multivitamin (Luo *et al.*, 2012b) or providing financial incentives to principals (Miller *et al.*, 2012) reduce child anaemia.

Learning from these early efforts, to better address undernutrition in poor areas, the NHFPC issued the Nutrition Improvement Program for Children in Poverty Areas in 2014. It introduces "nutrition package" (*ying yang bao* in Chinese) — soybean powder-based complementary food supplements containing vitamins A, D, B1, B2, B6, folic acid, calcium, iron and zinc. This package will be distributed to children aged between 6 and 24 months in nationally designated poor areas. The project aims to cover 80% of rural children in poor areas and to maintain the intake rate of these packages at above 60%. The final goal is to reduce the prevalence of child anaemia in poor rural areas by 20% and stunting by 5%. In 2014, the "nutrition package" was delivered to 1.37 million rural children in 341 counties in 21 provinces (Huo and Chen, 2015), covering all poor counties. These packages have been proved to be able to alleviate anaemia and undernutrition (Zhang *et al.*, 2015).

4. Overnutrition

While malnutrition has been persisting in China and other developing countries, overnutrition (namely, overweight and obesity) has turned up among Chinese children. It co-exists with malnutrition and has become more prominent in recent years as income rises.

4.1. *Overnutrition in Children Under 7 Years of Age*

Early in the 1980s, only 0.91% of children under 7 years of age were obese, while obesity quickly spread in the next two decades, approaching prevalence of 1.76% in 1996 and 3.44% in 2006 (Zong and Li, 2012). The CNNS in 2002 shows that 3.4% of children under 6 years of age were overweight and 2% were obese (Wu *et al.*, 2015). The average rural prevalence of overweight and obesity in 10 provinces in 2006 were 4.18% and 1.21%, respectively (Xie *et al.*, 2014). In the CHNS, prevalence of overweight and obesity for children aged 2–6 years were 7.7% and 6.6%, respectively, in 2009, and they increased rapidly to 10.1% and 12.4%, respectively, in 2011 (Piernas *et al.*, 2015). Another study in nine provinces shows that 15% of children aged 3–11 years in 2012 were overweight and 5.7% were obese under the IOTF standard, and the prevalence increased to 17.4% and 6.7%, respectively, under the WHO's criteria (Ning *et al.*, 2016).

Contrary to the gender disparity in many western countries (Ogden *et al.*, 1997; Chinn and Rona, 2001), Chinese boys are more likely to be overweight and obese than girls. There was no significant gender difference in obesity for preschool children in 1986, but after two decades, boys' prevalence (4.12%) was significantly higher than girls' (2.69%) in 2006 (Zong and Li, 2012).

Overnutrition has age-specific characteristics. Among preschool children, prevalence of overnutrition increases with age at the national level (Xie *et al.*, 2014) as well as at the regional level like southeast rural areas (Lyu *et al.*, 2013). The phenomenon is especially true in cities such as Beijing and Tianjin (Jiang *et al.*, 2006; Xiao *et al.*, 2015), while on the contrary, a negative association between overnutrition and child's age was observed in rural areas at the national level in 2005 (Lyu *et al.*, 2013) and 2006 (Xie *et al.*, 2014).

4.2. *Overnutrition for Children Above 7 Years of Age*

Overweight/obesity of older children also suggests a rapid and upward trend (Figure 7). By 2010, combining overweight and obesity, the proportion of overnutrition among children aged 7–18 years had approached 15%, which was equivalent to a moderate level among developed countries (Ma *et al.*, 2012). The CHNHS shows that in 2012, 9.2% of children

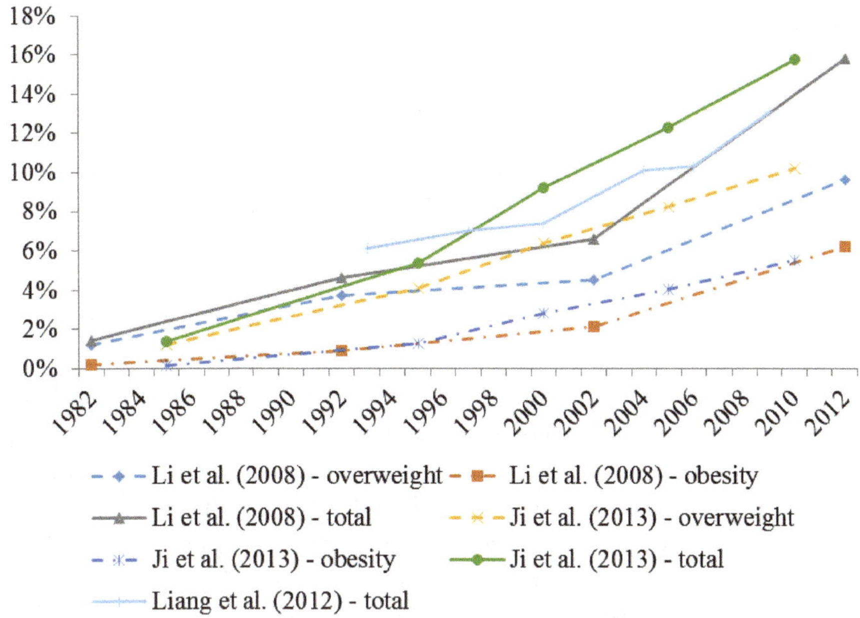

Figure 7. Estimates of child overnutrition in survey data (1982–2012).

Notes: Li *et al.* (2008) use the official survey, the CNNS, in 1982, 1992 and 2002, and study children aged 7–17 years. The lines denoted by Li *et al.* (2008) represent Li *et al.*'s (2008) estimates by 2002 and the estimates in 2012 based on the same data set are from Cheng and Li (2016). Ji *et al.* (2013) use the official survey, the CNSSCH, in 1985, 1990, 1995, 2000, 2005 and 2010, and study children aged 7–18 years. Liang *et al.* (2012) use the CHNS in 1993, 1997, 2000, 2004, 2006 and 2009, and study children aged 6–17 years.

Source: Authors' compilation of estimates in the literature.

aged 7–17 years were overweight and 6.2% were obese (Chang and Li, 2016). Figure 7 also shows that there is obviously a rapidly increasing trend in child overnutrition, especially since the early 2000s. Over the past decades, the average annual rate of increase in overweight and obesity was faster in China than in developed countries (Ma and Wu, 2009), such as the United States (Yu *et al.*, 2012).

Same as preschool children, there was no significant gender disparity in overnutrition in 1986 (Pan *et al.*, 2009; Song *et al.*, 2015). However, over the following three decades, gender disparity has been quickly expanding with boys being more likely to be in overnutrition

(Song *et al.*, 2013; Yu *et al.*, 2012). Reasons include differences in sex chromosome gene, patterns of weight gain and boys' more obesogenic lifestyle (Yu *et al.*, 2012; Song *et al.*, 2013; Sun *et al.*, 2014). Of them, an interesting point of view goes to social norms: sons' "privileges" in the Chinese tradition strengthens the gender disparity in overnutrition (Short *et al.*, 2001). The son-preferences endow boys with more family resources and better parenting than girls could have enjoyed (Sun *et al.*, 2014). Moreover, gender disparity in overnutrition is more obvious in adolescence than in early childhood. A possible reason is that girls prefer a slender body shape, especially during puberty, and they are more capable of controlling their weight than boys (Song *et al.*, 2013; Yu *et al.*, 2012).

Different from children under 7 years of age, data for school-age children suggest consistent results on age-specific prevalence of overnutrition. Younger children were more likely to be overweight than older ones in adolescence (Ji and Cheng, 2009; Zhang *et al.*, 2010; Su *et al.*, 2015). By cross-comparing children in different age cohorts, Yu *et al.* (2012) find that preschool children (5.3%) and school-aged children (5%) have higher prevalence of obesity compared with infant (4.8%), toddlers (3.8%) and adolescents (4.2%).

4.3. *Challenges*

4.3.1. *Severe child overweight/obesity*

The prevalence of obesity for school-aged children in Beijing was 15% in 2000, doubling the 1990 rate and exceeding that of developed countries for the first time (Ji, 2008). Adopting the Chinese national criteria to the CNSSCH in 2005 and 2010, Ji *et al.* (2013) and Ji and Cheng (2009) estimate that the prevalence of overweight (obese) children aged 7–18 years was 9.9% (5.1%) in 2010, as opposed to 7.73% (3.71%) in 2005. Although the US suggested higher prevalence of obesity of children aged 2–19 years (15.5% in 2004 and 15.9% in 2010, in Pan *et al.*, 2016), the speed of obesity epidemic was much faster in China than in the US Considering the size of affected young adolescents (aged 7–18 years), 20.08 (12.37) million were overweight (obese) in China in 2010, as opposed to 16.11 (9.91) million in 2000 (Ji *et al.*, 2013), registering an increase of a quarter over one decade. The authors also document concentration of overnutrition among males and in large coastal cities: in 2010, there were 12.37 (7.71) million overweight (obese) male (female) young; the prevalence of combined overweight and obesity was 32.6% for males and 19.1% for females in large coastal cities. Despite rapid epidemic of obesity, China has not yet issued any official policy or methods to address the problem. Efforts have been and will still be overwhelmingly put in addressing under- rather than overnutrition till 2030 according to the national blueprint "Healthy China 2030".

4.3.2. *Noticeable increases among rural children and migrant children*

Despite slightly higher prevalence of overweight and obesity in urban than in rural areas, rural children would bear the brunt of overnutrition, which is worth more attention from policymakers (Song *et al.*, 2015). The authors warn that the burden of overweight and obesity may be shifted from the rich to the poor given urban–rural inequality in health care (including access to medical facilities, the availability of medical insurance) and the quality of health services. Dividing the total population in 2010 into eight subgroups depending on social class, Ji *et al.* (2013) find that the prevalence of overweight/obesity of children aged 7–18 years in (affluent) rural upper class (24.4% for males and 14.7 for females) had exceeded that of the urban middle (23.4% for males and 12.8% for females) and urban lower classes (17.6% for males and 9.4% for females). An eminent feature documented among the rural upper class in their study and among the rich rural households in You *et al.* (2016) based on the CHNS over the period 2004–2009 is that many rural adolescents have strong preferences of fat-rich food like oily and fast food, pushing forward the already excessive intake of fat.

Ji *et al.* (2013) also observe an alarming phenomenon that migrating with families from rural to urban areas makes school-aged children in the rural upper class fall into an "obesogenic environment". Tough competitive environment and selection in higher level education added to students' heavy workloads, especially for these new emigrants: the 2005 National

Youth Risk Behavior Surveillance shows that 62.4% of the students in Grade 12 spent at least 3 hours a day (20.7% at least 4 to 5 hours a day) doing homework. This is accompanied by declining physical activities: 11.2% of students in Grades 10–12 did not take part in any physical education classes, as opposed to 6.6% for those in Grades 6–9; 3.3% of students in Grades 10–12 only had sufficient, intense physical exertion fewer than 3 days a week; 50.2% of them had fewer than 3 days of outdoor physical exercise, and 12.5% of them did not participate in any outdoor physical activities over the past month.

4.3.3. *Co-existence of under- and overnutrition and paradoxical malnutrition within one child*

The figures reviewed in previous sections unveil double burdens — under- and overnutrition facing Chinese children. UNICEF (2017) documents similar trends worldwide. By comparing Figure 4 and UNICEF (2017), China has lower levels of the prevalence of stunting than the average of upper middle-income countries, but our discussion in the previous subsection documents much severer child overweight and obesity in China than in other developing or even developed countries.

In addition to the macro-level double burdens of child malnutrition, it also seems paradoxical that stunting and overweight coexist for the same child. Wang *et al.* (2009) argued high prevalence of overweight among rural children could only be part of the truth, as children could be stunted overweight. Medical evidence has suggested that among nutritionally stunted children, adaption to nutritional insults that affect enzyme and hormone function is associated with impaired fat oxidation, which has proved to be a risk factor of excessive weight gain (Hoffman *et al.*, 2000).

Studies in China suggest that household income growth can generally improve diet adequacy, but it does not necessarily improve food quality because of strong preferences towards processed food, meat and fat at higher income (You *et al.*, 2016). This results in deficiencies of crucial micronutrients (Li and Shankar, 2007) and excessive consumption of high-fat low-fibre or protein diets (Du *et al.*, 2004). Children from medium household income are at increased risk to be stunted overweight

(Zhang *et al.*, 2016). Li *et al.* (2011) show that a lack of dietary diversity and high-energy-dense diets are related to a child falling into both stunting and overweight. Overall, excessive consumption of full-fat dairy and refined wheat flour products, while relatively lower consumption of high-protein foods such as dairy, vegetables, fruits and seafood, tend to give rise to the existence of stunting and overweight.

4.4. *Perspectives*

Despite the quickly expanded number of obesity, China has not yet made institutional arrangements in addressing this issue. By contrast, between 1980 and 2000 in the United States, the prevalence of overweight/obesity in children and adolescents rapidly increased, which led to growing public awareness of the obesity epidemic (Hedley *et al.*, 2004). The state-level childhood obesity-prevention legislation had been introduced in 2003 and has achieved great success in preventing overweight/obesity (Yu *et al.*, 2012). There has not been such legislation in China.

At the government level, the Ministry of Education issued the "Advice on Guaranteeing the Time of Daily Physical Activities for Primary and Secondary Students" in August 2005. Corresponding to this, the CDC initiated a program promoting classroom-based physical activities, "Happy 10 Minutes", in 2005. It requires the school sets up 10 minutes per day, in addition to the course of Physical Education, for students' physical activities. It should take the form of games with at least moderate activity amount. According to the CDC internal memo, more than 150 primary schools in 9 provinces had implemented the project by the end of 2009. Moreover, the Ministry of Education issued the No.7 document in 2007, including physical tests into the Senior High School Entrance Examination.[10] In 2015, the General Administration of Sport of China released the 13th Five-Year Plan on youth development.[11] The aims are to improve the youth sports attainment and encourage

[10]The official document can be found at http://www.moe.edu.cn/publicfiles/business/htmlfiles/moe/moe_1778/200710/27692.html [accessed June 20, 2017, in Chinese].

[11]The official document can be found at http://www.sport.gov.cn/n10503/c750118/content.html [accessed June 20, 2017, in Chinese].

adolescents to do more physical activities. Liu *et al.* (2008a) evaluate the impact of a 9-month "Happy 10 Minutes" project in two elementary schools in Beijing in 2005. While the average duration, intensity and energy expenditure of physical activities per day increased, only treated girls saw significant decreases in weight and BMI and, consequently, drops in the prevalence of overweight (from 15.3% to 12%) and obesity (from 16.9% to 11.3%). We have are not aware of more recent assessments with wider coverage for these government projects. Further, sustainability and gender differences are worth investigation. Li *et al.* (2008a) provide suggestive evidence that girls insist on physical activities more than boys, possibly because they are more concerned with body shape.

At the individual level, as mentioned in Section 2, the traditional social norm highlights a fat body shape for children rather than balanced diet or micronutrient intake. This makes the government's aforementioned efforts or any other policy intervention harder to implement at the bottom, i.e. the parental level. Effective efforts designed to suppress or prevent overweight among Chinese children need to involve parents and address traditional cultural factors (Zhang *et al.*, 2010).

In this respect, one may consider tackling child overnutrition (or undernutrition) problems by intervening with parents. This strand of literature is still under researched. For one thing, there appears to be weak intergenerational association of dietary intake — it varies between specific nutrients, foods and parent–child pairs (Wang *et al.*, 2011). For another, there have been no studies evaluating the impact of informing or educating parents about the potential health risk and problems caused by child obesity. The case of undernutrition puts doubts on such efforts, especially when traditional social norms still prevail.

5. Conclusion

This chapter reviews China's remarkable progress in child health and nutrition over the past three decades. China has already achieved the MDGs in health and nutrition (including for maternal and infant health). A nearly universal monitoring and health management system for children under 7 has been established. Infant and early-childhood mortality are no longer severe threats to mothers and children. The health facilities and national health insurance schemes have covered both urban and rural population, albeit to different extents, and the rural population is still facing problems relating to design and implementation of such social protection programs.

The main challenge appears to be a double burden along with dietary transition towards westernized life and eating styles — remaining undernutrition and rapidly growing overnutrition for children and even for the same child in his/her different life stages. In 2016, China set up ambitious goals to encourage physical activities and balanced diet and to improve national health by 2030. These fit into the 2030 Agenda for Sustainable Development, which is the world's ambitious and universal "plan of action for people, planet and prosperity", including 17 Goals, 169 targets and 231 initial indicators. With good intentions, efforts are claimed to be made to further reduce undernutrition and mortality, while the other side of the coin — overnutrition — appears to be shaded by traditional social norms and hedonia in westernized societal transition. Despite huge achievement in tackling undernutrition, China is still "on a slow boat" to the ultimate aim — freeing all children from malnutrition in all its forms.

References

Ban, L., Guo, S., Scherpbier, R. W., Wang, X., Zhou, H. and L. J. Tata (2017) "Child Feeding and Stunting Prevalence in Left-behind Children: A Descriptive Analysis of Data from a Central and Western Chinese Population", *International Journal of Public Health*, Vol. 62, pp. 143–151.

Chang, J. L. and Y. Wang (2016) *China Household Nutrition and Health Surveillance: Report of 2010–2013* (中国居民营养与健康监测 2010–2013 综合报告). Beijing: Peking University Medical Press [in Chinese].

Chang, S., He, W. and C. Chen (2006) "The Growth Characteristics of Children Under 5 in the Past 15 Years", *Journal of Hygiene Research,* Vol. 35, pp. 768–771.

Chen, C., He, W., Wang, Y., Deng, L. and F. Jia (2011) "Nutritional Status of Children During and Post-Global Economic Crisis in China", *Biomedical and Environmental Sciences,* Vol. 24, pp. 321–328.

Chen, J., Chen, W., Zeng, G. and G. Li (2016) "Secular Trends in Growth and Nutritional Outcomes of Children Under Five Years Old in Xiamen, China", *International Journal of Environmental Research and Public Health*, Vol. 13, p. e1104.

Chen, Y. (2012) "Impact of the Parental Rural–Urban Migration on the Health of Left-Behind Children in Rural China", *Chinese Journal of Health Policy*, Vol. 5, pp. 48–54.

Chinn, S. and R. J. Rona (2001) "Prevalence and Trends in Overweight and Obesity in Three Cross Sectional Studies of British Children, 1974–1994", *British Medical Journal*, Vol. 322, pp. 24–26.

de Brauw, A. and R. Mu (2011) "Migration and the Overweight and Underweight Status of Children in Rural China", *Food Policy*, Vol. 36, No. 1, pp. 88–100.

Dearth-Wesley, T., Wang, H. and B. M. Popkin (2008) "Under- and Overnutrition Dynamics in Chinese Children and Adults (1991–2004)", *European Journal of Clinical Nutrition*, Vol. 62, pp. 1302–1307.

Dearth-Wesley, T., Gordon-Larsen, P., Adair, L. S., Zhang, B. and B. M. Popkin (2012) "Longitudinal, Cross-Cohort Comparison of Physical Activity Patterns in Chinese Mothers and Children", *International Journal of Behavioral Nutrition and Physical Activity*, Vol. 9, http://www.biomedcentral.com/content/9/1/39 (open access).

Dong, Y., Wang, Z. and J. Ma (2016) "Analysis of Malnutrition Prevalence Among Children Aged 7–12 Years from 2005 to 2010 in China", *Acta Nutrimenta Sinica*, Vol. 38, No. 5, pp. 431–437 [in Chinese].

Du, S., Mroz, T. A., Zhai, F. and B. M. Popkin (2004) "Rapid Income Growth Adversely Affects Diet Quality in China — Particularly for the Poor!" *Social Science & Medicine*, Vol. 59, pp. 1505–1515.

Du, S., Wang, H., Zhang, B., Zhai, F. and B. M. Popkin (2014) "China in the Period of Transition from Scarcity and Extensive Undernutrition to Emerging Nutrition-Related Non-Communicable Diseases, 1949–1992", *Obesity Reviews*, Vol. 15, 8–15.

Hedley, A. A., Ogden, C. L., Johnson, C. L., Carroll, M. D., Curtin, L. R. and K. M. Flegal (2004) "Prevalence of Overweight and Obesity Among US Children, Adolescents, and Adults, 1999–2002", *Jama*, Vol. 291, pp. 2847–2850.

Hoffman, D. J., Sawaya, A. L., Verreschi, I., Tucker, K. L. and S. B. Roberts (2000) "Why are Nutritionally Stunted Children at Increased Risk of Obesity? Studies of Metabolic Rate and Fat Oxidation in Shantytown Children from Sao Paulo, Brazil", *American Journal of Clinical Nutrition*, Vol. 72, pp. 702–707.

Huo, J. and J. Chen (2015) "Ying Yang Bao: Improving Complementary Feeding for China's Children", *Journal of Nutritional Science and Vitaminology*, Vol. 61, pp. S186–S86.

Ji, C. (2008) "The Prevalence of Childhood Overweight/Obesity and the Epidemic Changes in 1985–2000 for Chinese School-Age Children and Adolescents", *Obesity Reviews*, Vol. 9, pp. 78–81.

Ji, C. (2009) "Changes of the Prevalence of Malnutrition in Chinese Rural Students from 1985 to 2005", *Chinese Journal of Child Health Care*, Vol. 17, No. 1, pp. 11–14 [in Chinese].

Ji, C., Chen, T. and Working Group on Obesity in China (WGOC) (2013) "Empirical Changes in the Prevalence of Overweight and Obesity Among Chinese Students from 1985 to 2010 and Corresponding Preventive Strategies", *Biomedical and Environmental Sciences*, Vol. 26, pp. 1–12.

Ji, C. and T. Cheng (2009) "Epidemic Increase in Overweight and Obesity in Chinese Children from 1985 to 2005", *International Journal of Cardiology*, Vol. 132, No. 1, pp. 1–10.

Jiang, J., Rosenqvist, U., Wang, H., Greiner, T., Ma, Y. and A. M. Toschke (2006) "Risk Factors for Overweight in 2- to 6-Year-Old Children in Beijing, China", *International Journal of Pediatric Obesity*, Vol. 1, pp. 103–108.

Kleiman-Weiner, M., Luo, R., Zhang, L., Shi, Y., Medina, A. and S. Rozelle (2013) "Eggs Versus Chewable Vitamins: Which Intervention Can Increase Nutrition and Test Scores in Rural China?" *China Economic Review*, Vol. 24, pp. 165–176.

Li, Q., Liu, G. and W. Zang (2015) "The Health of Left-Behind Children in Rural China", *China Economic Review*, Vol. 36, pp. 367–376.

Li, Y., Schouten, E. G., Hu, X., Cui, Z., Luan, D. and G. Ma (2008) "Obesity Prevalence and Time Trend Among Youngsters in China, 1982–2002", *Asia Pacific Journal of Clinical Nutrition*, Vol. 17, pp. 131–137.

Li, Y., Wedick, N. M., Lai, J., He, Y., Hu, X., Liu, A., Du, S., Zhang, J., Yang, X. and C. Chen (2011) "Lack of Dietary Diversity and Dyslipidemia Among Stunted Overweight Children: The 2002 China National Nutrition and Health Survey", *Public Health Nutrition*, Vol. 14, pp. 896–903.

Liang, Y., Xi, B., Song, A., Liu, J. and J. Mi (2012) "Trends in General and Abdominal Obesity Among Chinese Children and Adolescents 1993–2009", *Pediatric Obesity*, Vol. 7, pp. 355–364.

Liu, A., Hu, X., Ma, G., Cui, Z., Pan, P., Chang, S., Zhao, W. and C. Chen (2008a) "Evaluation of a Classroom-based Physical Activity Promoting Programme", *Obesity Reviews*, Vol. 9, pp. 130–134.

Liu, A., Zhao, L., Yu, D. and W. Yu (2008b) "Study on Malnutrition Status and Changing Trend of Children Under 5 Years Old in China", *Journal of Hygiene Research*, Vol. 37, pp. 324–326 [in Chinese].

Liu, H., Fang, H. and Z. Zhao (2013) "Urban–Rural Disparities of Child Health and Nutritional Status in China from 1989 to 2006", *Economics & Human Biology*, Vol. 11, pp. 294–309.

Liu, H., Rizzo, J. A. and H. Fang (2015) "Urban–Rural Disparities in Child Nutrition-Related Health Outcomes in China: The Role of Hukou Policy", *BMC Public Health*, Vol. 15, doi: 10.1186/s12889-015-2517-4 (open access).

Lu, S., Lin, Y., Vikse, J. H. and C. Huang (2016) "Well-being of Migrant and Left-Behind Children in China: Education, Health, Parenting, and Personal Values", *International Journal of Social Welfare*, Vol. 25, No. 1, pp. 58–68.

Luo, R., Shi, Y., Zhang, L., Liu, C., Rozelle, R. and B. Sharbono (2009) "Malnutrition in China's Rural Boarding Schools: The Case of Primary Schools in Shaanxi Province", *Asia Pacific Journal of Education*, Vol. 29, No. 4, pp. 481–501.

Luo, R., Shi, Y., Zhang, L., Liu, C., Rozelle, R., Sharbono, B., Yue, A., Zhao, Q. and R. Martorell (2012a) "Nutrition and Educational Performance in Rural China's Elementary Schools: Results of a Randomized Control Trial in Shaanxi Province", *Economic Development and Cultural Change*, Vol. 60, No. 4, pp. 735–772.

Luo, R., Shi, Y., Zhang, L., Zhang, H., Miller, G., Medina, A. and S. Rozelle (2012b) "The Limits of Health and Nutrition Education: Evidence from Three Randomized-Controlled Trails in Rural China", *CESifo Economic Studies*, Vol. 58, No. 2, pp. 385–404.

Luo, R., Shi, Y., Zhang, L., Zhao, Q. Shi, Y., Miller, G., Yu, E., Sharbono, B., Medina, A., Rozelle, S. and R. Martorell (2011) "Anaemia Among Students of Rural China's Elementary Schools: Prevalence and Correlates in Ningxia and Qinghai's Poor Counties", *Journal of Health, Population and Nutrition*, Vol. 29, No. 5, pp. 471–485.

Lyu, Y., Ouyang, F., Ye, X., Zhang, J., Lee, S. and Z. Li (2013) "Trends in Overweight and Obesity Among Rural Preschool Children in Southeast China from 1998 to 2005", *Public Health*, Vol. 127, pp. 1082–1089.

Ma, J., Cai, C., Wang, H., Dong, B., Song, Y., Hu, P. and B. Zhang (2012) "The trend Analysis of Overweight and Obesity in Chinese Students During 1985–2010", *Chinese Journal of Preventive Medicine*, Vol. 46, pp. 776–780 [in Chinese].

Ma, J. and S. Wu (2009) "Trend Analysis of the Prevalence of Obesity and Overweight Among School-Age Children and Adolescents in China", *Chinese Journal School Health*, Vol. 30, No. 3, pp. 195–200 [in Chinese].

Man, S. L. and Y. Guo (2016) "Research on the Social Determinants of Malnutrition among Children Under the Age of 5 in China", *Journal of Peking University (Health Sciences)*, Vol. 48, No. 3, pp. 418–423 [in Chinese].

MFA (2015) "Report on China's Implementation of the Millennium Development Goals (2000–2015)", Ministry of Foreign Affairs of P. R. China.

Miller, G., Luo, R., Zhang, L., Sylvia, S., Shi, Y., Foo, P., Zhao, Q., Martorell, R., Medina, A. and S. Rozelle (2012) "Effectiveness of provider Incentives for Anaemia Reduction in Rural China: A Cluster Randomised Trial", *British Medical Journal*, Vol. 345, doi: https://doi.org/10.1136/bmj.e4809 (open access).

Mo, X., Xu, L., Luo, H., Wang, X., Zhang, F. and R. Tobe (2016) "Do Different Parenting Patterns Impact the Health and Physical Growth of 'Left-Behind' Preschool-Aged Children? A Cross-Sectional Study in Rural China", *European Journal of Public Health*, Vol. 26, No. 1, pp. 18–23.

Mu, R. and A. de Brauw (2015) "Migration and Young Child Nutrition: Evidence from Rural China", *Journal of Population Economics*, Vol. 28, No. 3, pp. 631–657.

NHFPC (2012) "Nutrition Development Report for Children Under 6 Years Old", National Health and Family Planning Commission, internal memo [in Chinese].

NHFPC (2016). *2016 Development Report of China's Flowing Population*, National Health and Family Planning Commission (eds.). Beijing: China Population Publishing House [in Chinese].

Ning, K., Xue, Y. and T. He (2016) "Overweight and Obesity among 3–11 Years Old Chinese Children in 9 Regions: Prevalence and Comparison of Different Assessment Criteria", *Chinese Journal of Public Health*, Vol. 32, pp. 31–434 [in Chinese].

Ning, M. and C. Chang (2013) "Migration Decisions of Parents and the Nutrition Intakes of Children Left at Home in Rural China", *Agricultural Economics — Zemedelska Ekonomika*, Vol. 59, pp. 467–477.

Ogden, C. L., Troiano, R. P., Briefel, R. R., Kuczmarski, R. J., Flegal, K. M. and C. L. Johnson (1997) "Prevalence of Overweight Among Preschool Children in the United States, 1971 through 1994", *Pediatrics*, Vol. 99, p. e1.

Onis, M., Dewey, K. G., Borghi, E., Onyango, A. W., Blössner, M., Daelmans, B., Piwoz, E. and F. Branca (2013) "The World Health Organization's Global Target for Reducing Childhood Stunting by 2025: Rationale and Proposed Actions", *Maternal & Child Nutrition*, Vol. 9, pp. 6–26.

Pan, H., Jiang, Y., Jing, X., Fu, S., Jiang, Y., Lin, Z., Sheng, Z. and T. J. Cole (2009) "Child Body Mass Index in Four Cities of East China Compared to Western References", *Annals of Human Biology*, Vol. 36, pp. 98–109.

Pan, L., Freedman, D. S., Sharma, A. J., Castellanos-Brown, K., Park, S., Smith, R. B. and H. M. Blank (2016) "Trends in Obesity Among Participants Aged 2–4 Years in the Special Supplemental Nutrition Program for Women, Infants, and Children — United States, 2000–2014", *Morbidity and Mortality Weekly Report (MMWR)*, Vol. 65, No. 45, pp. 1256–1260.

Piernas, C., Wang, D., Du, S., Zhang, B., Wang, Z., Su, C. and B. M. Popkin (2015) "The Double Burden of Under- and Overnutrition and Nutrient Adequacy among Chinese Preschool and School-Aged Children in 2009–2011", *European Journal of Clinical Nutrition*, Vol. 69, No. 12, pp. 1323–1329.

Ren, W., Rammohan, A. and Y. Wu (2014) "Is There a Gender Gap in Child Nutritional Outcomes in Rural China?" *China Economic Review*, Vol. 31, pp. 145–155.

Seo, D. and J. Niu (2014) "Trends In Underweight And Overweight/Obesity Prevalence in Chinese Youth, 2004–2009", *International Journal of Behavioral Medicine*, Vol. 21, pp. 682–690.

Shi, Y., Bai, Y., Shen, Y., Kenny, K. and S. Rozelle (2016) "Effects of Parental Migration on Mental Health of Left-Behind Children: Evidence from Northwestern China", *China & World Economy*, Vol. 24, No. 3, pp. 105–122.

Short, S. E., Zhai, F., Xu, S. and M. Yang (2001) "China's One-Child Policy and the Care of Children: An Analysis Using Qualitative and Quantitative Data", *Social Forces*, Vol. 79, pp. 913–943.

Song, Y., Ma, J., Wang, H., Wang, Z., Hu, P., Zhang, B. and A. Agard (2015) "Secular Trends of Obesity Prevalence in Chinese Children from 1985 to 2010: Urban–Rural Disparity", *Obesity*, Vol. 23, pp. 448–53.

Song, Y., Wang, H., Ma, J. and Z. Wang (2013) "Secular Trends of Obesity Prevalence in Urban Chinese Children from 1985 to 2010: Gender Disparity", *PloS One*, Vol. 8, p. e53069.

Su, C., Zhang, B., Wang, Y., Jia, X., Xue, H. and H. Wang (2015) "Epidemics of Overweight and Obesity among Growing Childhood in China between 1997 and 2009: Impact of Family Income, Dietary Intake, and Physical Activity Dynamics", *Chinese Medical Journal*, Vol. 128, No. 14, pp. 1879–1886.

Sun, H., Ma, Y., Han, D., Pan, C. and Y. Xu (2014) "Prevalence and Trends in Obesity among China's Children and Adolescents 1985–2010", *PloS One*, Vol. 9, p. e105469.

UNICEF (2012) "Levels and Trends in Child Malnutrition: UNICEF-WHO-The World Bank Joint Child Malnutrition Estimates", UNICEF, New York; WHO, Geneva; the World Bank, Washington, DC.

UNICEF (2017) "Levels and Trends in Child Malnutrition: UNICEF-WHO-The World Bank Joint Child Malnutrition Estimates", UNICEF, New York; WHO, Geneva; the World Bank, Washington, DC.

Wang, X., Höjer, B., Guo, S., Luo, S., Zhou, W. and Y. Wang (2009) "Stunting and 'Overweight' in the WHO Child Growth Standards — Malnutrition among Children in a Poor Area of China", *Public Health Nutrition*, Vol. 12, pp. 1991–1998.

Wang, Y., Beydou, M. A., Li, J., Liu, Y. and L. A. Moreno (2011) "Do Children and Their Parents Eat a Similar Diet? Resemblance in Child and Parental Dietary Intake: Systematic Review and Meta-Analysis?", *Journal of Epidemiology & Community Health*, Vol. 65, No. 2, pp. 177–189.

Watson, J. L. (2000) "Food as a Lens: The Past, Present, and Future of Family Life in China", in *Feeding China's Little Emperors: Food, Children, and Social Change*, ed. Jun Jing. Stanford: Stanford University Press, pp. 199–212.

Wu, Y., and D. Qi (2016) "Urban-Rural and Provincial Disparities in Child Malnutrition in China", *Social Work in Public Health*, Vol. 31, pp. 574–588.

Wu, L., Yang, Z., Yin, S, Zhu, M. and H. Gao (2015) "The Relationship between Socioeconomic Development and Malnutrition in Children Younger than 5 Years in China During the Period 1990 to 2010", *Asia Pacific Journal of Clinical Nutrition*, Vol. 24, pp. 665–673.

Xue, H., Wu, Y., Wang, X. and Y. Wang (2016) "Time Trends in Fast Food Consumption and its Association with Obesity Among Children in China", *PloS One*, Vol. 11, p. e0151141.

Xiao, Y., Qiao, Y., Pan, L., Liu, J., Zhang, T., Li, N., Liu, E., Wang, Y., Liu, H. and G. Liu (2015) "Trends in the Prevalence of Overweight and Obesity among Chinese Preschool Children from 2006 to 2014", *PloS One*, Vol. 10, p. e0134466.

Xie, S., Wang, J., Li, N., Jiang, W., Yang, S., Li, X., Ling, Z. and J. Zhang (2014) "Survey on Overweight and Obesity of Preschool Children in Rural Areas from Ten Provinces of China", *Chinese Journal of Epidemiology*, Vol. 35, pp. 425–428 [in Chinese].

Yang, J. (2007) "China's One-Child Policy and Overweight Children in the 1990s", *Social Science & Medicine*, Vol. 64, pp. 2043–2057.

You, J. (2013) "The Role of Microcredit in Older Children's Nutrition: Quasi-Experimental Evidence from Rural China", *Food Policy*, Vol. 43, pp. 167–179.

You, J., Imai, K. and R. Gaiha (2016) "Declining Nutrient Intake in a Growing China: Does Household Heterogeneity Matter?" *World Development*, 77, 171–191.

You, J., Wang, S. and L. Roope (2017) "Intertemporal Deprivations in Rural China: Income and Nutrition", *Journal of Economic Inequality*, doi:1 0.1007/ s10888-017-9352-z.

Yu, D., Liu, A., Yu, W., Zhang, B., Zhang, J., Jia, F., Li, J. and L. Zhao (2011) "Prevalence of Malnutrition of Children Under 5 Years Old and Its Determinants in China's Poor Areas", *Journal of Hygiene Research*, 40(6), 714–718.

Yu, D., Zhao, L., Yang, Z., Chang, S., Yu, W., Fang, H., Wang, X., Yu, D., Guo, Q. and X. Xu (2016) "Comparison of Undernutrition Prevalence of Children under 5 Years in China between 2002 and 2013", *Biomedical and Environmental Sciences*, Vol. 29, pp. 165–176.

Yu, Z., Han, S., Chu, J., Xu, Z., Zhu, C. and X. Guo (2012) "Trends in Overweight and Obesity among Children and Adolescents in China from 1981 to 2010: A Meta-analysis", *PloS One*, Vol. 7, p. e51949.

Zhang, J., Seo, D., Kolbe, L., Middlestadt, S. and W. Zhao (2010) "Trends in Overweight Among School Children and Adolescents in Seven Chinese Provinces, from 1991–2004", *International Journal of Pediatric Obesity*, Vol. 5, pp. 375–382.

Zhang, J., Shi, J., Himes, J. H., Du, Y., Yang, S., Shi, S. and J. Zhang (2011a) "Undernutrition Status of Children Under 5 Years in Chinese Rural Areas-data from the National Rural Children Growth Standard Survey, 2006", *Asia Pacific Journal of Clinical Nutrition*, Vol. 20, pp. 584–592.

Zhang, J., Zhang, B., Liu, Wen-Wen, A. D. U., Chang, S., Ji, Z., Yu-Xia, M., Gao, G. and X. Shao-Ze (2011b) "Malnutrition Status of Children Under 5 Years Old in Western Poverty Rural Areas", *Chinese Journal of Health Education*, Vol. 27, pp. 403–405 [in Chinese].

Zhang, N., Bécares, L. and T. Chandola (2016) "Patterns and Determinants of Double-Burden of Malnutrition Among Rural Children: Evidence from China", *PloS One*, Vol. 11, p. e0158119.

Zhang, N., Bécares, L., Chandola, T. and P. Callery (2015) "Intergenerational Differences in Beliefs About Healthy Eating Among Carers of Left-Behind Children in Rural China: A Qualitative Study", *Appetite*, Vol. 95, pp. 484–491.

Zhou, C., Sylvia, S., Zhang, L., Luo, R., Yi, H., Liu, C., Shi, Y., Loyalka, P., Chu, J., Medina, A. and S. Rozelle (2015) "China's Left-Behind Children:

Impact of Parental Migration on Health, Nutrition, and Educational Outcomes", *Health Affairs*, Vol. 34, No. 11, pp. 1964–1971.

Zong, X. and H. Li (2012) "Secular Trends in Prevalence and Risk Factors of Obesity in Infants and Preschool Children in 9 Chinese Cities, 1986–2006", *PloS One*, Vol. 7, p. e46942.

Zong, X. and H. Li (2014) "Physical Growth of Children and Adolescents in China Over the Past 35 Years", *Bulletin of the World Health Organization*, Vol. 92, pp. 555–564.

Chapter 6

Food and Nutrition Security: The India Story

Shyam Khadka* **and Deepika Anand**[†]

FAO India Office, New Delhi, India
**Shyam.Khadka@fao.org*
[†]*deepika.anand@hotmail.com*

Abstract

Despite gains on the economic front, India is facing huge crisis especially in ensuring food and nutrition security for its citizens. The country has alarmingly high levels of poverty and undernutrition, warning, that the benefits of demographic dividend would otherwise become a challenge. The country has been undergoing nutrition transition over the past 30 years, resulting in the change of food baskets with decreasing intake of cereals, pulses, fruits and vegetables, and increasing intake of meat products, fat and salt. The situation is further worrisome as levels of physical activity are declining and mental stress is increasing, leading to high levels of obesity and non-communicable diseases. It is worthy that the country has numerous policies and programmes in place to correct the food and nutrition security situation; however, due to critical gaps, the results are not so encouraging. Only recently is the multi-dimensional and multi-causal nature of nutrition increasingly being realized, and nutrition is also seen as being critical to the development of human capital. Although, the recent strategy papers clearly articulate the action points for revolutionizing the nutrition sector of the country, there is a need to scale-up nutrition services and improve feeding and caring practices in the home, improve the efficiency and effectiveness of the safety nets and work towards increasing farm incomes especially for small and marginal farming households.

Keywords: Nutrition security, food security, India, undernutrition, agriculture.

1. Introduction

India, a country with a population of over 1.2 billion, is exceptionally placed, as the nation is home to the largest number of poor people in the world but also takes pride in having the largest number of people who have recently escaped poverty but are still vulnerable to falling back. In the last few decades, the country has witnessed economic improvement along with improvements in health and nutritional status of its population.

Between 2005 and 2010, India's share of global GDP increased from 1.8% to 2.7%, 53 million were lifted out of poverty, and it achieved an average annual growth rate of 7.6%, placing it in the top 10 of the world's fastest growing nations — on the other hand, it remains home to one-third of the global poor, and with a GDP per capita of US$1,709, India stands at 134 out of 178 countries and remains at the bottom of the group of middle-income countries. In the Fiscal Year (FY) 2014–2015, India's GDP grew by 7.3% following a 6.9% growth rate in the previous year. The International Monetary Fund (IMF) predicted that India would retain the status of fastest growing large economy until 2020 (Figure 1).

Similarly, while India's progress on human development has been remarkable with life expectancy having more than doubled from 31 years in 1947 to 65 years in 2012, and adult literacy more than quadrupled, from 18% in 1951 to 74% in 2011, India has some of the highest malnutrition rates in the world, children's learning outcomes remain poor, and inequalities in all dimensions including caste and gender, is a major concern.

The term *malnutrition* encompasses both undernutrition and overnutrition. Undernutrition is commonly measured by inadequate height-for-age

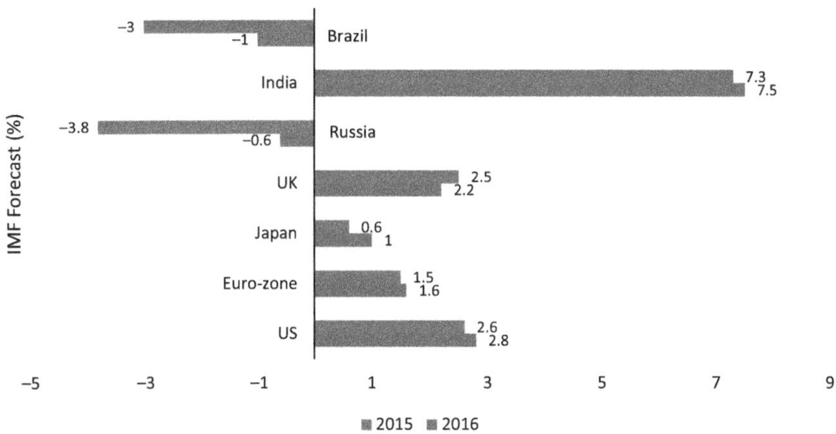

Figure 1. India: World's fastest growing large economy.

(stunting), by inadequate weight-for-height (wasting) or by deficiencies in micronutrients such as vitamin A, iodine, zinc and iron. Overnutrition is often measured as excessive weight-for-height (overweight and obesity) using growth reference standards for children and body mass index measurements (weight-for-height-squared, or kg/m^2) for adults.

2. Nutrition Transition in India

In the 1940s and 1950s, kwashiorkar (acute protein-energy malnutrition), keratomalacia (attributable to severe vitamin A deficiency), pellagra (nicotinic acid deficiency), beri-beri (arising from vitamin B1 deficiency) and anaemia were the major nutritional problems prevalent in large sections of populations (Gopalan, 2013). The major reasons for macro and micronutrient deficiencies were low and poor quality dietary intake because of poverty and low purchasing power, high prevalence of infection because of poor access to safe drinking water, sanitation and health care and poor utilization of available health facilities due to low literacy and lack of awareness (Ramachandran, 2007). By 1960s, along with high burden of macro and micronutrient deficiencies, India was faced with fast-emptying grain baskets and importing staples was observed to ward off famine (Djurfeldt *et al.*, 2005).

The era of late 1960s to 1980s was termed as the "Green Revolution" phase which revolutionized agriculture in India, replenished the Indian food basket and led to partial food security among Indian citizens. With the new fast-growing varieties of staples, especially wheat and rice, India could attain food self-sufficiency, but it failed to raise income in the rural areas of the country (Hazell, 2009). Phase of 1980s not only introduced high yielding varieties of grains but also played a critical role in preparing a wide market in rural areas for non-agricultural products and services (Fujita, 2010). The "Green Revolution" neglected pulses and horticultural products as means of ensuring food and nutrition security (Gopalan, 2013).

The period of 1990s saw added focus on the role of micronutrients. Deficiencies of vitamin A, iron and iodine were there but the roles of other micronutrients such as zinc, folic acid, magnesium, selenium and vitamin D started receiving greater attention. The term "hidden hunger" or deficiency of vitamins and minerals was widely used during this period as unlike the deficiency of macronutrients the deficiency of micronutrients was not clinically visible and hence remained unnoticed for long. It affected large percentage of vulnerable population especially children and women in the reproductive age group (Gopalan, 2013). According to IFPRI (2014), poor diet, increased micronutrient needs during certain life stages, such as pregnancy and lactation, and health problems such as diseases, infections, or parasites are prime factors contributing to hidden hunger.

According to Gopalan (2013), there is increasing evidence that micronutrients function synergistically within the human system and stand-alone supplementation or any other micronutrient will have limited benefits. Thus, enhanced focus on food-based approaches was suggested as an important strategy to ensure long-term food security. Even after years of iron supplementation programmes being in place for pregnant and lactating women, the levels of anaemia remain stubbornly high in the vulnerable groups (50.3%) (NFHS 4, 2015–2016). The decade of nineties saw a surge in population growth due to fall in death rates and high birth rates. There was migration from villages to cities because of better livelihood opportunities. The energy expenditures of almost all sections of population decreased as lifestyles became more sedentary (Gopalan, 2013).

3. Current Nutritional Scenario of India

Nutrition transition is defined as dietary changes which get reflected in nutritional outcomes including changes in average body stature and composition (Popkin and Ng, 2006). As per Stuckler *et al.* (2012), economic development has pushed the population from undernutrition to overnutrition, with food preferences changing from traditional low salt, saturated fat, and glycaemic indices to less healthy, complex western diets, thus causing "nutrition transition".

In the 21st century, India, along with the problems of undernutrition and communicable diseases faces additional challenges resulting from industrialization, urbanization and economic betterment (Ramachandran, 2006). The coexistence of undernutrition along with overweight and obesity, or diet-related Non-Communicable Diseases (NCDs), is now termed as "Double-burden of malnutrition" (Shrimpton and Rokx, 2012).

Undernutrition — "Not-so-hidden" anymore: While the rate of decline of undernutrition has almost doubled during the period 2007–2013 compared with the period 1999–2006, the levels remain unacceptably high (underweight: 29.4%, 35.7%; stunting: 38.7%, 38.4%; and wasting: 15.1%, 21%, respectively) (RSoC, 2014) (NFHS-4). India's ranking on undernutrition indicators is low: 114th out of 132 countries on under-5 stunting and 120th out of 130 countries on under-5 wasting (Global Nutrition Report, 2016). The burden of vitamin and mineral deficiencies or "hidden hunger" is also considerable. Iron deficiency is wide spread, exists across income quintiles and age groups. More than 50% of women of child bearing age, 75% of children below 5 years and 24% of men in the country are anaemic (NFHS-3). Around 62% of preschool children are deficient in vitamin A (Akhtar *et al.*, 2013). More than 13 million infants are susceptible to iodine deficiency disorders (UNICEF, 2009). Most importantly, these deficiencies do not occur in isolation. Other micronutrient deficiencies, such as vitamin B group, zinc and vitamin D are also prevalent and have overwhelming impact on the health and productivity of the population.

Overnutrition — "An emerging emergency for India": Dramatic changes in lifestyles and dietary patterns in the recent decades have contributed to an increasing prevalence of NCDs namely cardiovascular diseases (like heart attacks and stroke), cancers, diabetes and chronic respiratory diseases (such as chronic obstructive pulmonary disease and asthma) (WHO, 2017). According to WHO (2014), NCDs account for 60% of the total deaths in India and the probability of death in the age group of 30–70 years from the four main NCDs is 26.2%. Since this is the economically productive age group, if NCDs are not controlled, it can have serious implications on the economy of the country. As per Anchala *et al.* (2014), about 33% urban and 25% rural Indians were found to be hypertensive. The levels of hypercholesterolemia, hypertriglyceridemia, low HDL-C, high LDL-C were 13.9%, 29.5%, 72.3% and 11.8%, respectively (Joshi *et al.*, 2014). As per the latest estimates, India has 69.1 million (8.7%) people living with diabetes (IDF, 2015). Vitamin D deficiency ranges from 70% to 100% in the general population (Ritu and Gupta, 2014).

As per the recent findings of NFHS 4 (2015–2016), the BMI of 15.5% of urban women was found to be less than 18.5 kg/m^2 whereas 31.3% urban women were in the category of over-weight or obese (BMI $\geq$ 25.0 kg/m^2). Around 15% of urban men were underweight (BMI $<$ 18.5 kg/m^2) while 26.3% belonged to the category of overweight and obese (BMI $\geq$ 25.0 kg/m^2).

4. Dietary Consumption Patterns of India

The food consumption pattern in India has evolved over the past two decades due to income induced diet diversification, diet globalization, increasing urbanization and changing lifestyle of people (NCAER, 2014). In India, the share of food in total consumer expenditure has fallen from 73% to 55% in rural areas and from 64% to 42% in urban areas. The proportion of expenditure on non-food items has increased from 24% to 37.7% (Ramachandran, 2008). The change is occurring both among rural and urban households (NCAER, 2014).

Diets of a vast majority of Indians are predominantly cereal-based with insufficient intake of foods such as milk, pulses, fruits and vegetables.[1] Wheat and rice are the main staples consumed in India. The intake of cereals by adults is adequate ranging from 310 to 400 g/d. The intake

[1]As per NCAER (2014) and NNMB (2012).

of milk and milk products ranges from 66 to 165 mL/d which is below the recommendation of 300 mL/d. Similarly, the intake of pulses ranges from 22 to 34 g/d which is also much below the recommendation of 60–70 g/d. Fruits and vegetables (including roots and tubers) which are rich sources of micronutrients also fall short of the recommendation, with mean intake of mere 32 g/d for fruits and 208 g/d for vegetables as against the recommended 100 and 600 g/d intake. Data for intake of fat and sugar provides mixed picture as NNMB data shows that fat and sugar intake is lower than the recommendations while NCAER (2014) data reports the intake of fat meets the recommendations of 20–25 g/d, and a review paper has reported the sugar intake to be almost 2.5 times of the recommended 20 g/d (Gulati *et al.*, 2013).

Dietary intake of critical micronutrients such as iron, vitamin A and folate falls short of daily Recommended Allowances (RDA) (NNMB, 2012; ICMR, 2010). Even though required in minute amounts, dietary inadequacy of micronutrients can result in numerous ill-health effects. Women and children remain the most vulnerable to micronutrient deficiencies. Among adult women, average iron intake meets only 65% of the RDA; for pregnant women only about 40% of the RDA is met; and in lactating women about 75% of the RDA is met. Deficiency of iron in women not only reduces physical work capacity and causes fatigue, but could lead to depression, post-partum maternal haemorrhage; while in children it impairs growth and cognitive development. Dietary intake of folate is also below the RDA with adult females meeting only 60% of RDA while pregnant and lactating females meet only 25% and 45% of RDA, respectively. Low folate levels during pregnancy increases the risk of having a baby with neural tube defects. The dietary intakes of vitamin A by women (adult, pregnant and lactating) falls short of RDA by more than 50%, while 1–3 year old children met only around 35% of the RDA for vitamin A. Deficiency of vitamin A weakens the immunity and increases the susceptibility to infections.

5. Determinants of Nutritional Outcomes

India has a five-decade long history of programmes to deliver nutrition services at the community level to improve the nutrition status of women and children. Since the early 1960s, India has had a plethora of national schemes for providing maternal and child nutrition services. The Applied Nutrition Programme initiated in the early 1960s, followed by other programmes introduced in the 1970s, such as the Special Nutrition Programme and the Balwadi Feeding Programme, continued to provide nutrition services until the 1990s. However, despite being national in nature and covering most states, actual coverage of the programmes was patchy. Alongside these nutrition schemes, India, since the 1970s, has also implemented national programmes — vitamin A supplementation, iron-folate supplementation and salt iodization — to address micronutrient undernutrition. With the advent of the Integrated Child Development Services (ICDS) in 1975, all earlier schemes were phased out or merged with the ICDS (except MDM), and the micronutrient supplementation programmes continue through the maternal and child health programmes under the Ministry of Health and Family Welfare (MOHFW) (GoI). Both ICDS and the maternal and child health programmes have national coverage.

The population-based data from the recent National Family Health Survey-4 (NFHS-4) corroborates that despite substantial improvement in delivery of reproductive, new-born, child and maternal health services, there are huge coverage gaps. Only around 50% of pregnant women in the country received at least four Antenatal Care (ANC) visits. The coverage of full antenatal care remains low at 21% in 2015–2016, reflecting the need for improving the quality of care. The proportion of children aged 12–23 months, receiving all basic immunizations (BCG, measles, and 3 doses each of polio and DPT) has improved from 43.5% in 2005–2006 to 62% in 2015–2016. Breastfeeding, within one hour of birth and exclusive breastfeeding for the first 6 months, has shown some improvement but is still very low at 41.6% and 54.9%, respectively. Also, only around 30% of mothers consumed iron folic acid for 100 days or more when they were pregnant (as against 15% in NFHS-3).

Apart from the quality and quantity of diet consumed, there are many other indirect factors that affect the nutritional status of the population. Water, Sanitation and Hygiene (WASH) and Infant and Young Child Feeding (IYCF) are the two prime factors which are pertinent to India and should be seen as a priority.

- *Poor access to adequate and safe water and sanitation*: Access to adequate water and sanitation is critical to improving the quality of life and economic potential of all Indians. Of the 2.4 billion people lacking access to improved sanitation globally, about 776 million live in India (80% of them in rural India) and 946 million people practice open defecation in the country. World Health Organization (WHO) reports/estimates that one in every ten deaths in India is linked to poor sanitation and hygiene. Diarrhoea, a preventable disease, is the largest killer accounting for every 20th death. The deaths of nearly 210,000 children under 5 years of age were linked to Diarrhea alone in 2010, accounting for 13% of all under-five mortality. It is estimated that the total economic impact of inadequate sanitation in India is about US$53.8 billion a year, equivalent of 6.4% of India's GDP in 2006 or an annual loss of US$48 per person. Moreover, Open Defecation (OD) has had a sharp gender impact, negatively affecting the dignity and safety of women and girls. Despite the presence of national sanitation flagship programme, Swachh Bharat Mission Gramin (SBMG), only 130 districts out of 670 districts in the country have achieved Open Defecation Free (ODF) status since 2014. According to WHO estimates, about 38 million people are affected by water-borne diseases each year in India, of which over 75% are children (Forbes, 2015). An account estimates that sanitation saves about 200,000 lives a year of children below the age of 5 who die of illnesses related to diarrhoea.
- *Improper child feeding practices especially poor complementary feeding*: Adequate nutrition during early years of life plays an important role in achieving each child's full human potential. The period from birth to 2 years of age is known as a "critical window" for the promotion of optimal and healthy growth, proper organ formation and function, a strong immune system, and neurological and cognitive development. NFHS-4 (2015–2016) has reported that the complementary feeding practices among infants which are crucial for achieving adequate health and nutritional status still remain unsatisfactory in India. The results highlighted that only 42.7% of the children aged 6–8 months received solid or semi-solid foods along with breast-milk, decreasing from 52.6% which was reported in NFHS-3 (2005–2006).

It was found that only 8.7% of the breastfeeding children and 14.3% of the non-breastfeeding children in the age group of 6–23 months in urban and rural areas combined received an adequate diet. Only 9.6% of the total children (breastfeeding and non-breastfeeding) received an adequate diet.

- *Other determinants*: There is ample scientific evidence that poverty, caste and parental education are important determinants affecting the nutritional status of individuals. Living in resource-limited setting alone is associated with deficits in children's physical growth and psychological development, particularly language and cognition, mediated mostly through parental education and the home environment (Rubio-Codina *et al.*, 2015; Schady *et al.*, 2015; Hackman *et al.*, 2015; Fernald *et al.*, 2011). Table 1 shows the comparison of prevalence of stunting and underweight among children below 5 years of age belonging to different castes, wealth quintiles and rural–urban setting. It clearly indicates that the nutritional status of those belonging to lower-castes, poor wealth quintile and rural settings is more compromised.

Table 1. Living conditions and nutritional status of children below 5 years of age.

	Caste				**Wealth quintile**			**Setting**	
	SC	**ST**	**OBC**	**None of them**	**Lowest**	**Middle**	**Highest**	**Rural**	**Urban**
Stunting prevalence (%)									
NFHS-4 (2015–2016)	43	44	39	31	51	36	22	41.2	31
RSOC (2013–2014)	42.5	42.5	39.1	33.9 (others)	50.5		26.5	41.7	32.1
Underweight prevalence (%)									
NFHS-4 (2015–2016)	39	45	36	29	49	33	20	38.3	29.1
RSOC (2013–2014)	32.7	36.8	29.4	23.6 (other)	41.7		17.5	31.7	24.3

6. Poor Nutritional Outcomes in Selected Indian Districts

The recent national survey, NFHS-4 indicates that the burden of undernutrition (including stunting, underweight, wasting and anaemia among women and children) is concentrated in merely one sixth of the Indian districts. Analysis of the national data was undertaken to identify the districts with the maximum burden of undernutrition, primarily stunting and anaemia (among women and children). The 138 districts having stunting and anaemia prevalence figures above the national average are presented in Table A.1. The burden is concentrated in 12 Indian states, namely Uttar Pradesh (33 districts), Bihar (31 districts), Jharkhand (23 districts), Madhya Pradesh (15 districts), Rajasthan (9 districts), Gujarat and Odisha (7 each), Haryana (5 districts), West Bengal (3 districts), Chhattisgarh and Maharashtra (4 each) and Uttarakhand (1 district). Concerted multi-sectoral efforts addressing nutrition sensitive and nutrition-specific interventions would be required to fight the epidemic of macro and micronutrient malnutrition from the country. The need of the hour is to adopt the multi-sectoral convergence model.

7. Nutrition Targets

In 2012, the World Health Assembly unanimously endorsed (with 194 member countries) a set of six global nutrition targets (for stunting, anaemia, low birth weight, childhood overweight, breastfeeding and wasting) to be achieved by 2025 (Figure 2), to which India is committed, aiming to achieve these targets. Childhood stunting, an overarching measure of long-term malnutrition, has lifelong consequences not just for health but also for human capital and economic development, prosperity and equity. Being stunted in early childhood reduces schooling attainment, decreases adult wages, and makes children less likely to escape poverty as adults (Fink *et al.*, 2016; Hoddinott *et al.*, 2008, 2011). Conversely, reductions in stunting are estimated to potentially increase overall economic productivity, as measured by GDP per capita, by 4 to 11% in Africa and Asia (Horton and Steckel, 2013). For achieving WHA targets, it is estimated

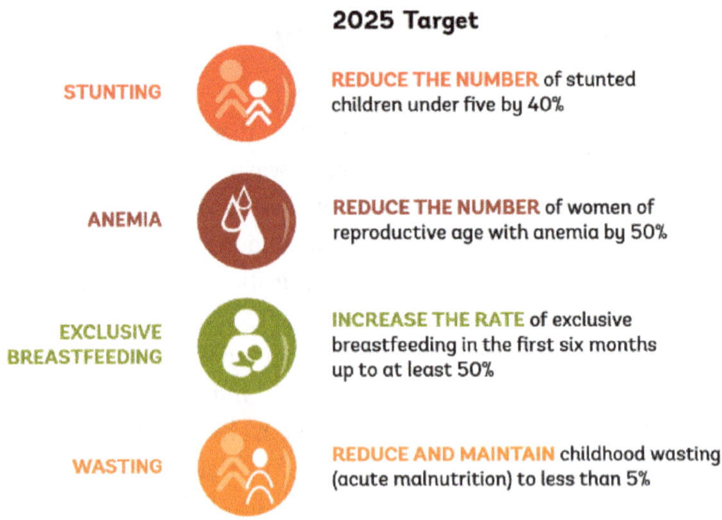

Figure 2. WHA targets 2025.

Source: WHO (2014).

that the country should consider investing 43,000 crores INR annually to fully finance the delivery of the recommended set of nutrition interventions,[2] at scale, which implies investment of 9,336 INR per year per child (0–24 months) (Chakrabarti *et al.*, 2017).

8. Role of Pro-nutrition Agriculture in Reducing Burden of Malnutrition

In India, agriculture and nutrition interact in a complex manner as agriculture is not only the mere source of food for the family but also

[2]Counselling during pregnancy, counselling for optimal breastfeeding, and counselling for complementary feeding and hand washing, vitamin A supplementation for children, Oral Rehydration Salts (ORS) and therapeutic zinc supplements for treatment of diarrhoea, deworming for children, adolescents and pregnant women, iron supplements for children, Iron-Folic Acid (IFA) supplements for adolescents, IFA and calcium supplements for pregnant and lactating women, complementary food supplements, supplementary food rations, additional food rations for severely malnourished children, facility-based treatment of severe acute malnutrition (SAM) children, insecticide-treated nets for pregnant women in malaria endemic areas, and maternity benefit for breastfeeding mothers.

income and affects the food prices and, hence, the availability of food in local market. With its close links to both the immediate causes of undernutrition (diets, feeding practices and health) and its underlying determinants (such as income, food security, education, access to WASH and health services, and gender equity), the agriculture sector can play a much stronger role than in the past in improving nutrition outcomes (Kadiyala *et al.*, 2014). The various ways through which agriculture and nutrition are linked include agriculture as a source of food for household consumption; as a source of income; effect of agricultural policy on food prices and food consumption; and women's employment in agriculture affecting childcare, child feeding and their own nutritional status are well established and accepted globally including India. Agriculture may impact the nutritional status by increasing the production and availability of nutrient rich foods (including biofortification) and their access and consumption.

9. The Coming Years

Food Demand Projections: For India, there is a strong disconnect between the rising per capita income and high levels of undernutrition and low levels of food consumption in the country. One of the explanations to this is that the food demand in India has not been growing at a rate the economic growth is happening in the country (Alexandratos and Bruinsma, 2012).

Figure 3 shows the projections for demand for certain food commodities by 2050 which are based on the following assumptions:

- Calorie projections (for 2050) are estimated to be 2,825 kcal/person/day, up from 2,300 in 2005/2007. This projected number is derived from Household Consumption Expenditure (HHCE) data between kcal from the FBS and HHCE per capita in 2005$ PPP from the World Bank data.
- Direct food consumption of cereals is anticipated to be lower in 2050 than in the base year: in 2050 they would provide 48% of total kcal, down from the 60% at present. Meat increases considerably to 9 kg in 2030 and to 18 kg in 2050, of which 12.5 kg is poultry meat. Food use of dairy products in milk equivalent to increase 63% from 2005–2007

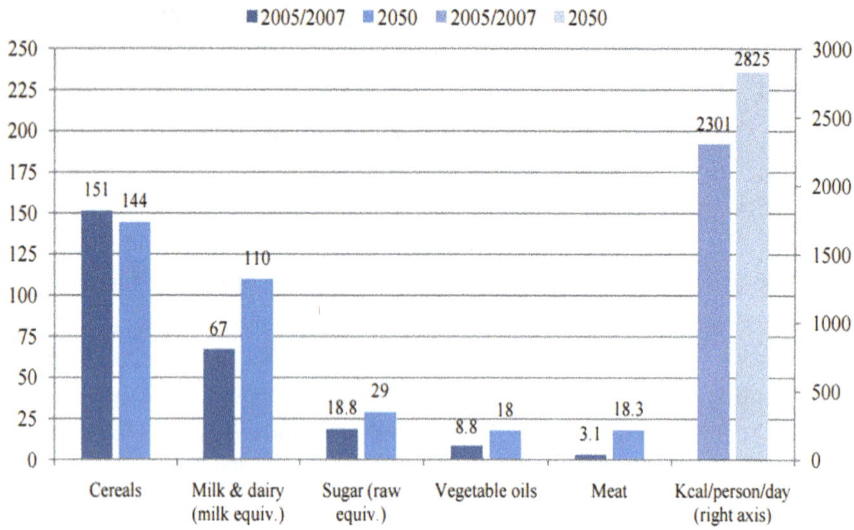

Figure 3. Food demand projections for India, 2050.

to 2050. Sugar, vegetable oils, fruit and vegetables all to increase considerably, but the first two ones to remain within nutritionally acceptable limits.

The Government is committed towards tackling the high rates of undernutrition: The recent Niti Aayog's, "Three-year action agenda: 2017–2018 to 2019–2020", conveys key health challenges very explicitly and also clearly articulates the action points for the same. Reform in institutional structures, leveraging technology for better monitoring and evaluation of collected data, harnessing the power of private sector for the benefit of community at large are some of the applaudable steps by the Government which may revolutionize the nutrition sector in the coming years.

Critical areas that may contribute to change in the nutrition scenario in the country include the following:

- Diversifying food crop production to improve access to nutrient rich foods especially for the vulnerable.

- Environment friendly post-harvest management may have a huge role to play considering the fast pace of urbanization happening in the country.
- Enhanced focus on women empowerment/protection through women-friendly policies/initiatives for accelerating reduction in undernutrition in India.
- Going back to the basics: Identifying and promoting expansion of food basket or dietary-diversity as the single long-term solution to fight both the macro and micronutrient malnutrition in the country; Educating or sensitizing the community, especially women and adolescent girls, about healthy dietary practices and cooking practices for preserving maximum nutrition; promoting traditional and indigenous varieties of crops; sensitizing community about importance of hygiene and sanitation for reducing the incidence of infections that may affect the nutritional status.

The Government of India has identified nutrition as being critical to the development of human capital. There are efforts and initiatives been undertaken to bring the malnutrition figures down. The highest body of the country, NITI Aayog has recently released the National Nutrition Strategy (Nourishing India) and has adopted the mission of a malnutrition free India. The multi-dimensional and multi-causal nature of nutrition is increasingly being realized. Although progress has been made, the degree of desired change is not yet being achieved. There is a need to understand why increased incomes, financial growth, urbanization and globalization has not resulted in better nutrition outcomes. There is a need to understand the reason why a host of agricultural developments, food security, poverty alleviation, health and other social improvement-related safety net programmes, some of which are world's largest, have not been successful to achieve their objectives. Some of the possible reasons could be that the horizontal linkages among programmes or policies are often missing the synergestic effects. In addition, nutrition lens is not always used in formulating development programmes. There could be many other contributory factors for the same which need to be identified and addressed on priority basis. It will be wiser to factor in new challenges as well, as we move ahead.

Annexure 1

Table A.1. List of nutritionally high-priority districts (Combining stunting and anaemia prevalence among children and women).

Total districts: 138		Name of the districts
State-wise breakup of districts		
Uttar Pradesh	33	Aligarh; Allahabad; Ambedkar Nagar; Auraiya; Azamgarh; Balrampur; Banda; Bareilly; Basti; Bijnor; Bulandshahr; Chandauli; Chitrakoot; Deoria; Faizabad; Ghazipur; Gonda; Jalaun; Jyotiba Phule Nagar; Kanpur Dehat; Kanpur Nagar; Kaushambi; Mahoba; Mau; Mirzapur; Moradabad; Muzaffarnagar; Pilibhit; Rampur; Sant Ravidas Nagar; Shahjahanpur; Siddharthnagar; Sultanpur
Bihar	31	Araria; Arwal; Banka; Begusarai; Bhagalpur; Bhojpur; Darbhanga; Gaya; Jamui; Jehanabad; Kaimur; Katihar; Khagaria; Kishanganj; Lakhisarai; Madhepura; Madhubani; Munger; Nalanda; Pashchim Champaran; Purba Champaran; Purnia; Rohtas; Saharsa; Samastipur; Saran; Sheikhpura; Sheohar; Sitamarhi; Supaul; Vaishali
Jharkhand	23	Bokaro; Chatra; Deoghar; Dhanbad; Dumka; Garhwa; Giridih; Godda; Gumla; Hazaribagh; Jamtara; Khunti; Kodarma; Lohardaga; Pakur; Palamu; Pashchimi Singhbhum; Purbi Singhbhum; Ramgarh; Ranchi; Sahibganj; Saraikela Kharsawan; Simdega
Madhya Pradesh	15	Alirajpur; Barwani; Bhind; Burhanpur; Datia; Dhar; Dindori; Gwalior; Jhabua; Khandwa (East Nimar); Khargone (West Nimar); Morena; Ratlam; Sheopur; Umaria
Rajasthan	9	Banswara; Baran; Bundi; Dungarpur; Jalor; Pratapgarh; Rajsamand; Sirohi; Udaipur
Gujarat	7	Bhavnagar; Dohad; Kachchh; Mahesena; Sabarkantha; Surendranagar; The Dangs
Odisha	7	Balangir; Bargarh; Koraput; Malkangiri; Nabarangapur; Sambalpur; Subarnapur
Haryana	5	Gurgaon; Karnal; Mewat; Panipat; Sonipat
West Bengal	3	Birbhum; Puruliya; Uttar Dinajpur
Chhattisgarh	2	Bastar; Dakshin Bastar Dantewada
Maharashtra	2	Dhule; Nandurbar
Uttarakhand	1	Haridwar

References

Akhtar, S., Ahmed, A., Randhawa, M. A., Atukorala, S., Arlappa, N., Ismail, T. and Z. Ali (2013) "Prevalence of Vitamin A Deficiency in South Asia: Causes, Outcomes, and Possible Remedies", *Journal of Health Population and Nutrition*, Vol. 31, No. 4, pp. 413–423.

Alexandratos, N. and J. Bruinsma (2012) "World Agriculture Towards 2030/2050: The 2012 Revision", ESA Working paper No. 12-03. Rome: FAO.

Anchala, R., Kannuri, N. K., Pant, H., Khan, H., Franco, O. H., Di Angelantonio, E. and D. Prabhakaran (2014) "Hypertension in India: A Systematic Review and Meta-Analysis of Prevalence, Awareness, and Control of Hypertension", *Journal of Hypertension*, Vol. 32, No. 6, pp. 1170–1177.

Chakrabarti, S., Kapur, A., Vaid, A. and P. Menon (2017) "Achieving the 2025 World Health Assembly Targets for Nutrition in India: What Will It Cost?" POSHAN Policy Note #2. New Delhi, India: International Food Policy Research Institute.

Djurfeldt Göran, H. H., Jirstrom, M. and R. Larsson (2005) "The Puzzle of the Policy Shift — The Early Green Revolution in India, Indonesia and the Philippines", in *The African Food Crisis: Lessons from the Asian Green Revolution*. ISBN 0 85199 998 0, CABI Publishing, CAB International, Wallingford, Oxon OX10 8DE, UK, pp. 49–51.

Fernald, L. C., Weber, A., Galasso, E. and L. Ratsifandrihamanana (2011) "Socioeconomic Gradients and Child Development in a Very Low Income Population: Evidence from Madagascar", *Developmental Science*, Vol. 14, pp. 832–847.

Fink, G., Peet, E., Danaei, G., Andrews, K., McCoy, D. C., Sudfeld, C. R., Smith Fawzi, M. C., Ezzati, M. and W. W. Fawzi (2016) "Schooling and Wage Income Losses Due to Early-Childhood Growth Faltering in Developing Countries: National, Regional, and Global Estimates", *The American Journal of Clinical Nutrition*, Vol. 104, No. 1, pp. 104–112.

Forbes (2015) "Ten Facts About Drinking Water in India That May Make You Sick". Available at: http://www.forbesindia.com/blog/economy-policy/ten-facts-about-drinking-water-in-india-that-may-make-you-sick/.

Fujita, K. (2010) *The Green Revolution and its Significance for Economic Development: The Indian Experience and its Implications for Sub-Saharan Africa*. JICA Research Institute.

Global Nutrition Report (2016) Available at: http://www.globalnutritionreport.org/.

Gopalan, C. (2013) "The Changing Nutrition Scenario", *Indian Journal of Medical Research,* Vol. 138, pp. 392–397.

Gulati, S., Misra, A., Colles, S. L., Kondal, D., Gupta, N., Goel, K., Bansal, S., Mishra, M., Madkaikar, V. and S. Bhardwaj (2013) "Dietary Intakes and Familial Correlates of Overweight/Obesity: A Four-cities Study in India". *Ann. Nutr. Metab.*, Vol. 62, pp. 279–290.

Gulati, S. and A. Misra (2014) "Sugar Intake, Obesity, and Diabetes in India", *Nutrients*, Vol. 6, pp. 5955–5974. DOI:10.3390/nu6125955.

Hackman, D. A., Gallop, R., Evans, G. W. and M. J. Farah (2015) "Socioeconomic Status and Executive Function: Developmental Trajectories and Mediation", *Developmental Science*, Vol. 18, pp. 686–702.

Hazell, P. B. R. (2009) "The Asian Green Revolution", *International Food Policy Research Institute*. IFPRI Discussion Paper 00911.

Hoddinott, J., Maluccio, J. A., Behrman, J. R., Flores, R. and R. Martorell (2008) "Effect of a Nutrition Intervention During Early Childhood on Economic Productivity in Guatemalan Adults", *Lancet*, Vol. 371, pp. 411–416.

Hoddinott, J., Maluccio, J., Behrman, J. R. *et al.* (2011) "The Consequences of Early Childhood Growth Failure Over the Life Course", IFPRI Discussion Paper 01073. Washington, DC: International Food Policy Research Institute.

Horton, S. and R. Steckel (2013) "Malnutrition: Global Economic Losses Attributable to Malnutrition 1900–2000 and Projections to 2050", in *The Economics of Human Challenges*, ed. B. Lomborg. Cambridge, U.K.: Cambridge University Press, pp. 247–272.

ICMR (2010). Recommended Dietary Allowances of Indians.

International Diabetes Federation (IDF) (2015) India. Available at: http://www.idf.org/membership/sea/india.

International Food Policy Research Institute (IFPRI) (2014) "Addressing the Challenge of Hidden Hunger", *Global Hunger Index*.

Joshi, S. R., Anjana, R. M., Deepa, M., Pradeepa, R., Bhansali, A., Dhandania, V. K., Joshi, P. P., Unnikrishnan, R., Nirmal, E., Subashini, R., Madhu, S. V., Rao, P. V., Das, A. K., Kaur, T., Shukla, D. K. and V. Mohan (2014) "Prevalence of Dyslipidemia in Urban and Rural India: The ICMR–INDIAB Study", *PLoS ONE*, Vol. 9, No. 5, p. e96808.

Kadiyala, S., Harris, J., Headey, D., Yosef, S. and S. Gillespie (2014) "Agriculture and Nutrition in India: Mapping Evidence to Pathways", *Annals of New York Academic Science*, Vol. 1331, pp. 43–56.

National Council of Applied Economic Research (NCAER) (2014) An Analysis of Changing Food Consumption Pattern in India.

National Family Health Survey (NFHS)-4 (2015–2016) India Fact Sheet. Ministry of Health and Family Welfare.

NNMB (2012) "Diet and Nutritional Status of Rural Population, Prevalence of Hypertension and Diabetes Among Adults and Infant and Young Child

Feeding Practices", Technical report no. 26. Report of third repeat survey. National institute of Nutrition.

Popkin, B. and S. W. Ng (2007) "The Nutrition Transition in High- and Low-Income Countries: What are the Policy Lessons?" *Agricultural Economics*, Vol. 37, pp. 199–211. DOI:10.1111/j.1574-0862.2007.00245.x.

Ramachandran, P. (2006) "The Double Burden of Malnutrition in India", in *The Double Burden of Malnutrition Case Studies from Six Developing Countries*. Food and Agricultural Organization of the United Nations.

Ramachandran, P. (2007) *Nutrition Transition in India 1947–2007*. Nutrition Foundation of India Publications. Available at: http://nutritionfoundationofindia.res.in/NutritionTransition.asp (accessed on January 22, 2017).

Ramachandran, P. (2008) "Changing Food Consumption Patterns in India", *Bulletin of the Nutrition Foundation of India*, Vol. 29, No. 2. Available at: http://www.nutritionfoundationofindia.res.in/pdfs/April%202008%20final.pdf.

Rapid Survey on Children (RSOC) (2014) Ministry of Women and Child Development, Government of India, Provisional — India Fact Sheet.

Ritu, G. and A. Gupta (2014) "Vitamin D Deficiency in India: Prevalence, Causalities and Interventions", *Nutrients*, Vol. 6, No. 2, pp. 729–775.

Rubio-Codina, M., Attanasio, O., Meghir, C., Varela, N. and S. Grantham-McGregor (2015) "The Socioeconomic Gradient of Child Development: Cross-Sectional Evidence from Children 6–42 Panel in Bogota", *Journal of Human Resources*, Vol. 50, pp. 464–683.

Schady, N., Behrman, J., Araujo, M. C. *et al.* (2015) "Wealth Gradients in Early Childhood Cognitive Development in Five Latin American Countries", *Journal of Human Resources*, Vol. 50, pp. 446–463.

Shrimpton, R. and C. Rokx (2012) "The Double Burden of Malnutrition: A Review of Global Evidence". HNP Discussion Paper, The World Bank.

Stuckler, D., McKee, M., Ebrahim, S. and S. Basu (2012) "Manufacturing Epidemics: The Role of Global Producers in Increased Consumption of Unhealthy Commodities Including Processed Foods, Alcohol, and Tobacco", *PLoS Med*, Vol. 9, No. 6, p. e1001235.

UNICEF (2009) "UNICEF Coverage Evaluation Survey 2009", All India Report. Ministry of Health and Family Welfare, Government of India, New Delhi.

World Health Organization (WHO) (2014) "Global Status Report on Noncommunicable Diseases". Available at: http://apps.who.int/iris/bitstream/10665/148114/1/9789241564854_eng.pdf?ua=1.

World Health Organization (WHO) (2017) "Noncommunicable Diseases Fact Sheet". Available at: http://www.who.int/mediacentre/factsheets/fs355/en/.

Chapter 7

Is Variety the Spice of Life? India's Nutrition Experience

Nidhi Kaicker,[*,§] **Vani S. Kulkarni**[†,¶] **and Raghav Gaiha**[‡,||]

[*]*Ambedkar University Delhi (AUD), India*
[†]*Yale University, US*
[‡]*University of Manchester, UK*
[§]*nidhi@aud.ac.in*
[¶]*vani.kulkarni@yale.edu*
[||]*raghavdasgaiha@gmail.com*

Abstract

This chapter departs from an influential study by Deaton and Dreze (2009), in which decline in calorie intake over the past few decades is attributed to lower calorie 'requirements' as a result of improvements in sanitation, health and more sedentary lifestyles, in order to address the central question of whether more diversified diets result in greater consumption of expensive calories and consequently in a reduction of calorie intake. We do so using the National Sample Survey (NSS) consumer expenditure data for 1993–1994, 2004–2005 and 2011–2012. Our analysis corroborates the fact that dietary diversification is associated with higher costs of calories, mainly because of reliance on more expensive calories (e.g., through a reduced dependence on cereals, which are the cheapest sources of calories), determined by a taste for variety in both rural and urban areas and across expenditure deciles over the period 1994–2012. Our analysis also confirms that higher costs of calories and greater affluence are associated with a reduction in calorie intake.

Keywords: Calories, diets, taste for variety, cost of calories, reduction in calorie intake, India.

1. Introduction

That India ranks 100 in a group of 119 countries in the Global Hunger Index in 2017 is abysmal enough regardless of how steeply it has deteriorated in recent years. The higher the rank, the worse is the state of hunger. India is currently undergoing a rapid economic and demographic transformation. Since 1980, average living standards have experienced a sustained and rapid rise. Rapid economic growth has been accompanied by rising urbanization.

A key feature of the economic transformation has been the change in the nature of the Indian diet — a shift away from cereals towards vanaspati-oil, eggs, meat, fish and poultry, fruits and vegetables — but with rural–urban variation. Some of the underlying factors of this dietary transition include expansion of the middle class, higher female labour force participation (with reduction in recent years), the emergence of nuclear two-income families, a sharp age divide in food preferences (with younger age groups more susceptible to new foods advertised in the media), and a rapid growth of supermarkets and fast food outlets.

What precisely is the impact of diet diversification on calorie intake is the focus of the present study. This is not to suggest that other nutrients (such as protein and fat) do not matter. Indeed, they do, but we have restricted much of our analysis to calories. It is worth emphasizing, however, that calorie deficiencies are regarded as the most basic and first-order problem, and often used to characterize widespread malnutrition, though other nutrient inadequacies also are found to be widespread.

In India, *despite* rising incomes, there has been a sustained decline in per capita calorie intake. One of the first examinations of this *puzzle* by Deaton and Dreze (2009) shows a decline in average calorie intake in the quarter century preceding 2005. The puzzle is essentially this: per capita calorie consumption is lower at a given level of per capita household expenditure, across the expenditure scale, at low levels of per capita expenditure as well as high. In other words, there is a steady downward *shift* of the calorie Engel curve, in a country which is undernourished! A contentious view offered in this study is that this is not attributable to changes in relative prices as an aggregate measure of the price of food — treated synonymous with the price of calories — changed little during the period in question. They are emphatic that assuming the elasticity of income with respect to nutrition is positive, the downward shift of the calorie Engel curve is due to the lower calorie "requirements", associated mainly with better health and lower activity levels.[1] As the evidence offered is fragmentary and patchy, this explanation is largely *conjectural.*

Another argument for the declining calorie intake is the lower expenditure on food as a proportion of the total expenditure, and voluntary choice of luxuries over food (Banerjee and Duflo, 2011; Basole and Basu, 2015; Sen, 2005). This argument is doubtful as a reduction of food expenditure (as proportion of the total expenditure), or the food budget squeeze, implies substitution of more expensive source of calories with cheaper source of calories to meet the energy "requirements", and the extant literature suggests that it is actually the reverse — even the poor are moving away from cheaper sources of calories to more expensive sources (Gaiha *et al.,* 2014; Kaicker *et al.,* 2016). Yet another argument for the lower calorie intake is the underreporting of food consumed, especially of eating out (Smith, 2015), but is far from conclusive.

Without rejecting the Deaton–Dreze view as implausible, we focus instead on a growing taste for variety as an important factor in lowering calorie intake during 1993–1994 to 2011–2012. As revealed by the 72nd round of the NSS for 2014–2015, there is considerable convergence between urban and rural lifestyles and consumption patterns. Of particular significance is pervasiveness of eating out in both urban and rural areas. Strong demand for processed and fried foods and snacks with attractive packaging and rich flavours, and sugary beverages, is fuelled by

[1] Srinivasan (1992) is deeply sceptical of such "requirements" on the grounds that energy expenditure adjusts to intake within a range. The question really is what the homeostatic range is within which this adjustment takes place.

aggressive advertising in mass media. The growing "taste" for variety is exhibited by not just the affluent but also by the lower economic strata.

The present study aims to build on two complementary and innovative contributions, Behrman and Deolalikar (1987, 1989). The first study, based on estimates for a relatively poor rural south Indian population, indicates that, although income elasticities of food expenditure are large, income elasticities of calorie intakes are much smaller.[2] A number of other recent studies report similar results for a wide range of developing country populations (e.g. Knudsen and Scandizzo (1979) for Sri Lanka, Morocco and India) with a few notable exceptions. Behrman and Deolalikar (1989) offer a quantifiable explanation of the phenomenon that calorie elasticities are substantially less than food expenditure elasticities: that food variety *per se* is valued so that people purchase increased food variety as their incomes increase even though that may not alter their calorie intakes much.

Variety is directly related to two characteristics of consumer preferences over various foods: the degree of curvature and the centrality (relative to the axes) of location of indifference curves. If concern for low-cost calories dominates food choices at very low incomes, it is expected that the food indifference curves will be relatively flat (so substitution among foods is considerable if relative food prices change) and located close to the axis for the traditional cheapest source of calories. Hence, there is a tendency towards high concentration on relatively cheap sources of calories. As incomes and food budgets increase, it is posited that food indifference curves across foods may become more sharply curved and centred further away from the axis for the low-cost calorie sources. For preferences characterized by such indifference curves, there will be less concentration on particular (cheap calorie-supplying) foods, greater variety of foods consumed for given food prices and less change in food composition in response to changes in relative food prices. This denotes a situation of greater curvature and locational centrality of food indifference curves and a taste for food variety. The cross-country analysis is based on ICP data for 1975 and 1980.

The estimates strongly suggest that, as their incomes and total expenditures on food increase from very low levels, consumers behave as if they

[2]These results appear to be somewhat exaggerated in light of more recent studies (Subramanian and Deaton, 1996; Jha *et al.*, 2009).

increasingly value food variety. It is implied that calorie intakes are likely to increase much less than expenditures on food with increased incomes for the poor because the poor use the additional income to purchase increased food variety. This implication is consistent with income elasticities of calorie intakes that are substantially less than food expenditure elasticities with respect to income at low levels of per capita income.

Based on an analysis of a decline in calorie intake between the 1993 and 1999 NSS rounds, Jha *et al.* (2009) corroborate that two sets of relationships are key to this result: one is the relative price effect, depending on the curvature of the food indifference curves for the poor and non-poor, and the second is the location of the indifference curves. The decline in calorie intake is thus a consequence of taste for variety associated with increasing curvature of food indifference curves and their increasing centrality. However, the curvature is higher among the non-poor but not substantially *vis-à-vis* the poor, although locational differences are pronounced for some food items.

The central question thus is: have more diversified diets resulted in greater consumption of expensive calories and consequently in reduction of calorie intake? We address this in what follows, using the National Sample Survey (NSS) consumer expenditure data for 1993–1994, 2004–2005 and 2011–2012.

1.1. *Scheme*

In Section 2, we sketch changes in calorie intake, undernourishment and costs of calories. We discuss salient features of the NSS data and conversion of food expenditure into nutrients' intakes in Section 3. This is followed by a discussion in Section 4 of changes in calorie, protein and fat intakes and in their distribution during 1994–2012 in greater detail. Section 5 discusses changes in calorie, protein and fat deprivation. Section 6 offers a detailed discussion of the rise in the cost of calories by expenditure decile and over time. Section 7 examines diet diversification by expenditure decile, and how it evolved over the period 1994–2012. A composite index of diet diversification is constructed which is an improvement over indices used in earlier studies. Section 8 specifies the model which is estimated using instrument variable regression with fixed state effects. Section 9 is devoted to discussion of the econometric results.

Section 10 discusses the significance of our contribution relative to the pioneering contribution of Behrman and Deolalikar (1989) and its elaboration and validation in India's context by Jha *et al.* (2009), and from a broader policy perspective. Section 11 offers concluding observations on specific policy concerns and imperatives.

2. Changes in Calorie Intake, Undernourishment and Cost of Calories

The fact that average calorie intake was slightly higher in 2011–2012 than in 2004–2005 is seen as a *reversal* of the declining intake of calories over 1983–2005. We offer a more nuanced view based on a disaggregated analysis that in part refutes this interpretation.

The *base* year matters. The average calorie intake was lower in 2005 compared to 1994 in Rural India. It was also lower in 2012 relative to 1994. However, the calorie intake in 2012 was higher than in 2004–2005. So, if the comparison is confined to 1994–2012, there was no reversal. A different pattern is revealed for urban India. The average calorie intake was lower in 2005 compared to 1994. It rose between 2005 and 2012. However, it declined between 1994 and 2012.

Some related statistics of undernourishment are appalling. The proportion of undernourished among rural poor has risen over time and accounted for a larger majority of the poor (about 84% in 2011–2012 *vis-à-vis* 75% in 1993–1994). The proportion of undernourished among urban poor rose, but moderately (from 64% in 1993 to 68% in 2011). The poor are thus more likely to be undernourished.

(Real) cost of calories rose consistently between 1994 and 2005, and between 2005 and 2011, across per capita expenditure deciles in both rural (Rural India) and urban areas (Urban India).

3. Data

The empirical analysis uses household level data from three recent thick rounds of the quinquennial Consumer Expenditure Survey (CES) conducted by the NSSO: 1993–1994 (50th Round), 2004–2005 (61st Round) and 2011–2012 (68th Round). The thick rounds of the CES are large scale, nationally representative surveys of households, conducted approximately every 5 years, which collect detailed data about the level and pattern of consumption expenditure.

Each survey round contains approximately 80,000 rural households (located in 8,000 villages) and 45,000 urban households (located in 4,500 urban blocks). Survey weights are used to make the sample nationally representative. The surveys record household expenditures and quantities of each food item consumed in the last 30 days (with home grown foods and gifts both valued at the prevailing local prices) or uniform recall period. There are 169 different food items, including 12 products made from rice or wheat, 9 types of pulses, 7 milk products and many vegetables, spices and meats. Their conversion into calories, proteins and fats is done using the Gopalan *et al.* (1971) and ICMR (1990) ratios. Food prices are based on unit values that are aggregated into Public Sector Undertakings (PSU) averages. Nominal prices are adjusted to 2004–2005 Consumer Prices for Agricultural Labourers for Rural Areas and Consumer Price Index for Industrial Workers (CPIIW).

4. Changes in Intake and Distribution of Calories, Protein and Fat

4.1. *Aggregate*

Table 1 gives comparisons of calorie intake in 1994, 2005 and 2012, using *t*-tests for significant differences. As both rural and urban comparisons reveal, the intake was significantly lower in 2005 relative to 1994; however, it rose significantly during 2005–2012. Between 1994 and 2012, there was a decline.

So inference of *reversal* of declining calorie intake based on comparisons during 2005–2012 is potentially misleading.

In Table 2, comparisons of protein intake during the corresponding periods are given with tests of significance. Average protein intake in Rural India declined significantly during 1994–2005; it remained unchanged during 2005–2012; however, it fell significantly during 1994–2012. In Urban India, it recorded a significant reduction during 1994–2005, but rose significantly during 2005–2012. However, as in Rural India, it fell significantly during 1994–2012.

Table 1. Changes in calorie intake, 1994–2012.

	RURAL INDIA			URBAN INDIA		
	1994 & 2005	**2005 & 2012**	**1994 & 2012**	**1994 & 2005**	**2005 & 2012**	**1994 & 2012**
1993–1994	2284.44		2284.44	2279.18		2279.18
2004–2005	2186.46	2186.46		2147.13	2147.13	
2011–2012		2220.29	2220.29		2211.84	2211.84
Difference	97.98	−33.83	64.15	132.05	−64.71	67.34
t-statistic	14.96	−5.20	14.66	15.92	−8.19	12.13
p-value	0.00	0.00	0.00	0.00	0.00	0.00

Source: Authors' calculations from various rounds of the NSS.

Table 2. Changes in protein intake, 1994–2012.

	RURAL INDIA			URBAN INDIA		
	1994 & 2005	**2005 & 2012**	**1994 & 2012**	**1994 & 2005**	**2005 & 2012**	**1994 & 2012**
1993–1994	63.72		62.07	62.07		62.07
2004–2005	59.00	59.00		57.73	57.73	
2011–2012		59.10	59.04		59.04	59.04
Difference	4.72	−0.10	3.03	4.34	−1.31	3.03
t-statistic	23.09	−0.53	20.89	19.38	−5.92	20.89
p-value	0.00	0.59	0.00	0.00	0.00	0.00

Source: Authors' calculations from various rounds of the NSS.

The average fat intake was significantly higher in 2005 compared to 1994 in Rural India, as also in 2012 relative to 2005, and in 2012 relative to 1994. Thus, in sharp contrast to calorie and protein intakes, fat recorded a consistent rise throughout (Table 3).

4.2. *Disaggregation by MPCE Deciles*

Calorie intake rose by Monthly Per Capita Consumption Expenditure (MPCE) deciles in Rural India in 1994, 2005 and 2012, as shown in

Table 3. Changes in fat intake, 1994–2012.

	RURAL INDIA			URBAN INDIA		
	1994 & 2005	**2005 & 2012**	**1994 & 2012**	**1994 & 2005**	**2005 & 2012**	**1994 & 2012**
1993–1994	34.98		34.98	47.85		47.85
2004–2005	40.13	40.13		48.61	48.61	
2011–2012		45.28	45.28		53.27	53.27
Difference	−5.14	−5.16	−10.30	−0.75	−4.66	−5.42
t-statistic	−13.64	−12.91	−68.54	−1.20	−7.77	−17.01
p-value	0.00	0.00	0.00	0.23	0.00	0.00

Source: Authors' calculations from various rounds of the NSS.

Table 4. To avoid tedious details, our comments are confined to the differences between 1994 and 2012. In the lowest 4 expenditure deciles in Rural India, calorie intake was significantly higher in 2012 relative to 1994. In all higher expenditure deciles, calorie intakes were significantly lower. As in Rural India, calorie intake by expenditure decile in Urban India rose in 1994, 2005 and 2012. Between 1994 and 2012, except for the two lowest expenditure deciles in which calorie intake was significantly higher in 2012, in all higher expenditure deciles it was significantly lower.

4.2.1. *Protein*

In Rural India, protein intake by expenditure decile rose in 1994, 2005 and 2012. Except for the lowest decile in which there was a significant rise, in all higher expenditure deciles there were significant reductions between 1994 and 2012. Urban India witnessed a similar pattern: higher protein intake by decile in 1994, 2005 and 2012. Besides, except for the lowest expenditure decile, which saw a significant increase, all higher deciles recorded significant reductions (Table 5).

4.2.2. *Fat*

As shown in Table 6, in Rural India, fat intake by expenditure decile rose in 1994, 2005 and 2012. Between 1994 and 2012, each decile witnessed

Table 4. Calorie intake by deciles of MPCE.

Deciles of MPCE	Mean value			Difference			Wald (F statistic)		
	1993–1994	2004–2005	2011–2012	1994 & 2005	1994 & 2012	2005 & 2012	1994 & 2005	1994 & 2012	2005 & 2012
				RURAL					
1	1465.4	1484.7	1679.7	19.30 (1.3%)	214.30 (14.6%)	195.00 (13.1%)	4.0	344.1	279.8
2	1731.3	1681.2	1823.8	−50.10 (−2.9%)	92.50 (5.3%)	142.60 (8.5%)	32.6	56.5	132.3
3	1851.7	1801.9	1915.1	−49.80 (−2.7%)	63.40 (3.4%)	113.20 (6.3%)	12.5	28.2	47.7
4	1975.5	1881.4	1981.6	−94.10 (−4.8%)	6.10 (0.3%)	100.20 (5.3%)	92.3	**0.2 (NS)**	64.1
5	2057.4	1961.7	2041.5	−95.70 (−4.7%)	−15.90 (−0.8%)	79.80 (4.1%)	81.3	**1.7 (NS)**	36.6
6	2165.3	2044.2	2115.8	−121.10 (−5.6%)	−49.50 (−2.3%)	71.60 (3.5%)	126.2	14.8	31.6
7	2276.6	2157.4	2188.6	−119.20 (−5.2%)	−88.00 (−3.9%)	31.20 (1.4%)	44.0	43.2	**2.6 (NS)**
8	2411.5	2291.8	2272.0	−119.70 (−5.0%)	−139.50 (−5.8%)	−19.80 (−0.9%)	13.2	108.6	**0.4 (NS)**
9	2590.0	2377.4	2352.1	−212.60 (−8.2%)	−237.90 (−9.2%)	−25.30 (−1.1%)	229.2	261.8	**2.7 (NS)**
10	3036.9	2791.7	2649.6	−245.20 (−8.1%)	−387.30 (−12.8%)	−142.10 (−5.1%)	76.5	251.9	30.4

				URBAN					
1	1527.3	1512.6	1636.8	−14.70 (−1.0%)	109.50 (7.2%)	124.20 (8.2%)	**1.4 (NS)**	84.5	92.0
2	1759.7	1686.5	1763.2	−73.20 (−4.2%)	3.50 (0.2%)	76.70 (4.5%)	35.4	**0.1 (NS)**	33.9
3	1888.0	1835.7	1858.5	−52.30 (−2.8%)	−29.50 (−1.6%)	22.80 (1.2%)	**1.4 (NS)**	5.0	**0.3 (NS)**
4	1992.3	1856.7	1920.5	−135.60 (−6.8%)	−71.80 (−3.6%)	63.80 (3.4%)	96.2	23.9	17.7
5	2096.1	1945.9	1980.5	−150.20 (−7.2%)	−115.60 (−5.5%)	34.60 (1.8%)	99.9	68.9	4.7
6	2193.7	2021.6	2052.0	−172.10 (−7.8%)	−141.70 (−6.5%)	30.40 (1.5%)	61.2	87.4	**2.0 (NS)**
7	2315.3	2108.5	2129.7	−206.80 (−8.9%)	−185.60 (−8.0%)	21.20 (1.0%)	79.8	107.8	**1.0 (NS)**
8	2450.0	2212.6	2246.5	−237.40 (−9.7%)	−203.50 (−8.3%)	33.90 (1.5%)	123.9	129.8	**2.6 (NS)**
9	2674.0	2338.3	2379.8	−335.70 (−12.6%)	−294.20 (−11.0%)	41.50 (1.8%)	180.2	154.8	**3.2 (NS)**
10	3043.7	2690.7	2608.3	−353.00 (−11.6%)	−435.40 (−14.3%)	−82.40 (−3.1%)	33.3	106.2	**2.3 (NS)**

Source: Authors' calculations from various rounds of the NSS.

Table 5. Protein intake by deciles of MPCE.

	Mean value			Difference			Wald (F statistic)		
Deciles of MPCE	**1993–1994**	**2004–2005**	**2011–2012**	**1994 & 2005**	**1994 & 2012**	**2005 & 2012**	**1994 & 2005**	**1994 & 2012**	**2005 & 2012**
				RURAL					
1	41.40	39.64	43.67	–1.76 (–4.3%)	2.27 (5.5%)	4.03 (10.2%)	22.24	33.76	113.01
2	47.94	45.13	47.86	–2.81 (–5.9%)	–0.08 (–0.2%)	2.73 (6.0%)	94.61	**0.04 (NS)**	52.91
3	51.03	49.09	50.54	–1.94 (–3.8%)	–0.49 (–1.0%)	1.45 (3.0%)	10.96	**1.61 (NS)**	5.21
4	54.19	51.16	52.98	–3.03 (–5.6%)	–1.21 (–2.2%)	1.82 (3.6%)	80.63	9.42	20.02
5	56.88	53.13	54.41	–3.75 (–6.6%)	–2.47 (–4.3%)	1.28 (2.4%)	128.53	38.31	10.85
6	60.20	56.00	57.16	–4.20 (–7.0%)	–3.04 (–5.0%)	1.16 (2.1%)	104.65	40.84	7.25
7	63.35	58.61	59.28	–4.74 (–7.5%)	–4.07 (–6.4%)	0.67 (1.1%)	153.69	89.98	**2.34 (NS)**
8	67.63	62.04	61.59	–5.59 (–8.3%)	–6.04 (–8.9%)	–0.45 (–0.7%)	132.88	198.99	**0.78 (NS)**
9	73.54	66.18	64.88	–7.36 (–10.0%)	–8.66 (–11.8%)	–1.30 (–2.0%)	136.96	322.03	**3.97 (NS)**
10	86.53	77.33	73.44	–9.20 (–10.6%)	–13.09 (–15.1%)	–3.89 (–5.0%)	159.76	347.36	31.83

URBAN									
1	42.85	42.07	44.05	−0.78 (−1.8%)	1.20 (2.8%)	1.98 (4.7%)	**3.70 (NS)**	9.94	24.81
2	48.66	46.47	47.82	−2.19 (−4.5%)	−0.84 (−1.7%)	1.35 (2.9%)	28.07	4.22	10.25
3	52.30	51.63	50.26	−0.67 (−1.3%)	−2.04 (−3.9%)	−1.37 (−2.7%)	**0.12 (NS)**	23.78	**0.49 (NS)**
4	55.38	50.83	51.87	−4.55 (−8.2%)	−3.51 (−6.3%)	1.04 (2.0%)	92.20	52.62	4.31
5	57.72	53.76	53.38	−3.96 (−6.9%)	−4.34 (−7.5%)	−0.38 (−0.7%)	55.57	103.28	**0.49 (NS)**
6	60.41	55.03	55.62	−5.38 (−8.9%)	−4.79 (−7.9%)	0.59 (1.1%)	103.80	104.36	**1.37 (NS)**
7	63.64	57.60	57.22	−6.04 (−9.5%)	−6.42 (−10.1%)	−0.38 (−0.7%)	87.33	165.29	**0.38 (NS)**
8	67.59	60.35	60.67	−7.24 (−10.7%)	−6.92 (−10.2%)	0.32 (0.5%)	116.66	164.12	**0.25 (NS)**
9	73.22	63.39	64.47	−9.83 (−13.4%)	−8.75 (−12.0%)	1.08 (1.7%)	204.60	162.43	**2.43 (NS)**
10	83.63	73.05	71.02	−10.58 (−12.7%)	−12.61 (−15.1%)	−2.03 (−2.8%)	40.78	100.62	**2.02 (NS)**

Source: Authors' calculations from various rounds of the NSS.

Table 6. Fat intake by deciles of MPCE.

Deciles of MPCE	Mean value 1993–1994	Mean value 2004–2005	Mean value 2011–2012	Difference 1994 & 2005	Difference 1994 & 2012	Difference 2005 & 2012	Wald (F statistic) 1994 & 2005	Wald (F statistic) 1994 & 2012	Wald (F statistic) 2005 & 2012
RURAL									
1	14.04	16.14	22.13	2.10 (15.0%)	8.09 (57.6%)	5.99 (37.1%)	62.05	693.44	515.32
2	17.76	21.25	28.05	3.49 (19.7%)	10.29 (57.9%)	6.80 (32.0%)	213.54	1325.03	489.14
3	20.59	25.10	31.78	4.51 (21.9%)	11.19 (54.3%)	6.68 (26.6%)	31.27	1356.47	63.43
4	23.25	27.90	35.63	4.65 (20.0%)	12.38 (53.2%)	7.73 (27.7%)	214.03	1301.57	352.20
5	26.51	30.84	38.30	4.33 (16.3%)	11.79 (44.5%)	7.46 (24.2%)	76.99	1002.94	173.43
6	29.91	34.14	41.92	4.23 (14.1%)	12.01 (40.2%)	7.78 (22.8%)	170.88	935.19	341.81
7	33.51	39.91	45.98	6.40 (19.1%)	12.47 (37.2%)	6.07 (15.2%)	15.38	983.83	13.56
8	38.69	43.39	50.30	4.70 (12.1%)	11.61 (30.0%)	6.91 (15.9%)	24.71	643.76	48.80
9	46.61	48.98	55.65	2.37 (5.1%)	9.04 (19.4%)	6.67 (13.6%)	21.44	310.84	128.63
10	63.82	66.58	68.67	2.76 (4.3%)	4.85 (7.6%)	2.09 (3.1%)	9.39	34.96	5.64

				URBAN					
1	19.41	22.13	28.84	2.72 (14.0%)	9.43 (48.6%)	6.71 (30.3%)	117.75	1154.49	459.39
2	26.48	28.81	36.36	2.33 (8.8%)	9.88 (37.3%)	7.55 (26.2%)	35.67	889.97	294.51
3	31.61	36.53	41.49	4.92 (15.6%)	9.88 (31.3%)	4.96 (13.6%)	**2.92** **(NS)**	702.11	**2.96** **(NS)**
4	37.30	37.74	45.77	0.44 (1.2%)	8.47 (22.7%)	8.03 (21.3%)	**0.62** **(NS)**	219.91	294.53
5	42.21	41.43	49.44	–0.78 (–1.8%)	7.23 (17.1%)	8.01 (19.3%)	**2.49** **(NS)**	217.86	218.10
6	47.22	47.53	53.54	0.31 (0.7%)	6.32 (13.4%)	6.01 (12.6%)	**0.05** **(NS)**	148.80	18.79
7	53.44	51.90	57.46	–1.54 (–2.9%)	4.02 (7.5%)	5.56 (10.7%)	**2.26** **(NS)**	45.07	28.80
8	60.78	57.55	62.55	–3.23 (–5.3%)	1.77 (2.9%)	5.00 (8.7%)	10.14	6.96	22.58
9	71.80	65.12	69.50	–6.68 (–9.3%)	–2.30 (–3.2%)	4.38 (6.7%)	23.06	**3.33** **(NS)**	18.23
10	86.72	85.60	80.01	–1.12 (–1.3%)	–6.71 (–7.7%)	–5.59 (–6.5%)	**0.10** **(NS)**	19.01	**2.66** **(NS)**

Source: Authors' calculations from various rounds of the NSS.

a significant increase. In Urban India, the pattern was somewhat dissimilar: while fat intake rose by decile in 1994, 2005 and 2012, except for the 9th and 10th deciles which witnessed reductions in fat intake in 1994–2012, all other expenditure deciles recorded significant increases.

4.3. *Engel Curves*

As a supplement to disaggregated analysis of changes in calorie, protein and fat intake by expenditure decile, we examine below how their intakes vary by MPCE, based on Engel curves. These are shown in Figure 1.

4.3.1. *Calories*

The Engel curve for Rural India for 1994 lies above that for 2012, further confirming that at the same level of MPCE, calorie intake was lower in 2012. The gap also widened — especially at higher MPCE. At low MPCE the Engel curve for 1994 rises at a faster rate than the 2012 curve, but the former dips at a high MPCE and then rises steadily. In contrast, the 2012 curve at low MPCE rises slowly and dips at high MPCE and rises at a slow rate at higher MPCE. Between 2005 and 2012, except for low MPCE, at all other higher MPCE, the 2012 Engel curve lies below that for 2005.

In Urban India, except at low MPCE, the 2012 curve was above the corresponding curves for 1994 and 2005, it is lower at all higher MPCE. The gap between the 1994 and 2012 curves also widened at higher MPCE, with a steady but faster rise of the former relative to the latter.

4.3.2. *Protein*

The protein Engel curve for 2012 in Urban India lies consistently below that for 1994, as also below that for 2005, except at low MPCE. This is a striking illustration of reduction of protein intake between 1994 and 2012. The Urban India Engel curves for protein present a contrast. Except for lowest MPCE at which the 2012 curve lies above that for 2005 but below the 1994 curve, at higher MPCE the 2012 curve lies below those for 1994 and 2005.

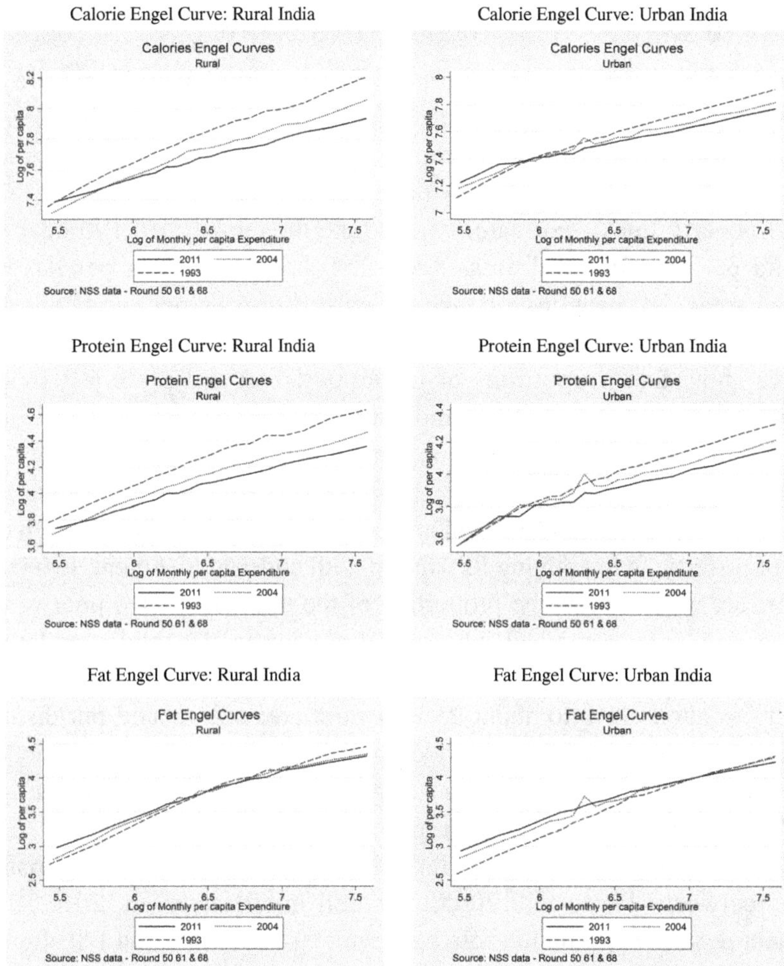

Figure 1. Engel curves.

4.3.3. *Fat*

The fat Engel curves are more revealing than the decile-wise analysis. The 2012 curve for Rural India lies above those for 1994 and 2005 over a large segment, but at higher MPCE it lies just below the 2005 curve and well below the 1994 curve. In Urban India, a large segment of the Engel curve for 2012 lay above both 1994 and 2005 curves, but at higher MPCE it overlapped with the 2005 curve and lay below the 1994 curve.

5. Changes in Nutritional Deprivation

If we take the nutritional norms as valid, the overall picture of nutritional deprivation worsened considerably over the period 1994–2012. Table 7 for Rural India shows the shares of calorie, protein and fat deficient populations, and by poverty status (using Tendulkar's state level poverty lines). For calories, we take the cut-off of 2100 kcal per capita per day for rural areas and 1,800 kcal per capita per day for urban areas. For proteins we take the cut-off of 60 g per capita per day and, for fats, we take the cut-off of 30 g per capita per day. The estimates show that proportions of undernourished and protein-deficient population rose between 1994 and 2005, but declined subsequently and the proportion of the fat-deficient population declined consistently during 1994–2012.

Using NSS data, and Tendulkar's poverty lines, there was a near halving of poverty. In examining its overlap with undernourishment, two indicators are used. One is the proportion of the undernourished poor or the number of undernourished who are also poor in the total population. Given the sharp decline in poverty, it is not surprising that this proportion fell from about 41% to about 25% in rural areas. A related but distinct indicator is the proportion of undernourished among the poor. This has risen over time and accounted for a larger majority of the poor (about 84% in 2012 *vis-à-vis* 75% in 1994 in rural areas).

In Urban India, as shown in Table 8, the proportion of undernourished rose between 1994 and 2005, but fell moderately in 2012. The protein-deficient population rose between 1994 and 2005, but fell slightly in 2012. The fat-deficient population fell consistently and was barely one third of that in 1994.

The proportion of undernourished poor reduced from 23% to 11% between 1994 and 2012 due to sharp reduction in the share of urban poor; but the proportion of poor who are undernourished rose from 64% in 1993 to 68% in 2011. The poor are thus more likely to be undernourished.

As shown in Table 9, the mean differences in proportion of undernourished differ significantly by caste, whether poor or not in both Rural and Urban India between 1994–2005, 2005–2012 and 1994–2012.

Table 7. Proportion of undernourished, protein and fat deficient Rural India.

	RURAL								
	1993–1994			2004–2005			2011–2012		
	Poor	**Non-poor**	**Total**	**Poor**	**Non-poor**	**Total**	**Poor**	**Non-poor**	**Total**
Undernourished	41.2%	11.5%	52.7%	40.8%	20.5%	61.3%	24.8%	30.0%	54.8%
Not undernourished	14.1%	33.2%	47.3%	7.7%	31.0%	38.7%	4.9%	40.4%	45.3%
Total	55.3%	44.7%	100%	48.5%	51.5%	100%	29.7%	70.3%	100%
Protein deficient	41.9%	15.7%	57.6%	41.4%	25.4%	66.9%	26.6%	38.3%	64.9%
Not protein deficient	13.4%	29.0%	42.4%	7.0%	26.1%	33.1%	3.1%	32.0%	35.1%
Total	55.3%	44.7%	100%	48.5%	51.5%	100%	29.7%	70.3%	100%
Fat deficient	44.5%	14.9%	59.4%	36.4%	13.4%	49.8%	17.8%	11.9%	29.7%
Not fat deficient	10.8%	29.9%	40.6%	12.1%	38.1%	50.2%	11.8%	58.4%	70.3%
Total	55.3%	44.7%	100%	48.5%	51.5%	100%	29.7%	70.3%	100%

Source: Authors' calculations from NSS data.

Table 8. Proportion of undernourished, protein and fat deficient urban India.

	URBAN								
	1993–1994			2004–2005			2011–2012		
	Poor	**Non-poor**	**Total**	**Poor**	**Non-poor**	**Total**	**Poor**	**Non-poor**	**Total**
Undernourished	23.2%	12.3%	35.5%	20.8%	17.3%	38.1%	10.9%	21.5%	32.4%
Not undernourished	12.9%	51.7%	64.5%	9.2%	52.7%	61.9%	5.0%	62.6%	67.6%
Total	36.0%	64.0%	100%	29.9%	70.1%	100%	16.0%	84.0%	100%
Protein deficient	30.9%	31.8%	62.7%	26.9%	41.8%	68.7%	14.9%	52.2%	67.1%
Not protein deficient	5.2%	32.2%	37.3%	3.0%	28.2%	31.3%	1.1%	31.8%	32.9%
Total	36.0%	64.0%	100%	29.9%	70.1%	100%	16.0%	84.0%	100%
Fat deficient	26.0%	9.6%	35.6%	18.3%	7.2%	25.4%	7.4%	5.2%	12.5%
Not fat deficient	10.1%	54.4%	64.4%	11.7%	62.9%	74.6%	8.6%	78.9%	87.5%
Total	36.0%	64.0%	100%	29.9%	70.1%	100%	16.0%	84.0%	100%

Source: Authors' calculations from various rounds of NSS.

Table 9. t-Tests of differences in mean proportion of undernourished.

	Mean value			Difference			t-Value		
	1993–1994	2004–2005	2011–2012	1994 & 2005	1994 & 2012	2005 & 2012	1994 & 2005	1994 & 2012	2005 & 2012
RURAL									
Total	0.46	0.53	0.47	–0.07	–0.01	0.06	–27.40	–2.81	23.42
SC	0.55	0.60	0.57	–0.05	–0.02	0.03	–8.12	–2.78	5.12
ST	0.54	0.61	0.49	–0.07	0.05	0.11	–11.09	7.10	17.56
Others	0.42	0.49	0.43	–0.08	–0.02	0.06	–24.26	–5.53	17.60
Poor	0.73	0.83	0.82	–0.10	–0.09	0.01	–29.96	–19.84	2.19
Non-poor	0.23	0.36	0.38	–0.13	–0.15	–0.02	–41.28	–46.78	–6.58
URBAN									
Total	0.27	0.34	0.26	–0.07	0.02	0.08	–21.48	5.80	26.68
SC	0.23	0.32	0.27	–0.09	–0.04	0.05	–8.08	–3.44	4.90
ST	0.38	0.43	0.31	–0.05	0.07	0.12	–5.63	7.49	13.46
Others	0.26	0.33	0.25	–0.06	0.02	0.08	–18.56	4.92	22.69
Poor	0.61	0.65	0.62	–0.04	–0.01	0.03	–6.86	–1.99	3.67
Non-poor	0.15	0.20	0.19	–0.05	–0.04	0.01	–17.06	–13.82	3.68

Aggregate proportion of undernourished in Rural India rose slightly but significantly during 1994–2012. While it rose slightly but significantly among the Scheduled Castes (SCs), it reduced significantly among the Scheduled Tribes (STs). Among Others, it rose slightly but significantly during this period. It rose sharply and significantly among the poor, as also among the non-poor.

Aggregate proportion of undernourished in Urban India fell slightly but significantly during 1994–2012. Among the SCs there was a significant increase while among the STs there was a significant decrease. Others recorded a slight but significant reduction. There was a slight but significant increase among the poor as well as the non-poor.

6. Costs of Calories

One of the key hypotheses here is whether individuals/households are switching to more expensive sources of calories driven by a taste for variety. We first look at cross-tabulations of costs of calories by MPCE deciles in Table 10. (Real) cost of calories rose across expenditure deciles in both Rural and Urban India in 1994, 2005 and 2012. For each decile the cost of calories rose over time, 1994–2005 and 1994–2012. Average cost of calories rose 3.5 times in Rural India and 3.6 times in Urban India between 1994–2012. Whether the mean decile-wise differences are statistically different is tested using the *t*-test (at the 1% level).

Using LOWESS — a non-parametric data smoothing technique — we further investigate the relationships between cost of calories and MPCE.[3] These are shown in Figure 2.

While costs of calories rose by expenditure decile in both Rural and Urban India in 1994, the rise was much steeper at high MPCE in the latter. The 2005 graphs show a much steeper rise at high MPCE in both Rural and Urban India — especially in the latter. The 2012 graphs are distinguishable from the 2005 graphs in two respects: (i) over a large range of MPCE — including the lowest — there was a steep rise in the costs of

[3]For an admirably clear exposition, see Deaton (1996).

Table 10. *t*-Tests of differences in costs of calories by expenditure decile.

Deciles of MPCE	Mean value			Difference			*t*-value		
	1993–1994	2004–2005	2011–2012	1994 & 2005	1994 & 2012	2005 & 2012	1994 & 2005	1994 & 2012	2005 & 2012
				RURAL					
1	2.39	3.79	6.82	−1.40	−4.43	−3.03	−14.55	−22.26	−25.60
2	2.39	4.10	7.52	−1.70	−5.12	−3.42	−34.42	−46.77	−46.81
3	2.55	4.30	8.29	−1.76	−5.75	−3.99	−35.90	−59.42	−56.07
4	2.64	4.52	8.52	−1.88	−5.88	−3.99	−50.18	−78.50	−66.98
5	2.71	4.75	9.03	−2.04	−6.32	−4.28	−62.22	−98.69	−82.51
6	2.86	4.91	9.49	−2.06	−6.63	−4.57	−67.82	−110.00	−93.24
7	3.00	5.26	10.12	−2.27	−7.13	−4.86	−59.46	−120.00	−97.15
8	3.16	5.59	10.66	−2.43	−7.50	−5.07	−78.05	−140.00	−120.00
9	3.39	6.01	11.60	−2.63	−8.21	−5.58	−88.86	−160.00	−130.00
10	3.97	7.22	13.98	−3.25	−10.01	−6.76	−96.96	−160.00	−130.00

(Continued)

Table 10. (*Continued*)

	Mean value			Difference			*t*-value		
Deciles of MPCE	**1993–1994**	**2004–2005**	**2011–2012**	**1994 & 2005**	**1994 & 2012**	**2005 & 2012**	**1994 & 2005**	**1994 & 2012**	**2005 & 2012**
				URBAN					
1	2.78	4.55	8.35	−1.77	−5.56	−3.80	−44.95	−73.56	−54.10
2	3.03	5.08	9.64	−2.05	−6.61	−4.56	−59.63	−99.92	−75.26
3	3.27	5.55	10.63	−2.28	−7.36	−5.08	−60.67	−120.00	−77.01
4	3.50	6.02	11.41	−2.52	−7.92	−5.39	−41.37	−130.00	−64.13
5	3.74	6.26	12.12	−2.52	−8.38	−5.86	−61.75	−130.00	−80.72
6	3.95	6.79	12.98	−2.84	−9.03	−6.18	−59.02	−130.00	−74.78
7	4.24	7.14	13.92	−2.90	−9.68	−6.78	−71.37	−140.00	−88.67
8	4.59	7.65	14.91	−3.06	−10.32	−7.25	−69.44	−130.00	−94.37
9	5.09	8.38	16.32	−3.30	−11.23	−7.94	−72.15	−130.00	−97.64
10	5.91	9.93	19.04	−4.02	−13.13	−9.11	−62.80	−110.00	−81.50

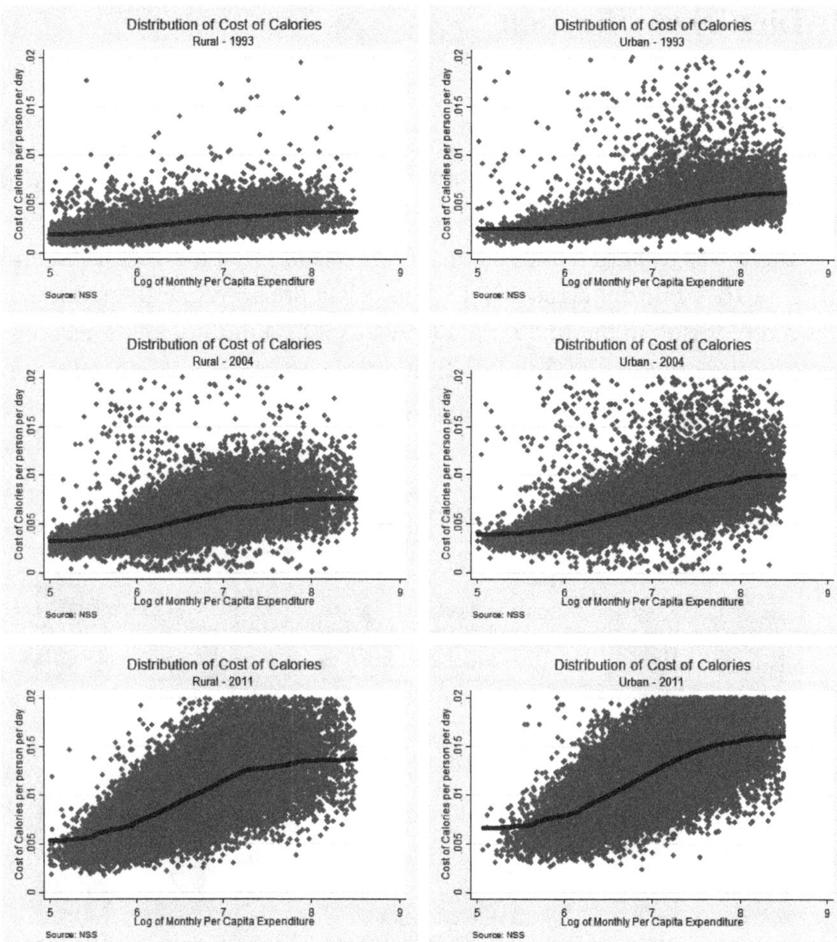

Figure 2. LOWESS of cost of calories on MPCE.

calories with a further rise which nearly flattened in the highest range of MPCE in Rural India; and (ii) in Urban India, the slope was steeper with a smaller flat segment at the highest range of MPCE.

In brief, the LOWESS graphs further corroborate that the costs of calories rise with higher MPCE, with rates varying between Rural and Urban India, and over time.

7. Diet Diversification

7.1. *Changes in Diets*

Let us first consider changes in consumption of various food items in rural and urban areas between 1993–1994 and 2011–2012, as shown in Figure 3.

There was a sharp reduction in cereal consumption between 1994 and 2012 — 16% in rural areas and 13% in urban areas. While the reduction was more drastic in the first period (1994 to 2005) in rural areas, as compared to the second (2005 to 2012), in urban areas, the rate of reduction was almost equal in both the periods.

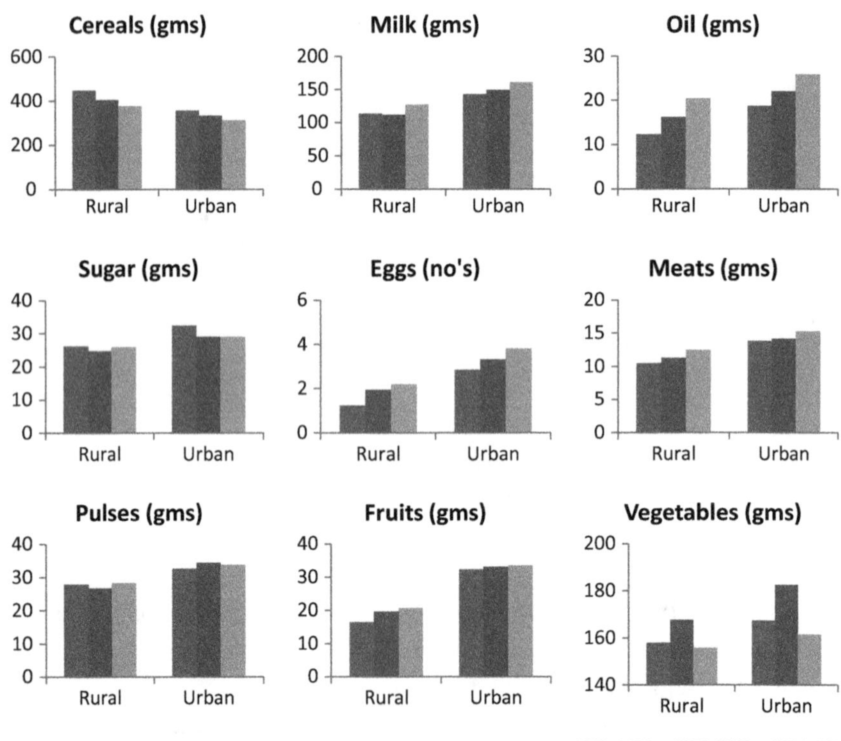

Figure 3. Changes in diets in India (1994–2012) — daily per capita consumption.

Source: Authors' calculations from various rounds of the NSS.

In rural areas, pulses/nuts/dry fruits recorded a sharp drop between 1994 and 2005, but their intake increased substantially in the second period. The consumption of sugar decreased too, in both the sectors in the first period, followed by a slight increase. By contrast, intakes of vanaspati-oil rose sharply in both rural and urban areas, especially in the first period. The consumption of milk and milk products increased, and, more substantially, for urban areas (by about 12% between 1994 and 2012), especially in the second period. Intakes of meat/fish/poultry increased significantly in rural areas (by 19%) and in urban areas (by 10%) between 1994 and 2012. Vegetable intakes increased moderately in the first period in both rural and urban areas, but declined by a greater amount in the second, leaving a net decline between 1994 and 2012. Fruit consumption increased. There are marked differences in the intakes of various food commodities among various income classes, too (Kaicker *et al.*, 2016).

These dietary shifts are linked to intakes of calories, proteins and fats with varying importance, as shown in Kaicker *et al.* (2016).[4]

7.2. *Disaggregation by MPCE Deciles*

To capture diversification in diets, i.e. a move from a cereal dominated diet to more variety in food consumption basket, we use a Food Diversity Index (FDI). The FDI is calculated as the sum of squares of the shares of the various food items in the food consumption basket. Algebraically,

$$FDI_{it} = \sum_{j=1}^{5} S_{jit}^2 \tag{1}$$

where FDI_{it} is the food diversity index for household i at time t, S_{jit} is the share of commodity j in the food consumption basket of ith household in time t. This is similar to the Herfindahl index used to measure the competitiveness of an industry. High value of the index implies a monopolistic market (or, in our case, a more concentrated food basket) and low value implies a nearly perfect competitive market (in our case, a more diverse food basket). We use five food groups to construct the FDI: (i) cereals and

[4] See Annex 1 for a graphical illustration of changes in sources of calories, protein and fat.

pulses; (ii) milk, milk products, eggs, and meats; (iii) oil; (iv) sugar; and (v) fruits and vegetables. Figure 4 shows the variation in FDI by expenditure decile for rural and urban areas in 1994, 2005 and 2012.

FDI for Rural India fell consistently across expenditure deciles in 1994, 2005 and 2012, except the 9th decile which saw a rise. The 1994 curve was above that for 2005, and the latter was above that for 2012. There are two implications: (i) diet diversification was greater at successively higher expenditure deciles; and (ii) diet diversification rose between 1994–2005 and between 2005–2012 (except for the 9th and 10th deciles) but with a narrowing of the gap between 2005–2012. This implies slowing of diet diversification during 2005–2012 (between the 6th and 9th deciles).

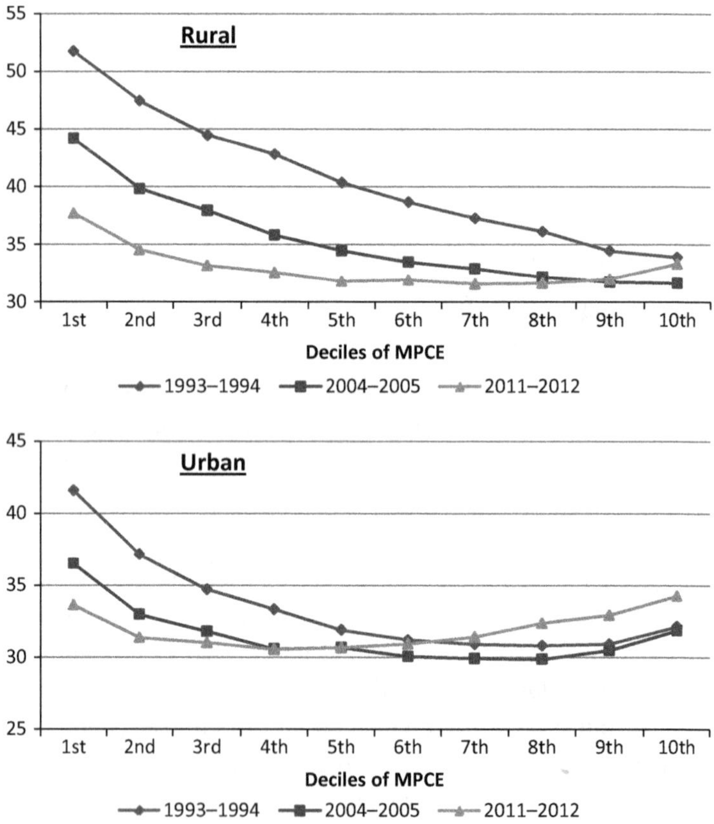

Figure 4. Herfindahl index for rural and urban India.

Source: Authors' calculations based on various rounds of the NSS.

The FDI graphs for Urban India differ markedly. FDI curves for 1994 and 2005 fell with expenditure deciles and the latter lay below the former. So the implications are: (i) diet diversity was greater at successively higher MPCE; and (ii) diet diversification was greater in 2005 than in 1994. (ii) The 2012 curve lay below the 2005 curve and crosses over at the 4th decile, and also crosses over the 1994 curve between the 6th and 7th deciles, pointing to a reduction in diet diversity above these expenditure deciles.

Often diet diversity is taken to be synonymous with diet quality. In a recent contribution (Rashid *et al.*, 2011), for example, one of the two measures of diet quality is diet diversity. The latter is defined as the number of different foods or food groups consumed over a given reference period. It is rationalized that increasing the variety of foods across and within groups ensures adequate intake of essential nutrients that promote good health. In fact, it is pointed out that there is a strong positive association between diet diversity and nutrient adequacy (Ruel, 2002). But another study (SOFI, 2012) takes a broader view that dietary changes in the past two decades have had both positive and negative impacts on nutrition. On the positive side, the quality of diets at the aggregate global level has improved, and nutritional outcomes have improved in most parts of the world. On the negative side, diets increasingly contain more energy-dense, semi-processed foods, saturated fats and sugars. These dietary shifts/changes are associated with an increase in overnutrition and obesity. The latter are causally linked to higher prevalence rates of non-communicable diseases (NCDs) such as diabetes, cardiovascular disease and cancer (Gaiha *et al.*, 2014, 2015). So whether the nutritional implications are positive or negative is essentially an empirical issue.

8. Econometric Methodology

An IV regression model with fixed effects is estimated as specified below:

$$CC_{it} = \alpha_0 + \alpha_1 FDI_{kt} + \boldsymbol{P}_{jkt}\boldsymbol{\beta} + X_{it}\gamma + u_i + \varepsilon_{it} \tag{2}$$

$$CL_{it} = c_0 + c_1 \widehat{CC}_{it} + \boldsymbol{X}_{it}\boldsymbol{\theta} + \pi_i + \boldsymbol{e}_{it}. \tag{3}$$

In the first stage regression (or the reduced form), the dependent variable is the cost of calories for the ith household in year t, FDI denotes the food diversity index constructed at the PSU level for the kth PSU, P denotes a vector of food prices (j^{th} food commodity price relative to cereal price at the kth PSU level), X household characteristics that very over time (such as household size, number of male adults with education above middle level, adult females with education above middle level, MPCE, and u denoting a state dummy, and the error term, ε. In the second stage (structural equation), the dependent variable is calorie intake per capita in ith household and year t, and the explanatory variables include the predicted cost of calories from the first equation and all household characteristics, excluding the relative food prices and FDI (at the PSU level) as instruments in the first equation. The identification strategy relies on the direct effect of relative food prices and diet diversity on the cost of calories which in turn impacts calorie intake.[5] Two features are noteworthy: (i) to circumvent the endogeneity of relative food prices and diet diversification at the household level, these variables are constructed at the PSU level; and (ii) in order to capture the unobserved heterogeneity (say, cultural diversity leading to diet diversity), we have used states as fixed effects.[6]

9. Results

The results are given in Table 11. Let us first consider the reduced form results.

Since FDI and diet diversification are inversely related, the negative coefficient of FDI implies that less diversified diets are associated with lower costs of calories. Or, in other words, households more dependent on, say, cereals have a weaker taste for variety, and tend to rely on cheaper sources of calories. The effect of MPCE is significantly positive, but the magnitude is negligible. All (relative) food prices (relative to price of

[5]An important insight from Subramanian and Deaton (1996) is that when food prices change there are more significant shifts between different grades of food commodities (e.g. different grades of rice) than between food commodities. We are grateful to K. Imai for raising this concern.

[6]For an exposition of merits of fixed effects in panel data at the state level, see Wooldridge (2013).

Table 11. Fixed effect IV regression results.

	First stage dep variable: Cost of calories			**Second stage dep variable: Log calorie intake**		
Number of observations			**315874**			
	F **(48, 315825) = 3271.47**			F **(40, 315825) = 761.36**		
	Adj R – Squared = 0.332					
	Coef.	***t*-Values**	$P > t$	**Coef.**	z	$P > z$
Cost of calories				−23.37	−25.10	0.000
Diet diversification	−2.13	−16.98	0.000			
Price ratios	0.00	2.69	0.010			
Price ratio (Milk to Cereal)	−1.13	−153.21	0.000			
Price ratio (Oil to Cereal)	−0.25	−11.42	0.000			
Price ratio (Sugar to Cereal)	0.02	15.14	0.000			
Price ratio (Eggs to Cereal)	0.11	46.91	0.000			
Price ratio (Meat to Cereal)	0.70	135.38	0.000			
Price ratio (Pulses to Cereal)	0.25	35.93	0.000			
Price ratio (Fruits to Cereal)	2.17	76.82	0.000			

(*Continued*)

Table 11. (*Continued*)

	First stage dep variable: Cost of calories			**Second stage dep variable: Log calorie intake**		
Number of observations			**315874**			
	F (48, 315825) = 3271.47			**F (40, 315825) = 761.36**		
	Adj R – Squared = 0.332					
	Coef.	***t*-Values**	$P > t$	**Coef.**	z	$P > z$
Price ratio (Vegetables to Cereal)	0.00	2.69	0.000			
Household size	–0.29	–81.14	0.000	–102.96	–106.92	0.000
Number of male adults with education above middle level	0.33	35.33	0.000	123.33	50.51	0.000
Number of female adults with education above middle level	0.52	44.90	0.000	44.93	14.72	0.000
MPCE	0.00	87.81	0.000	0.15	98.91	0.000
Sector (0 = rural, 1 = Urban)	0.86	48.20	0.000	–134.26	–30.74	0.000
Constant	9.00	107.86	0.000	2944.16	188.92	0.000
Test of excluded instruments	F (9, 315825) = 8261.09					
Sargan statistic	518.738; Chi–2 (P value) = 0.000					

cereals) have significant effects, with two negative (milk to cereals and oil to cereals) and the rest positive. Household characteristics matter too. The larger the household, the lower is the cost of calories presumably because of economies of scale in buying food.

The larger the numbers of adult males and females, the higher the costs. Location also makes a difference. The costs of calories were higher in urban areas (Urban India) relative to rural areas (Rural India). The joint significance of multiple instruments (diet diversification, and relative food prices, both at PSU level) is confirmed by the F-test at the 1% level. So the relevance of these instruments is validated. As there are multiple instruments, we test for the over-identifying restrictions using the Sargan test. The Chi-square statistics reject the null that all IVs are uncorrelated with the error term. This implies that some of the IVs are not exogenous and therefore the results must be interpreted with caution.

In the structural equation, the dependent variable is log of per capita calorie intake. For expositional convenience, we will refer to it as calorie intake since the two are monotonically related. The higher the MPCE, the larger the calorie intake. The effect is significant and large. The higher the cost of calories, the lower the calorie intake. This effect is also significant and large. The larger the household size, the lower the calorie intake. It is puzzling that lower cost of calories among larger households doesn't translate into higher calorie intake. Whether there is greater food wastage in such households needs investigation. That more educated adult males and females are better aware of healthier diets is consistent with significant positive coefficients of these two variables. Also, it is confirmed that urban areas are more likely to consume tastier, better flavoured and packaged food, fried meats and vegetables which are low in calorific content.

In brief, the results validate the central hypothesis that diet diversification and affluence are significantly linked to higher costs of calories — especially the former — and these in turn lower calorie intake.

10. Discussion

An influential study by Deaton and Dreze (2009) shows that, despite rising incomes in India, there has been a sustained decline in per capita calorie intake over the period 1983–2004, primarily due to lower calorie "requirements". The reduction in calorie requirements is attributed mainly to better health environment and less strenuous activity levels. Departing from this focus but encompassing it in an alternative demand theory-based explanation of dietary changes, Gaiha *et al.* (2014) analyzed first the factors associated with dietary diversification; and (ii) in the second stage, the effect of dietary diversification on calorie intake. Dietary diversification is associated with food prices, income/expenditure, household characteristics — especially whether it belongs to a middle class — and its location, and time-related changes transmitted through prices and expenditure, and residually through lifestyle, activity patterns and epidemiology of disease environment. The more important result, however, is the lowering of calorie intake as a result of dietary diversification, controlling for the effects of food prices, expenditure, household characteristics (other than middle class affiliation), urban location, and time-related changes. The latter add an important dimension to food and health policies.

In a classic (Behrman and Deolalikar, 1989), the authors offer a quantifiable explanation of the phenomenon that calorie elasticities are substantially less than food expenditure elasticities: specifically, food variety *per se* is valued so that people purchase increased food variety as their incomes increase even though that may not alter their calorie intakes much. In an extension, Jha *et al.* (2009), based on an analysis of a decline in calorie intake between the 1993 and 1999 NSS rounds in India, corroborate that two sets of relationships are key to this result: one is the relative price effect, depending on the curvature of the food indifference curves for the poor and non-poor, and the second is the location of the indifference curves. The decline in calorie intake is thus a consequence of taste for variety associated with increasing curvature of food indifference curves and their increasing centrality. However, the curvature is higher among the non-poor but not substantially *vis-à-vis* the poor, although locational differences are pronounced for some food items.

In the present study, the first of its kind in so far as it relies on three recent rounds of NSS for 1993–1994, 2004–2005 and 2011–2012 with detailed cost of calorie estimates, we build on these previous studies.[7] Our central question is: have more diversified diets resulted in greater

[7]In an earlier study, Kaicker *et al.* (2016) examine the role of dietary diversification in lowering the calorie intake over the period 1994–2012 but without taking into account the role of rising costs of calories.

consumption of expensive calories and consequently in reduction of calorie intake?

The main findings are that diet diversification is associated with higher costs of calories mainly because of reliance on more expensive calories (e.g. through reduced dependence on calories, which are the cheapest sources of calories), determined by a taste for variety in both rural and urban areas and across expenditure deciles over the period 1994–2012. Our analysis also corroborates that higher costs of calories and greater affluence are associated with reduction in calorie intake. These findings have considerable significance from a policy perspective.

Drawing upon an earlier analysis (Gaiha *et al.*, 2015), based on *India Human Development Survey* for 2005, eating out is pervasive going by the fact that about 30% of the households did so. Eating out is a feature not just of the metros or urban areas but also of urban slums and rural areas, though it is less pervasive in the last two areas. In the six largest metros (Mumbai, Delhi, Kolkata, Chennai, Bangalore, and Hyderabad), about 34% of the households ate out, as compared to about 27% elsewhere. Eating out was thus more pervasive among the metro residents, who also spent larger amounts.

About 25% of the Scheduled Castes (SCs), about 27% of the Scheduled Tribes (STs), and about 31% of the Other Backward Castes (OBCs), and Others ate out. Even some of the most deprived and socially excluded groups — especially the SCs and STs — have switched from traditional staples to fast foods and opted for greater variety in food consumption. This is further corroborated when the sample is split into the poor and non-poor households using the official poverty line. While a much larger proportion of the non-poor households (about 32%) ate out, those among the poor (about 12.5%) were far from negligible. A more disaggregated classification of the households into four MPCE classes (less than Rs 300, between Rs 300–500, between Rs 500 and 1,000, and greater than Rs 1,000) further *dispels* any doubts that eating out as a manifestation of dietary transition is mostly *a middle-class phenomenon.*[8] Our (preliminary analysis with more recent IHDS data) for 2011–2012 not only confirms a rapid growth in eating out but also larger (real) expenditures.

[8]These expenditure estimates are based on 2004–2005 prices.

The health implications of the changes in dietary patterns are not clear cut. There is a trade-off — while a nutritionally balanced diet is associated with better health, processed and fried foods are responsible for higher prevalence of non-communicable diseases (NCDs) such as heart disease, cancer and diabetes. Since there are signs of an epidemiological transition in India — higher mortality from these diseases compensating for decline in mortality from infectious diseases — enhancing awareness of healthy diets is important from a policy perspective (Gaiha *et al.*, 2014, 2015). As consumer preferences for flavour, packaging and variety evolve in complex ways in the context of rapidly integrating food markets, a careful scrutiny of policy interventions (e.g. labelling of food quality, consumer awareness campaigns through the media and other channels) may help understand better how to influence food choices.

11. Concluding Observations

While concerns for poverty and hunger must dominate the policy agenda, the options for dealing with obesity and the upsurge in non-communicable diseases can only be neglected at the peril of millions of lives that may suffer their worst consequences. Although shifts in diet and physical activities are desirable in many ways — arguably varied and pleasurable — it will be a mistake to overlook the onerous nutritional and health effects and the tragic but avoidable loss of well-being.

A challenge is to raise awareness of the health implications of the dietary transition *despite* its slowing down in more recent years. As growing affluence, lifestyle changes and urbanization are *irreversible*, the focus must shift to provision of public goods (e.g. rural infrastructure) to facilitate participation of smallholders in high-value chains, regulation of food safety standards, nutrition labelling, food and nutrition supplementation, stringent restrictions on tobacco and alcohol consumption, nutritional education — especially of women — and active involvement of the private sector in adhering to regulatory standards and nutritional norms. The latter is largely a question of designing appropriate incentives for the private sector to collaborate better with the public sector. Whether these regulatory measures and norms alone will suffice is unclear as food preferences are shaped in complex ways by some irreversible changes taking place.

Acknowledgement

We greatly appreciate Raj Bhatia's expert advice in data preparation, and Radhika Agarwal's valuable research assistance. We are indebted to K.L. Krishna, Katsushi Imai and Anil Deolalikar for insightful suggestions on the econometric analysis; and the editor, Raghbendra Jha, for his gracious invitation to contribute this chapter and his meticulous advice on sharpening the focus. Any errors are, however, the sole responsibility of the authors.

Annex 1

Food composition changes are associated with the decline in nutrient intakes. Figures A.1–A.3 show the distribution of calories, protein and fat intake by food commodities for rural and urban areas between 1994 and 2012.

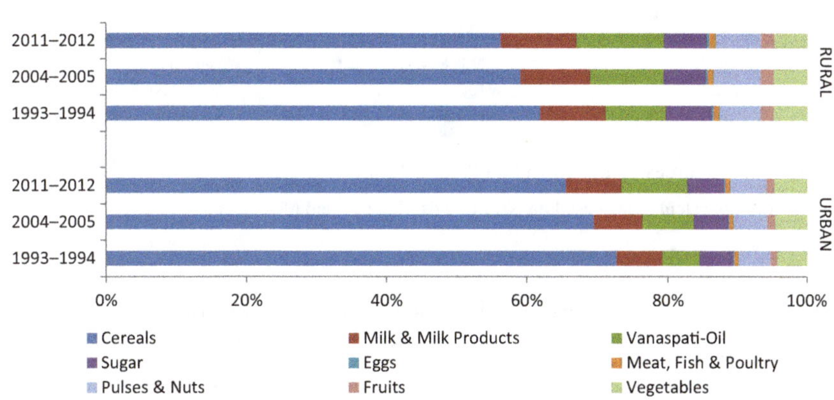

Figure A.1. Source of calories in India (1993–2012).

Source: Authors' calculations based on NSS rounds 50th, 61st and 68th.

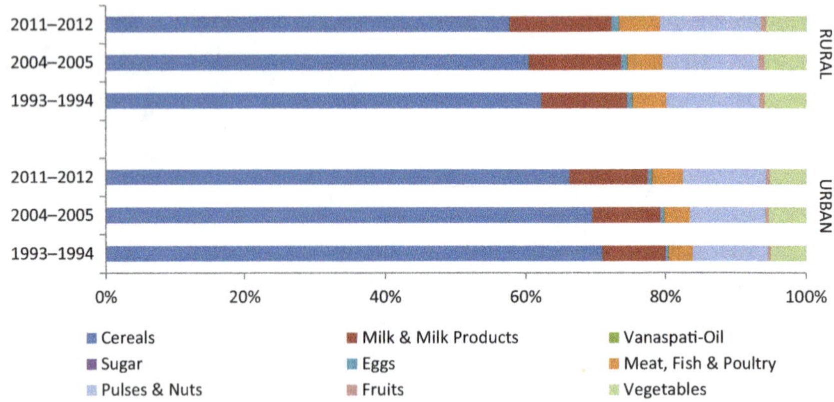

Figure A.2. Sources of protein in India (1993–2012).

Source: Authors' Calculations based on NSS Rounds 50th, 61st and 68th.

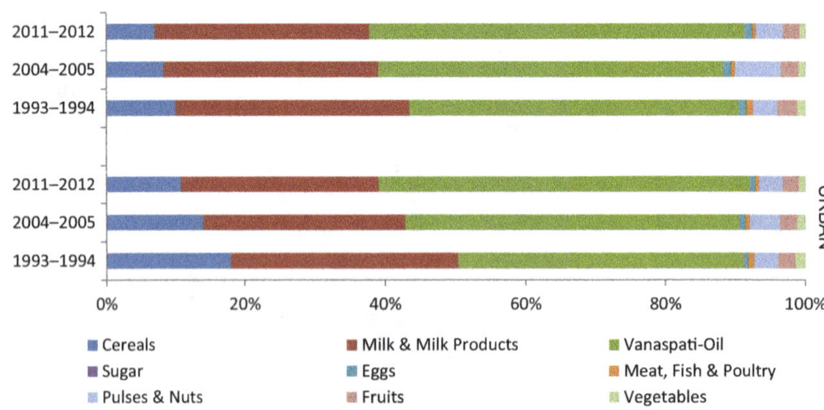

Figure A.3. Sources of fats in India (1993–2012).

Source: Authors calculations based on NSS rounds 50th, 61st and 68th.

In Rural India, as discussed earlier, calorie intakes declined between 1994 and 2012. Most of it is attributable to the decline in calories from cereals. Calories from cereals reduced from 1530 in 1993 to 1383 in 2004 and 1282 in 2011. The contribution of milk/milk products, sugar, pulses, fruits and vegetables remained largely unchanged between 1993 and 2011. The contribution of vanaspati-oil to the calorie intake increased substantially. Calories obtained from oil increased from 111 in 1994 to 145 in 2004 and 184 in 2012. Similar results are found for Urban India as well.

In both Rural and Urban India, protein intake declined between 1994 and 2005, and slightly increased thereafter. Much of the initial decline is reflected in a reduction in protein intake from cereals and slightly from pulses. In Rural India, the protein intake from cereals decreased from 42 gms in 1994 to 38 gms in 2005 and 35 gms in 2012. The corresponding numbers for Urban India are 34 gms (1994), 32 gms (2005) and 30 gms (2012). Intake from dairy products. (milk, eggs and meats) increased moderately. Proteins from other sources are a very small fraction and largely remained unchanged between 1994 and 2012.

Between 1994 and 2012 fat intake rose in both rural and urban areas. Vanaspati-oil has the maximum share in total fat intakes, and its contribution rose over the period 1993 and 2011. In Rural India, fat intake from vanaspati-oil rose from 12 gms in 1994 to 16 gms in 2005 and 20 gms in 2012. In Urban India, the share of vanaspati-oil rose from 19 gms in 1994 to 22 gms in 2005 and 26 gms in 2012. The other significant contributor to fat intake are cereals, pulses and milk products (including ghee and butter), but their contribution reduced between 1993 and 2011. Declining intake of fats from these commodities were more than offset by the increased intake of fat from vanaspati-oil (Kaicker *et al.*, 2016).

References

Banerjee, A. and E. Duflo (2011) *Poor Economics: A Radical Rethinking of the Way to Fight Global Poverty*. New York: Public Affairs.

Basole, A. and D. Basu (2015) "Fuelling Calorie Intake Decline: Household-level Evidence from Rural India", *World Development*, pp. 82–95.

Behrman, J. and A. Deolalikar (1987) "Will Developing Country Nutrition Improve with Income: A Case Study for Rural South India", *Journal of Political Economy*, Vol. 95, pp. 108–138.

Behrman, J. and A. Deolalikar (1989) "Is Variety the Spice of Life? Implications for Calorie Intake", *The Review of Economics and Statistics*, Vol. 71, No. 4, pp. 666–672.

Deaton, A. (1996) *The Analysis of Household Surveys: A Microeconometric Approach in Development Policy*. Baltimore: Johns Hopkins University Press.

Deaton, A., and J. Dreze (2009) "Food and Nutrition in India: Facts and Interpretations", *Economic and Political Weekly*, Vol. XLIV, No. 7, pp. 42–65.

FAO (Food and Agriculture Organisation) (2012) *The State of Food Insecurity in the World* (SOFI, 2012), Rome: Food and Agriculture Organisation.

Gaiha, R., Jha, R. and V. S. Kulkarni (2014) *Diets, Malnutrition and Disease, The Indian Experience*. New Delhi: Oxford University Press.

Gaiha, R., Jha, R., Kulkarni, V. S. and N. Kaicker (2015) "Diets, Nutrition and Poverty in India", in *Handbook on Food, Politics and Society*, ed. R. Herring. New York: Oxford University Press.

Gopalan, C., Sastri, B. and S. Balasubramanian (1971) *Nutrition Values of Indian Foods*. Hyderabad: Institute for Nutrition, Indian Council of Medical Research.

Indian Council of Medical Research (ICMR) (1990) *Nutrition Requirements and Recommended Dietary Allowances for Indians*. New Delhi: ICMR.

Jha, R., Gaiha, R. and A. Sharma (2009) "Modelling Variety in Consumption Expenditure on Food in India", *International Review of Applied Economics*, Vol. 23, No. 4.

Kaicker, N., Kulkarni, V. S. and R. Gaiha (2016) "Demand for Nutrients in India: An Analysis based on the 50th, 61st and 68th Rounds of the NSS", Second International Conference on South Asian Economic Development, South Asian University, New Delhi.

Knudsen, O. and P. Scandizzo (1979) "Nutrition and Food Needs in Developing Countries", SWP328, Washington DC: World Bank.

Rashid, D. A., Smith, L. C. and T. Rahman (2011) "Determinants of Dietary Quality: Evidence from Bangladesh", *World Development*, Vol. 39, No. 12, pp. 2221–2231.

Ruel, M. (2002) *Is Dietary Diversity an Indicator of Food Security or Dietary Quality? Do the Determinants of Diet Quantity and Quality Differ?* Washington, DC: International Food Policy Research Institute, mimeo.

Sen, A. (2005) "Description as Choice", *Oxford Economic Papers*, Vol. 32, No. 3, pp. 353–369.

Srinivasan, T. N. (1992) "Undernutrition: Concepts, Measurements and Policy Implications", in *Nutrition and Poverty*, ed. S. R. Osmani. Oxford: Clarendon Press.

Subramanian, S. and A. Deaton (1996) "The Demand for Food and Calories", *Journal of Political Economy,* Vol. 104, pp. 133–162.

Wooldridge, J. M. (2013) *Introductory Econometrics*, 5th edn. Mason, OH: Thomson South Western.

Chapter 8

Agriculture and Female Malnutrition in India

Priya Rampal*,‡ and Ranjula Bali Swain†

**Leveraging Agriculture for Nutrition in South Asia (LANSA), M. S. Swaminathan Research Foundation, Chennai, India*
†Misum, Stockholm School of Economics and Department of Economics, Södertörn University, Stockholm, Sweden
‡priyarampal@mssrf.res.in

Abstract

It is widely recognized that combating malnutrition for women is central not only for their own health but also for the attainment of nutritional adequacy for future generations, including infants, children and adolescents. Attaining adequate nutrition for women is necessary throughout their life, but particularly so before, during and after pregnancy, if intergenerational nutritional adequacy is to be attained. Adequacy of nutrition also helps an individual become more productive and saves medical treatment costs that may otherwise have occurred. However, India's less than satisfactory record of female, infant and child nutrition underscores the need to take urgent steps, particularly if the Sustainable Development Goals (SDGs) are to be attained. With this as the background the present chapter focuses on the role of agriculture in providing adequate nutrition for women and the methods through which women in the rural sector can leverage existing institutions and programs to ameliorate nutritional inadequacy. This would require the design of informative indices of nutritional attainment and close cooperation in policy between governments, civil society organizations and international advisory groups. The chapter reviews some ways in which these can be attained.

Keywords: Maternal nutrition, individual productivity, infant survival, women's role in agriculture, drinking water, health and sanitation facilities, India.

1. Introduction

The United Nations Secretary General Ban Ki-moon launched the Zero Hunger Challenge in 2012 which has been absorbed in the Sustainable Development Goals (SDG) agenda to be achieved by 2030. The SDGs, which aim at transforming the world through sustainable development, are a set of 17 "Global Goals". These include ending poverty and hunger (SDGs 1 and 2), improving health, nutrition and education (SDGs 3 and 4), making cities more sustainable, combating climate change, and protecting oceans and forests (SDGs 11, 13 and 14). The focus of the fifth SDG is gender equality. Since women comprise approximately half the global population, it is important that they are integrated in all the SDGs, especially the first four goals which focus on reducing poverty and hunger, promoting good health and well-being, and providing quality education (United Nations, 2017).

Women are not just primary caregivers, they also contribute to national income in their capacity to earn. Women are the backbone of rural economies. According to the FAO, more than 70% of the economically active women work in agriculture in the least developed countries (Mucavele, 2017). Women play an important role in almost all stages of food production. In the rural areas, the food consumed is mostly grown by women. However, this does not cover other basic needs, such as health care, paying for the education of their children or other daily expenses since they have limited financial resources due to an inefficient supply chain and poor savings. Their contribution could be much greater if they had equal access to essential resources and services, such as land, credit and training (FAO, 2003). Further, malnutrition poses many problems for women. It weakens their ability to survive childbirth, makes them more susceptible to disease and infections, and lowers immunity (Ransom and Elder, 2003).

In the life cycle of an individual, the first 1,000 days from the time of conception are recognized as the Window of Opportunity. The first 270 days are *in utero,* i.e. directly related to a mother's health and nutrition. The nutritional status inside this window of opportunity is a strong determinant of later nutritional outcomes (Rampal, 2013). Malnutrition in early childhood, especially in the first thousand days impedes motor, sensory, cognitive, social and emotional development of children undermining educational outcomes and future income (Gragnolati *et al.*, 2005; Smith and Haddad, 2000; UNICEF, 2011). Malnourished children are at a higher risk of disease and are more likely to grow into malnourished adults (Horton, 1999; Alderman *et al.*, 2006). Several studies point out that investing in child nutrition and health leads to gains in the future (Strauss and Thomas, 1998; Alderman *et al.*, 2006; FOCUS, 2006; Behrman, 2009). These gains are of three kinds: First, productivity gains which work directly by enhancing the physical capacity to perform tasks and indirectly by increasing school enrollment, attendance and cognitive scores (Thomas and Strauss, 1997; Behrman *et al.*, 2004; Case and Paxson, 2008). The second is through saving of costs that otherwise could be spent on caring for unhealthy children (Almond *et al.*, 2005). Third, there may be intergenerational benefits through which subsequent generations become more productive (Ramakrishnan *et al.*, 1999; Hoddinott *et al.*, 2011).[1]

It is important to give adequate attention to women's health and nutrition from the early childhood itself to break the intergenerational aspect of malnutrition. This chapter aims to shed light on this strong link between maternal and child nutrition. Further, it showcases the important role that women play in agrarian economies. Greater involvement and empowerment of women can potentially lead to better nutrition for women and their children. In the following section, we discuss the intergenerational aspect of malnutrition in detail. Section 3 focuses on the current nutritional situation of women and children in India, and on how it links to

[1] For details, refer to FOCUS (2006).

child nutrition. Section 4 discusses the role of women in agriculture and the ways in which agriculture can lead to better nutritional status. Section 5 discusses important national policies and priorities for women in India, including microfinance, while Section 6 concludes.

2. Intergenerational Aspect of Malnutrition

As discussed in the previous section, combating malnutrition for women can lead to better nutrition for future generations. These are referred to as intergenerational benefits (Ramakrishnan *et al.*, 1999; Hoddinott *et al.*, 2011). Poor nutrition starts *in utero* and extends, particularly for females, till adulthood (United Nations ACC/SCN, 2000). Inadequate food, health and care and a lack of WASH (Water, Sanitation and Hygiene), leads to the growth of more malnourished adults (UNICEF, 1990). Undernutrition that occurs during childhood, adolescence and pregnancy for women has an adverse impact on the birthweight of infants. When undernourished women are pregnant, they are unable to provide the right environment for the foetus in the first 270 days of the window of opportunity when children are completely dependent on their mothers to get essential energy, protein, fats and micronutrients (Martorell, 1999). These infants might be born with a Low Birthweight (LBW) and also suffer from Intrauterine Growth Retardation (IUGR). If these infants survive, it is quite probable that they suffer from undernutrition. Low birthweight is associated with higher probability of the child being stunted or underweight especially in the first 1,000 days (ACC/SCN, 2000). Such children are more likely to face poor cognition, low nutritional outcomes, lower immunity and a higher risk of disease and infections throughout their lives (Gragnolati *et al.*, 2005; Smith and Haddad, 2000).

Breastfeeding is an important intervention in reducing child mortality (UNICEF, 2011). Improvement of complementary feeding has been shown to be most effective to improve child growth, and together with maternal nutrition interventions help improve child nutritional status (WHO, 2003). Breast milk is the perfect food for babies as it has nutrients and antibodies that are essential for a baby (WHO, 2003; UNICEF, 2011). The incidence of diarrhoea and respiratory diseases is very high in developing countries. A mother's knowledge of taking care of the child during illness and otherwise is of paramount importance. First 6 months of exclusive breastfeeding have a significant effect in the reduction of mortality from diarrhoea and pneumonia, as well as other factors (Black *et al.*, 2008; Richard *et al.*, 2012). Only a healthy woman can produce the right amount and quality of breast milk. Optimal complementary feeding practices from 6 and 24 months of age in addition to breast milk are needed for children to reach their true growth potential and prolonged protection from diarrhoea and pneumonia (WHO, 2013). Hygienic and nutrient rich complementary foods are often prepared by the mothers to meet their children's nutritional needs. Timely consumption of these by the children is important to prevent them from getting dehydrated and losing weight when they are sick.[2]

Adolescence is now recognized as a second window of opportunity for compensating for early childhood growth failure due to rapid growth in this time (Proos and Gustafsson, 2012). However, the effects of early childhood undernutrition on future outcomes such as cognitive development and earnings may not be fully redressed (Case and Paxson, 2008). It is important to prevent foetal and early childhood undernutrition. Investing in maternal and childhood nutrition has the potential benefits of increased adult productivity and reduced health costs throughout the life cycle (Almond *et al.*, 2005).

3. Child and Maternal Malnutrition in India

Levels of child and maternal malnutrition are extremely high in India. Table 1 shows the important health and nutrition indicators for women and children over the four rounds collected by the National Family and Health Survey (NFHS) in 1992–1993, 1998–1999, 2005–2006 and 2015–2016. The NFHS is a large-scale, multi-round survey conducted in a representative sample of households throughout India. According to the NFHS-4, in 2015–2016, almost 40% of India's children under the age of five were stunted. Stunting or low height-for-age is a long-term measure of undernutrition. Wasting, i.e. low weight-for-height indicates the prevalence of acute malnutrition. In 2015–2016, 21% of the children under the age of five were wasting while in 2005–2006, about 23% of the children under three were wasting. The third indicator, weight-for-age (underweight),

[2]For more details, refer to http://www.gainhealth.org/programs/maternal-infant-and-young-child-nutrition/.

Table 1. Nutritional status of women and children over the years.

	2015–2016			2005–2006			1998–1999	1992–1993
	All-India	Urban	Rural	All-India	Urban	Rural	All-India	All-India
Treatment of childhood diseases								
Children with diarrhea in the last 2 weeks who received ORS (%)	50.6	58.5	47.9	26.2	32.7	24	26.9	17.8
Children with diarrhea in the last 2 weeks taken to a health facility (%)	67.9	74.1	65.8	61.5	65.4	60.2	65.3	61.9
Children with acute respiratory infection or fever in the last 2 weeks taken to a health facility (%)	73.2	80	70.8	70.5	80.1	67.5	na	na
Child Feeding Practices and Nutritional Status of Children								
Children under 3 years breastfed within one hour of birth (%)	41.6	42.8	41.1	23.4	28.9	21.5	16	9.5
Children age 0–5 months exclusively breastfed (%)	54.9	52.1	56	46.3	40.3	48.3	na	na
Children age 6–9 months receiving solid or semi-solid food and breastmilk (%)	42.7	50.1	39.9	55.8	62.1	53.8	na	na
Children who are stunted (%)	38.4	31	41.2	44.9	37.4	47.2	51	na
Children who are wasted (%)	21	20	21.5	22.9	19	24.1	19.7	na
Children who are underweight (%)	35.7	29.1	38.3	40.4	30.1	43.7	42.7	51.5

Nutritional Status of Adults (age 15–49 years)								
Women whose BMI is below normal (BMI < 18.5 kg/m²) (%)	22.9	15.5	26.7	33	19.8	38.8	36.2	na
Men whose BMI is below normal (BMI < 18.5 kg/m²) (%)	20.2	15.3	23	28.1	17.5	33.1	na	na
Women who are overweight or obese (BMI ≥ 25.0 kg/m²) (%)	20.7	31.3	15	14.8	28.9	8.6	10.6	na
Men who are overweight or obese (BMI ≥ 25.0 kg/m²) (%)	18.6	26.3	14.3	12.1	22.2	7.3	na	na
Anaemia among Children and Adults								
Children age 6–59 months who are anaemic (<11 g/dL) (%)	58.4	55.9	59.4	78.9	72.2	80.9	74.2	na
Non-pregnant women age 15–49 years who are anaemic (<12 g/dL)	53.1	50.9	54.3	56.2	51.5	58.2	51.8	na
Pregnant women age 15–49 years who are anaemic (<11 g/dL) (%)	50.3	45.7	52.1	57.9	54.6	59	49.7	na
Men age 15–49 years who are anaemic (<13 g/dL) (%)	22.7	18.4	25.2	24.3	17.2	27.7	na	na

Note: Data is of children below 5 years in the year 2015–2016 and of children below 3 years for previous years.
Source: NFHS-4 factsheets.

captures elements of both stunting and wasting. There is a reduction in underweight children from 40% to 36% between 2015–2016 and 2005–2006. However, per year this is an improvement of mere 0.5% which is not in proportion to the level of economic growth. Around a quarter of women in India suffered from low Body Mass Index (BMI) in 2015–2016. This has reduced from almost one third in 2005–2006. Concurrently, the percentage of obese women has increased from 15% to 21%. This phenomenon of a stunted child and an overweight mother is emerging especially in developing countries (Garrett and Ruel, 2003). This is because women do not eat nutritious food and don't take care of their own health. Women do much worse than men on all health and nutrition indicators. There are still stark differences between urban and rural areas with the urban sector doing much better than the rural sector.

Almost 53% of women (as opposed to 23% men) suffered from anaemia in 2015–2016. There is very little improvement from 2005 to 2006 when 55% women were anaemic. Anaemia in women can result from poor dietary intake, low birth weight, infections and deficient WASH (Water, Sanitation and Hygiene), early age at marriage, high fertility, short birth intervals. Anaemia has dire consequences. It leads to reduced work capacity, poor child development and decreased learning, increased maternal, neonatal and infant mortality, risk of miscarriages, and low birth weight for the child. It is a form of hidden malnutrition which needs to be tackled to reduce malnutrition levels.[3]

The high percentage of children born with low birth weight in India confirms the intergenerational transfer of malnutrition. Almost a third of babies weighed less than 2.5 kg at birth in 2005–2006 (NFHS-3). Only 26% of children with diarrhoea were given oral rehydration salts in 2005–2006 and this percentage increased to 50.6% in 2015–2016. There is some improvement in the outreach of public health messages. Over the years the percentage of completely immunised children has increased. In 1992–1993, 35.5% children were completely immunized. The percent improved to 42% in 1998–1999 while only marginal improvement was noted in 2005–2006, when only 44% of children aged 12–23 months were fully immunized. This percentage increased to 64% in 2015–2016.

[3]For further details, refer to http://www.healthline.com/health/iron-deficiency-anemia#causes accessed in July 2017.

There is a need to ensure proper care for pregnant and lactating women by ensuring proper nutrition and reduced burden of work for them. Breastfeeding and appropriate feeding are important for preventing malnutrition. Only 23% of children under the age of three were breastfed within one hour of birth in 2005–2006 and this percentage increased to 42% in 2015–2016. Forty six percent of babies less than 5 months old were exclusively breastfed in 2005–2006 and the percentage increased to 55% in 2015–2016. During the same time period, the percentage of children aged 6–9 months who received solid or semi-solid food and breast milk decreased from 55% to 50%. The awareness of mothers for breastfeeding, complementary feeding and child care during disease is important. Malnutrition among children born to illiterate mothers is higher than the children born to women who have completed 10 or more years of schooling (Shivakumar, 2007). Fifty one percent of the children born to illiterate mothers are stunted as opposed to 31% who are born to mothers with 10 or more years of education (NFHS-4).

India is a diverse country and there is state-wise variation in the level of malnutrition. States such as Tamil Nadu, Kerala, and Andhra Pradesh do much better on nutrition indicators as compared to states like Madhya Pradesh, Bihar, Odisha and Maharashtra. The former states have the least percentages of undernourished children and women. In Kerala, only about 10% of women have low BMI while 16% children are underweight (NFHS-4). In the latter states, more than 35% of the children are underweight and more than 20% of the women have low BMI (NFHS-4).

4. Women and Agriculture

A large proportion of the population affected by malnutrition live in developing countries where agriculture and allied activities are the main source of livelihood. A majority of India's population continues to be dependent on agriculture for their livelihoods with close to 60% of the rural households in 2012–2013 classified as agricultural households (GoI, 2014). Women are the backbone of rural economies. Women work for longer hours than men, especially in developing countries (Mucavele, 2015). In some communities, four hours a day is taken up by activities such as gathering fuel and carrying water (UNDP, 2006). The FAO also claims that the contribution of women in agriculture could be higher if they had equal access to essential resources and assets (FAO, 2003).[4]

Food Security has many dimensions beyond production and demand. It includes "availability", "accessibility" and "utilization" which includes "absorption" and bioavailability of food, making it inclusive of "Nutrition Security" (Rainer *et al.*, 2000; Dev and Sharma, 2010). A nutrition focus can help address the problem of malnutrition. It is crucial that the poor have access to diversified and nutritious foods which can provide macronutrients such as energy, fat, protein and micronutrients such as iron, vitamins and minerals. Agriculture is the primary source of food and nutrients, a source of income, has effects on food prices and influences women's work burden. For example, the time they spend working on the field, or in taking care of very young children. (Gillespie and Kadiyala, 2011; Kadiyala *et al.*, 2014). Given these links and the fact that it remains the major activity of a majority of the region's population (Hazell *et al.*, 2011), agriculture can potentially be a strong driver of nutrition, giving adequate importance to women's role. However, agriculture growth rates in South Asia are slowing (Hazell *et al.*, 2011). Agricultural growth tends to be more poverty reducing than other forms of growth and sluggish growth in agriculture means slower reduction in poverty levels (Swaminathan, 2010; De Janvry and Sadoulet, 2009). This is of even greater concern for South Asia, because of the agriculture-nutrition disconnects (MSSRF/WFP 2004; Headey, 2011). The focus is on growing cash crops or profitable crops such as wheat and rice which have a higher Minimum Support Price. The focus on growing nutritious crops is lacking.

Greater women empowerment can be achieved by increasing maternal education, economic empowerment, intra-household decision making power, and community level empowerment (Jones *et al.*, 2007). Therefore, it becomes important to recognize the role of women in agriculture given a majority of them work in agriculture and allied activities. Ensuring equal land rights (Rao, 2006), investing in female human capital (Rao, 2006), and providing more opportunities for women off the farm (Misra, 2000) are a few suggestions. Few studies have concluded that women play a critical role in projects which improve dietary intake or nutritional status (Leroy and Frongillo, 2007; Mullins *et al.*, 1996; World Bank, 2007).

---

[4]Refer to http://www.fao.org/worldfoodsummit/english/fsheets/women.pdf for more details.

"Cultivation and consumption of own production" is a pathway that can bring about direct changes in the food production system enhancing availability, access and consumption of nutritious food for farming households. This approach is referred to as Farming System for Nutrition (FSN). FSN is a farmer led strategy, defined by Prof. M. S. Swaminathan, who is recognized as the Father of the Green Revolution in India, as:

> The introduction of agricultural remedies to the nutritional maladies prevailing in an area through mainstreaming nutritional criteria in the selection of the components of a farming system involving crops, farm animals and, wherever feasible, fish (Nagarajan *et al.*, 2014).

Box 1 gives a case study of a project on home gardens being undertaken by the M. S. Swaminathan Research Foundation (MSSRF) where women play a vital role in increasing household nutrition.

Box 1: Home Gardens: An Intervention to Link Agriculture to Nutrition

MSSRF has been leading a study since mid-2013 to demonstrate the feasibility of an FSN approach in the states of Odisha and Maharashtra in India, under a research programme on Leveraging Agriculture for Nutrition in South Asia (LANSA).[5] Both Maharashtra and Odisha are states in India which have high levels of malnutrition. Within the states, high burden or high priority districts in terms of malnutrition were chosen. To ensure equitable health and nutrition, and to bring about sharper improvements in health and nutrition outcomes, the bottom 25% of the districts in every state according to the ranking of districts based on composite health index have been identified as High Priority Districts (HPDs). The current study is underway in a core set of seven villages (658 households with population of 2,845) in Koraput District of Odisha and five villages (556 households with population of 2,254) in Wardha District in Vidarbha region of Maharashtra. In both the locations, percentage of women (47%) with Chronic Energy Deficiency (CED) and low BMI (<18.5) was found to be

(*Continued*)

[5]Visit www.lansasouthasia.org for further details.

Box 1: (*Continued*)

higher than for the men (40%) (Bhaskar *et al.*, 2017). The percentage of Non-Pregnant Non-Lactating (NPNL) women having anaemia was 85.9% in Wardha, and 62% in Koraput. In both Wardha and Koraput, about 55–60% of pregnant women and 75% of lactating women were anaemic (Bhaskar *et al.*, 2017). The diet of people is cereal dominated with consumption of all other food groups being less than the Recommended Dietary Intake (RDI) levels. The baseline analysis is that existing cropping system at both the study locations have very less area under nutrient rich crops, with low production and narrow on-farm crop diversity especially of millets and pulses.

The study investigated how to design location-specific FSN interventions to improve household diet diversity and nutrition outcomes. Three strategies were focused on:

(a) Increasing the availability of cereals and pulses for household food requirement by enhancing production.
(b) Widening the on-farm crop diversity to improve the dietary diversity.
(c) Promoting vegetable cultivation through household and community level gardens with naturally biofortified fruits and vegetable species and nutri-dense varieties especially green leafy vegetables to address micronutrient malnutrition.

The third strategy required greater participation from the women. These interventions were designed at two levels (i) Household level, managed by individuals, mostly women and (ii) Common area in the village, managed by a group of members in the community (to meet the space constraint in certain households).

Household nutrition garden: Households with backyard area and with incidence of anaemia and vitamin A deficiency among members were targeted for cultivating nutrient-rich vegetables and fruits (206 in Koraput and 246 in Wardha). The average area of backyard land available is low, ranging from 6.3 sqm to 15.9 sqm. Many households preferred to cultivate vegetables on a patch in the field itself and were encouraged to do so. A seasonal calendar of locally available vegetables was prepared and seeds

(*Continued*)

Box 1: (*Continued*)

were distributed accordingly. Besides, saplings of naturally fortified plants, viz., moringa, mango, guava, sapota, pomegranate, lemon, papaya, were also distributed to the households. The produce mainly goes for own consumption with the surplus being distributed to neighbours.

Community nutrition garden: Community nutrition gardens on common or land leased without rental have been operating in about 0.1 acre each in Saheli, Heti and Borgaon Gondi since late 2013 in Wardha. Leafy vegetables such as spinach, amaranth (rajgira and chavalai), fenugreek, coriander and cabbage; roots and tubers such as carrot, radish, beetroot and garlic; other vegetables such as chillies, tomato, brinjal, lady's finger, cauliflower, cucumber and ridge gourd; and cereals such as maize were planted. They are maintained by a group of women in each village and the produce shared among them. Surplus produce is given to neighbours, relatives or to the village school for inclusion in the mid-day meal. The community initiative is an effort to create greater awareness of the importance of cultivating and consuming vegetables.

The FSN approach also has to be backed by an enabling environment. "...non-food factors influencing nutrition security like clean drinking water, environmental hygiene and sanitation should get concurrent attention through ensuring convergence in the delivery of health and other infrastructure and services" (Rao and Swaminathan, 2017).

— Farming System for Nutrition (MSSRF, 2017)

4.1. *WASH and Nutrition*

Water, Sanitation and Hygiene (WASH) or non-food factors can have a large impact on health and nutrition. In India, open defecation has declined very slowly. However, other countries show faster improvements in WASH, which contribute to improvements in child nutrition (Spears and Haddad, 2015). A lack of access to WASH affects women disproportionally. Women and girls spend a lot of their time collecting water for their families (United Nations, 2010). For women, this time could be used to undertake income generating activities, housework or childcare. Girls could spend this time at school (Lenton *et al.*, 2005). Menstruating adolescent girls and female school staff might not feel comfortable using school sanitation facilities, which results in absenteeism 10–20% of the time. (Lopez-Quintero *et al.*, 2009; Blanton, 2010).

Further, collecting and carrying water during pregnancy can cause reproductive health consequences. Women who lack safe water are more prone to WASH-related illnesses, such as hookworm infestation. If the woman is pregnant, this also leads to low birth weight for their child and, therefore, intergenerational malnutrition. Improving access to WASH, and increasing awareness of pregnant mothers about maintaining general hygiene is vital to reduce maternal mortality and infant mortality. Giving birth in an environment which lacks proper WASH has a negative impact on the health and survival of both mother and baby (Narayan, 1993).

5. National Priorities and Policies for Women in Agriculture

The Indian government has several policies that focus on women, health and agriculture. We discuss a few of these in this section. First, the National Policy of Farmers in 2007, which pays special attention to women farmers. Second, the National Policy for Women in Agriculture in 2008 to address the needs of women working in agriculture. Third, National Policy for Women in 2016 which further strengthens the policies for women. Fourth, we discuss the Self-Help Group Bank Linkage Program. Last, we discuss The Mahila Kisan Sashaktikaran Pariyojana and the Kudumbashree programme started by the Kerala government.

5.1. *National Policy for Farmers*

The National Policy for Farmers, 2007, on recommendations of National Commission on Farmers (GoI, 2007), provided for a holistic approach to increase the net income of farmers. The broad areas of its coverage include economic well-being of the farmers in addition to increased production and productivity, asset reforms with respect to land, water, livestock, fisheries and bioresources; supply of good quality seeds and disease-free planting material, integrated pest management system; region and crop specific implements, machinery and technology; timely, adequate and easy reach of institutional credit at reasonable interest rates. The policy also covers strengthening the extension services, implementing Minimum Support Prices, providing appropriate social security schemes and enlarging the food security basket to include nutritious foods. The policy gives due importance to women farmers. It has a clause that appropriate support services like creches, child care centres and adequate nutrition needed by women working in fields would be funded.

5.2. *National Policy for Women in Agriculture*

In 2008, the National Commission for Women prepared the draft National Policy for women in agriculture with the aim to address the gender inequalities and social disadvantages faced by women working in agriculture and allied sectors. The policy aims to ensure women's access to and control over resources, adequate and equal availability of services like irrigation, credit, insurance, technology, extension, information, training and markets for women in agriculture sector, recognize single women in all rural households as farmers/agricultural workers and give them equal rights, safeguard the food security of the country by providing sufficient food grains at affordable prices for all, so that malnutrition particularly among women and children may be eliminated.

5.3. *National Policy for Women 2016*

The draft National Policy for women 2016 seeks to strengthen policies for women to enable them to enjoy their fundamental rights and realize their full potential (GoI, 2016). The policy aims to do this by mainstreaming gender in all sectors and programmes such as health, education, employment and an enabling environment which includes WASH and political participation. It also addresses violence against women. In terms of health, the policy focuses on health, food security and nutrition by recognizing women's reproductive rights, addressing health and nutrition challenges of girls from adolescence to adulthood to tackle the intergenerational aspect of malnutrition, geriatric health care and expansion of health insurance schemes and addressing the intergenerational cycle of undernutrition. It takes the draft policy for women farmers in 2008 further by ensuring schemes and programmes for their training in soil conservation, dairy development and other allied sectors. The policy aims to involve Self-Help Groups, and cooperatives will be encouraged to follow sustainable agricultural practices. Agriculture for nutrition campaigns will be launched in high priority districts to encourage cultivation of nutritional crops, horticultural products and traditional varieties. Procurement of such crops will be encouraged so they can be served in the anganwadis as supplementary nutrition or in schools in the mid-day meal programme.

5.4. *Self-Help Group Bank Linkage Programme*

Self-Help Groups (SHG) programme which has made substantial contribution to achieving better nutritional status for women and their families is empowering women. After the success of Grameen Bank, which was launched in Bangladesh by Muhammad Yunus in the 1980s, microfinance has been recognized as a potential poverty alleviation tool which also leads to women empowerment. Microfinance helps empower women from poor households to contribute to economic growth and sustainable livelihoods along with increased decision-making power which in turn leads to better nutrition, education and health (Bali Swain, 2012; Bali Swain and Wallentin, 2009, 2012; Pitt and Khandker, 1998; Pitt *et al.*, 2006).

In India, the SHG Bank Linkage programme (SBLP) was the prime strategy for women's empowerment in the Ninth Plan (1997–2002) and Tenth Plan (2002–2007) of the Government of India. The SBLP is a microfinance programme initiated in the early 1990s as a pilot programme by the National Bank for Agriculture and Rural Development (NABARD)[6] that links the SHG of 10 to 20 members to a bank for savings or credit. The SHGs are supported and linked to banks through the Self-Help

[6]National Bank for Agriculture and Rural Development (NABARD) is an apex development financial institution in India entrusted with "matters concerning policy, planning and operations in the field of credit for agriculture and other economic activities in rural areas in India".

Promoting Institutions (SHPIs) like Non-Governmental Organisations (NGOs), banks or government organizations, among others. About 75% of the groups were formed by NGOs and financed directly by banks (NABARD, 2006). The development of the SBLP has also been regionally imbalanced with the southern states of Andhra Pradesh, Tamil Nadu and Karnataka accounting for 54% of the SHGs and 75% of the bank credit (Sinha, 2009). Bali Swain and Wallentin (2012) find that for the SHG members, the economic factor is the most effective in empowering women. Greater autonomy and social attitudes also have a significant women-empowerment impact. In a separate study, Floro and Bali Swain (2013) focused on self-employed women and men in 14 predominantly slum communities in Bolivia, Ecuador, Philippines and Thailand. Their findings suggest that urban low-income households can mitigate food shortage through undertaking an enterprise activity that earns income and is also a direct source of food. Since food consumption is directly linked to nutritional status, it is important to work towards greater woman empowerment as it has a direct impact on nutritional outcomes for the whole household, especially children. Bali Swain and Wallentin (2017) suggest that if women's empowerment is to be pursued as a serious objective, the expansion of SBLP to the other states has to remain focused on the effective economic empowerment of women through livelihood creation. Greater emphasis also needs to be placed on creating awareness about empowerment-related issues.

5.5. *Other Government Programmes*

Another government programme called The Mahila Kisan Sashaktikaran Pariyojana (MKSP) was launched in 2010–2011 under the National Rural Livelihood Mission (NRLM) to improve the current status of women in agriculture and to enhance opportunities for their earning and empowerment.[7] It facilitates small-scale projects with regular investments to improve women's participation, skill and productivity in agriculture and allied activities. Sustainable practices like community-managed

---

[7] https://www.indiahub.com/schemes/women/mahila-kisan-sashaktikaran-pariyojana accessed in August 2017.

agriculture, zero-budget farming and non-pesticide management, and creation of Community Resource Persons (CRPs) and Pashu Sakhis selected from the community of women farmers are promoted.

A state specific programme called Kudumbashree is a community network implemented by the State Poverty Eradication Mission (SPEM) of the Government of Kerala in 1997.[8] It consists of a three-tier structure with Neighbourhood Groups (NHGs) as primary level units, Area Development Societies (ADS) at the ward level and Community Development Societies (CDS) at the local government level. While the community network is formed around the central themes of poverty eradication and women empowerment, its main features include democratic leadership, and support structures formed from the "Kudumbashree family".

The Kudumbashree network by March 15, 2017 had 2,77,175 NHGs affiliated to 19,854 ADSs and 1073 CDSs with a total membership of 43,06,976 women. Kudumbashree membership is open to all adult women, limited to one membership per family. In 2011, the Ministry of Rural Development (MoRD), Government of India, recognized Kudumbashree as the State Rural Livelihoods Mission (SRLM) under the National Rural Livelihoods Mission (NRLM).

6. Conclusion

Adequate nutrition is important for everyone. For women, it is even more so. This is because of two kinds of effects: first, the direct effect that nutrition has on increasing an individual's productivity and saving costs which otherwise might be spent on improving health and nutrition. This effect is gender neutral. Second, the impact that maternal nutrition might have on future generations. Here, women form the link between transferring malnutrition from one generation to the next, referred to as the intergenerational aspect of malnutrition. Maternal malnutrition's toll on maternal and infant survival stands in the way of countries' work towards the SDGs. The high percentage of children born with low birth weight in India confirms the intergenerational transfer of malnutrition. India's high levels of child and maternal malnutrition reflect the inadequate diet, the lack of

[8] Kudumbashree (2017) accessed at http://www.kudumbashree.org/pages/171 accessed in September 2017.

proper health and child care services. It is important to give adequate attention to women's health and nutrition from early childhood itself to break this intergenerational aspect of malnutrition.

Women's role in agriculture is an important pathway to link agriculture to the nutritional status of the population. In this chapter we have showcased an important case study through which encouraging women to plant nutritious crops in home gardens can lead to better nutrition outcomes for the whole household and even community. There is a need to ensure proper care and increased awareness for pregnant women by ensuring proper nutrition and reduced burden of work for them. An enabling environment with proper drinking water, hygiene, sanitation, health services is important for nutrition security. The Government recognizes the importance of women in the economy and has come up with policies at regular intervals to achieve gender parity and improve the status of women. However, the implementation of the policies needs to be better.

There is a dearth of proper indicators to measure women empowerment and its link to nutrition in literature. International Food Policy Research Institute (IFPRI, 2012) has come out with the Women's Empowerment in Agriculture Index (WEAI) which measures the empowerment, agency and inclusion of women in the agriculture sector in an effort to identify ways to overcome those obstacles and constraints. The Index measures the roles and extent of women's engagement in the agriculture sector in five domains: decisions about agricultural production, access to and decision-making power over productive resources, control over use of income, leadership in the community and time use. It also measures women's empowerment relative to men within their households. Innovative Methods and Metrics for Agriculture and Nutrition Actions (IMMANA, 2016) is undertaking a study to develop a Women's Empowerment in Nutrition Index (WENI) that reflects nutritional empowerment across agrarian contexts in South Asia. These two would be useful tools to study the link between nutrition and agriculture with a special focus on women.

Acknowledgements

The authors are thankful to Dr. R.V. Bhavani, Project Manager, LANSA, for her valuable feedback. All errors remain our own.

References

Alderman, H., Hoddinott, J. and B. H. Kinsey (2006) "Long Term Consequences of Early Childhood Malnutrition", *Oxford Economic Papers*, Vol. 58, No. 3, pp. 450–474.

Almond, D., Chay, K. Y. and D. S. Lee (2005) "The Costs of Low Birth Weight", *The Quarterly Journal of Economics*, Vol. 120, No. 3, pp. 1031–1083, MIT Press.

Behrman, J. (2009) "Early Life Nutrition and Subsequent Education, Health, Wage, and Intergenerational Effects", in *Health and Growth, Commission on Growth and Development*, ed. Spence and Lewis. Accessed at www.growthcommission.org.

Behrman, J., Alderman, H. and J. Hoddinott (2004) "Hunger and Malnutrition", in *Global Crises, Global Solutions*, ed. Bjørn Lomborg. Cambridge, UK: Cambridge University Press. Accessed at http://siteresources.worldbank.org/INTPOVRES/Resources/477227-1142020443961/2311843-1163084618556/MODULE6_2007_HungerandMalnutrition.pdf accessed in August 2017.

Bali Swain, R. and F. Y. Wallentin (2017) "The Impact of Microfinance on Factors Empowering Women: Differences in Regional and Delivery Mechanisms in India's SHG Programme", *The Journal of Development Studies*, Vol. 53, No. 5, pp 1–16.

Bali Swain, R. and F. Y. Wallentin (2012) "Factors Empowering Women in Indian Self-help Group Programs", *International Review of Applied Economics*, Vol. 26, No. 4, pp. 425–444.

Bali Swain, R. (2012) *The Microfinance Impact*. Routledge, London and New York: Taylor and Francis Books.

Bali Swain, R. and F. Y. Wallentin (2009) "Does Microfinance Empower Women? Evidence from Self-help Groups in India", *International Review of Applied Economics*, Vol. 23, No. 5, pp. 541–556.

Bhaskar, V., Nithya, D. J., Raju, S. and R. V. Bhavani (2017) "Establishing Integrated Agriculture-Nutrition Programmes to Diversify Household Food and Diets in Rural India", *Food Security*, Vol. 9, pp. 981–999.

Blanton, E. (2010) "Evaluation of the Role of School Children in the Promotion of Point-of-Use Water Treatment and Handwashing in Schools and Households—Nyanza Province, Western Kenya, 2007", *American Journal of Tropical Medicine and Hygiene*, Vol. 82, No.4, pp. 664–671.

Black, R. E., Allen, L. H., Bhutta, Z. A., Caulfield, L. E., de Onis, M., Ezzati, M., Mathers, C., Rivera, J. and for the Maternal and Child Undernutrition Study

Group (2008) "Maternal and Child Undernutrition: Global and Regional Exposures and Health Consequences", *Lancet*, Vol. 371, pp. 243–260.

Case, A. and C. Paxson (2008) "Stature and Status: Height, Ability, and Labor Market Outcomes", *Journal of Political Economy*, Vol. 116, No. 3, pp. 499–531.

De Janvry, A. and E. Sadoulet (2009) "Agricultural Growth and Poverty Reduction: Additional Evidence", *World Bank Research Observer*, Vol. 25, No. 1, pp. 1–20.

Dev, S. M. and A. Sharma (2010) "Food Security in India: Performance, Challenges and Policies", Oxfam Working Papers accessed at http://policy-practice.oxfam.org.uk/publications/food-security-in-india-performance-challenges-and-policies-346637 in July 2017.

FAO (2003) "Gender: Key to Sustainability and Food Security", accessed at ftp://ftp.fao.org/docrep/fao/005/y3969e/y3969e00.pdf in July 2017.

Floro, M. S. and R. Bali Swain (2013) "Food Security, Gender, and Occupational Choice Among Urban Low-Income Household", *World Development*, Vol. 42, pp. 89–99.

FOCUS (2006) "Focus on Children Under Six", Citizen's Initiative for the Rights of Children Under Six (CIRCUS).

Garrett, J. L. and M. T. Ruel (2003) "Stunted Child-Overweight Mother Pairs: An Emerging Policy Concern?", Food Consumption and Nutrition Division, IFPRI Discussion Paper No. 148 accessed at http://pdf.usaid.gov/pdf_docs/Pnact013.pdf in July 2017.

Gillespie, S. and S. Kadiyala (2011) "Exploring the Agriculture-Nutrition Disconnect in India, 2020" Conference Brief 20, for the conference — *Leveraging Agriculture for Improving Nutrition and Health* organized by the International Food Policy Research Institute (IFPRI), New Delhi, February 10–12.

Government of India (GoI) (2007) Department of Agriculture & Cooperation Ministry of Agriculture "National Policy for Farmers", accessed at http://agricoop.nic.in/sites/default/files/npff2007%20%281%29.pdf in August 2017.

GoI (2014) Key Indicators of Situation of Agricultural Households in India, NSSO 70th Round, Ministry of Statistics and Programme Implementation, Government of India, New Delhi.

GoI (2016) Ministry of Women and Child Development "National Policy for Women", accessed at http://wcd.nic.in/sites/default/files/draft%20national%20policy%20for%20women%202016_0.pdf in July 2017.

Gragnolati, M., Shekar, M., Dasgupta, M., Bredenkamp, C. and Y. Lee (2005) "India's Undernourished Children: A Call for Reform and Action", Health,

Nutrition and Population (HNP) Discussion Paper. Washington DC: World Bank.

Hazell, P., Headey, D., Pratt, A. and D. Byerlee (2011) "Structural Imbalances and Farm and Nonfarm Employment Prospects in Rural South Asia", Background Paper for World Bank Report: More and Better Jobs in South Asia, Washington, DC: The World Bank.

Hoddinott, J., Maluccio, J., Behrman, J., Martorell, R., Melgar, P., Quisumbing, A., Ramirez-Zea, M., Stein, A. and K. Yount (2011) "The Consequences of Early Childhood Growth Failure Over the Life Course", Washington, DC: Mimeo, International Food Policy Research Institute.

Horton, S. (1999) "Opportunities for Investments in Nutrition in Low-income Asia", *Asian Development Review*, Vol. 17, Nos. 1, 2, pp. 246–273.

Headey, D. (2011) "Pro-Nutrition Economic Growth: What is it, and How do I Achieve it?" Background paper for the conference — *Leveraging Agriculture for Improving Nutrition and Health*, organized by the International Food Policy Research Institute (IFPRI), New Delhi, February 10–12.

IMMANA (2016) "Women's Empowerment in Nutrition Index(WENI) Measuring nutritional Empowerment to Better Link Agriculture to Nutrition", accessed at http://anh-academy.org/sites/default/files/3.%20Narayanan.pdf.

IFPRI (2012) "Women's Empowerment in Agriculture Index", accessed at http://www.ifpri.org/publication/womens-empowerment-agriculture-index in June 2017.

Indian Institute of Population Sciences (IIPS) and Ministry of Health and Family Welfare (MHFW) (1995) "National Family Health Survey-1 (NFHS-1)", 1992–93, International Institute for Population Sciences, Mumbai.

IIPS and MHFW (2000) "National Family Health Survey-2 (NFHS-2)", 1998–99, International Institute for Population Sciences, Mumbai.

IIPS and Macro International (2007) "National Family Health Survey-3 (NFHS-3)", 2005–2006, International Institute for Population Sciences, Mumbai.

IIPS and Macro International (2016) "National Family Health Survey-4 (NFHS-4)", 2015–2016, International Institute for Population Sciences, Mumbai accessed at http://rchiips.org/nfhs/factsheet_NFHS-4.shtml in August 2017.

Jones, N., Mukherjee, M. and S. Galab (2007) "Ripple Effects or Deliberate Intentions? Assessing Linkages between Women's Empowerment and Childhood Poverty", UNICEF/Young Lives Social Policy Paper 002, May.

Kadiyala, S., Harris, J., Headey, D., Yosef, S. and S. Gillespie (2014) "Agriculture and Nutrition in India: Mapping Evidence to Pathways", *Annals of the New York Academy of Sciences*, Vol. 1331, pp. 43–56.

Lenton, R., Wright, A. and K. Lewis (2005) "Health, Dignity, and Development: What Will it Take?" UN Millennium Project Report, p. 25 accessed at http://www.unmillenniumproject.org/documents/WaterComplete-lowres.pdf in August 2017.

Leroy, J. and E. Frongillo (2007) "Can interventions to promote animal production ameliorate undernutrition?" *Journal of Nutrition*, Vol. 137, No. 1, pp. 2311–2316.

Lopez-Quintero, C., Freeman, P. and Y. Neumark (2009) "Hand Washing Among School Children in Bogotá, Colombia", *American Journal of Public Health*, Vol. 99, No.1, pp. 94–101.

Martorell, R. (1999) "The Nature of Child Malnutrition and its Long-term Implications", *Food and Nutrition Bulletin*, Vol. 20, pp. 288–292.

Misra, V. N. (2000) "Role of Female Labour Force Participation in Rural Poverty and Non-farm Employment: Indian Experience", *Indian Journal of Labour Economics*, Vol. 43, No. 2, pp. 221–246.

Mullins, G., Wahome, L., Tsangari, P. and L. Maarse (1996) "Impacts of Intensive Dairy Production on Smallholder Farm Women in Coastal Kenya", *Human Ecology*, Vol. 24, pp. 231–253.

Mucavele, S. (2017) "The Role of Rural Women in Agriculture", accessed at http://www.wfo-oma.org/women-in-agriculture/articles/the-role-of-rural-women-in-agriculture.html in July 2017.

MSSRF (2017) "Farming System for Nutrition", MSSRF/OP/2017/6.

MSSRF/WFP (2004) "Atlas of the Sustainability of Food Security in India", M. S. Swaminathan Research Foundation, Chennai.

National Commission of Women (2008) "Draft National Policy for Women in Agriculture", accessed at http://ncw.nic.in/Comments/Agricultural_Policy.pdf in July 2017.

Narayan, D. (1993) "Participatory Evaluation: Tools for Managing Change in Water and Sanitation", World Bank Technical Paper No. 207, accessed at http://www.bvsde.paho.org/bvsarg/i/fulltext/partici/partici.pdf in July 2017.

NABARD (National Bank of Agriculture and Rural Development) (2006) "Progress of SHG–bank linkage in India: 2005–2006", Working Paper NABARD.

Nagarajan, S., Bhavani, R. V. and M. S. Swaminathan (2014) "Operationalizing the Concept of Farming System for Nutrition Through the Promotion of Nutrition-Sensitive Agriculture", *Current Science*, Vol. 107, No. 6, pp. 959–964.

Pitt, M. and S. R. Khandker (1998) "The Impact of Group-based Credit Programs on Poor Households in Bangladesh: Does the Gender of the Participant Matter?" *Journal of Political Economy*, Vol. 106, pp. 958–996.

Pitt, M., Khandker, S. R. and J. Cartwright (2006) "Empowering Women with Microfinance: Evidence from Bangladesh", *Economic Development and Cultural Change*, Vol. 54, No. 4, pp. 791–831.

Proos, L. and J. Gustafsson (2012) "Is Early Puberty Triggered by Catch-Up Growth Following Undernutrition?" *International Journal of Environmental Research and Public Health*, Vol. 9, pp. 1791–1809.

Rao, N. (2006) "Land Rights, Gender Equality, and Household Food Security: Exploring the Conceptual Links in the Case of India", *Food Policy*, Vol. 31, No. 2, pp. 180–193.

Rao, N. and M. S. Swaminathan (2017) "A Farmer-led Approach to Achieving a Malnutrition-Free India", *Agricultural Research*, Vol. 6, No. 1, pp. 1–7.

Rampal, P. (2013) "Dynamics of Changing Nutritional Status of Children in Andhra Pradesh", Young Lives Working Paper accessed on http://younglives.qeh.ox.ac.uk/files/others/inequalities-conference-papers/rampal-dynamicschangingnutritionalstatuschildrenandhrapradesh in May 2017.

Ransom, I. E. and K. L. Elder (2003) "Nutrition of Women and Adolescent Girls: Why it Matters?" Population Reference Bureau accessed at http://www.prb.org/Publications/Articles/2003/NutritionofWomenandAdolescentGirlsWhyItMatters.aspx in August 2017.

Ramakrishnan, U., Barnhart, H., Schroeder, D. G., Stein, A. D. and R. Martorell (1999) "Early Childhood Nutrition, Education and Fertility Milestones in Guatemala", *Journal of Nutrition*, Vol. 129, pp. 2199–2202.

Rainer, G., Hans, S., Hans, P. and A. P. Hans-Joachim (2000) "The Four Dimensions of Food and Nutrition Security: Definitions and Concepts", European Union and FAO accessed at http://www.foodsec.org/DL/course/shortcourseFA/en/pdf/P-01_RG_Concept.pdf

Richard, S. A., Black, R. E., Gilman, R. H., Guerrant, R. L., Kang, G., Lanata, C. F., Mølbak, K., Rasmussen, Z. A., Sack, R. B., Valentiner-Branth, P., Checkley, W. and Childhood Infection and Malnutrition Network (2012) "Wasting is Associated with Stunting in Early Childhood", *The Journal of Nutrition,* Vol. 142, No. 7, pp. 1291–1296.

Spears, D. and L. Haddad (2015) "Why Sanitation Matters for Nutrition", Chapter 3 in *Global Food Policy Report* accessed at http://motherchildnutrition.org/pdf/Why-sanitation-matters-for-nutrition-IFPRI-2015.pdf.

Sinha, F. (2009) *Microfinance Self Help Groups in India: Living up to Their Promise*? Essex: Practical Action Publishing.

Shivakumar, A. K. (2007) "Why Are Levels of Child Malnutrition Not Improving?" *Economic and Political Weekly*, Vol. 42, No. 15, pp. 1337–1345.

Swaminathan, M. S. (2010) "Science and Sustainable Food Security", Selected Papers of M. S. Swaminathan. IISc. Centenary Lecture Series. in Tjan Kwang. Wei (ed.), Vol. 3, World Scientific Publishing. Co. Pte. Ltd.

Smith, L. and L. Haddad (2000) "Explaining Child Malnutrition in Developing Countries", International Food Policy Research Institute Research Monograph 111. IFPRI, Washington DC.

Strauss, J. and D. Thomas (1998) "Health, Nutrition and Economic Development", *Journal of Economic Literature*, Vol. 36, No. 2, pp. 766–817.

Thomas, D. and J. Strauss (1997) "Health and Wages: Evidence on Men and Women in Urban Brazil", *Journal of Econometrics*, Vol. 77, No. 1, pp. 159–185.

United Nations Development Programme (UNDP) (2006) "Mainstreaming Gender in Water Management, Resource Guide", Gender and Water Alliance (GWA).

United Nations (2017) "Sustainable Development Goals", accessed at http://www.un.org/sustainabledevelopment/sustainable-development-goals/ in August 2017.

United Nations, OHCHR, UN-HABITAT, WHO (2010) The Right to Water, Fact Sheet No. 35. (OHCHR report, p. 10) accessed at http://www.ohchr.org/Documents/Publications/FactSheet35en.pdf.in July 2017.

United Nations Administrative Committee on Coordination Sub–Committee on Nutrition (ACC/SCN) (2000) 4th Report — The World Nutrition Situation: Nutrition throughout the Life Cycle accessed on https://www.unscn.org/web/archives_resources/files/rwns4.pdf in July 2017.

UNICEF (United Nations Children's Fund) (1990) "Strategy for Improved Nutrition of Children and Women in Developing Countries", A policy review, New York.

UNICEF (2011) "The Situation of Children in India: A Profile", accessed at http://www.unicef.org/sitan/files/SitAn_India_May_2011.pdf in March 2015.

WHO (World Health Organization). (2003) "Global Strategy for Infant and Young Child Feeding. Geneva: WHO", accessed at http://www.who.int/nutrition/topics/global_strategy/en/ in August 2017.

WHO (2013) "Essential Nutrition Actions: Improving Maternal, Newborn, Infant and Young Child Health and Nutrition", accessed at http://www.who.int/nutrition/publications/infantfeeding/essential_nutrition_actions.pdf.

World Bank (2007) "From Agriculture to Nutrition: Pathways, Synergies, and Outcomes", Report No. 40196-GLB. Washington, DC: The World Bank.

Part III
Food Security Issues in Africa

Chapter 9

Africa's Food Insecurity and Its Determinants

Manoj K. Pandey

Development Policy Centre, Crawford School of Public Policy, College of Asia and the Pacific, Australian National University, Canberra, Australian Capital Territory, Australia
manoj.pandey@anu.edu.au

Abstract

Despite impressive reduction in global hunger, a growing undernourished population with inadequate food security poses a serious challenge for Africa. In this chapter, I seek to examine progress of food insecurity in Africa and its determinants. I use fixed-effect panel data regression approach to analyse annual data during 1990–2016 for 59 African countries. The chapter finds that expansion of food production and agricultural output are strongly associated with reduced prevalence of undernourishment, depth of food deficit and prevalence of food inadequacy. While a higher aggregate income growth is associated with improved food security, rising rate of inflation and faster population growth have opposite effects. Remittances received by countries help to reduce prevalence and depth of food insecurity. Though not very consistent, better access to electricity, improved water sources and better road infrastructure are significant factors associated with better food security. The results add to the growing evidence on the importance of food self-sufficiency, rising aggregate and agricultural growth that could compensate for negative effects of rising rate of aggregate inflation and population growth.

Keywords: Agriculture, economic growth, food inadequacy, food security, undernourishment.

1. Introduction

Despite impressive global economic progress over the last decade, Africa and some parts of Asia have not made significant progress in achieving food security and ending hunger from its population. As per United Nations Organization for Food and Agriculture (FAO) 2016 estimates, about 793 million people are hungry and an additional 2 billion people are expected to enter extreme hunger and malnutrition trap. As priority goal 2 of United Nations' Sustainable Development Goals (SDGs 2) to "end hunger, achieve food security and improved nutrition, and promote sustainable agriculture", extreme hunger and malnutrition remains a barrier to sustainable development.[1] It has both direct and indirect consequences ranging from loss of work hours and productivity to poor health and diseases, loss of earnings and risk of falling in the poverty trap. Decades of sustained poor diet and nutrition have resulted in 45% of deaths in children under 5 — 3.1 million children each year — and one quarter of the world's children suffer stunted growth. The food security situation is even worse in developing countries with large concentrations in Africa and Asia.

While the hunger target of the first Millennium Development Goal (MDG 1) was within reach globally, Africa had made only modest progress (FAO, International Fund for Agricultural Development (IFAD) and World Food Programme (WFP), 2014). The annual reduction in the proportion of the population facing hunger is still slow across Africa and as the African population continues to grow, much more effort and innovation will be urgently needed to improve food security. United Nations' Target 2.1 of SDG 2 is to "end hunger and ensure access by all people, in particular the poor and people in vulnerable situations including infants, to safe, nutritious and sufficient

[1]A detailed discussion on Sustainable Development Goal 2 is provided at http://www.un.org/sustainabledevelopment/hunger/.

food all year round by 2030". This will require increase in the availability and access to nutritious food through agricultural production and productivity, improved global supply chain and reduction in food losses and wastage.

In this chapter, I review status of food insecurity in Africa and examine the factors associated with changes in the food insecurity situation. In other words, I examine gravity of food insecurity and its association with food supply, growth, remittances, infrastructure and prices. Based on the classifications provided by FAO, IFAD and WFP (2015), three proxies, namely the Prevalence of Undernourishment (PoU), the Depth of Food Deficit (DoFD) and the Prevalence of Food Inadequacy (PoFA), are used to capture access dimension of food insecurity. The data used for the analysis is from 59 African countries covering the period from 1990–2016. I use country-specific fixed effect panel data regression approach to estimate the reduced form food insecurity equation.

The analysis reveals that, on the one hand, expansion of food supply through agricultural production, a higher aggregate economic growth, increased inflow of personal remittances, better electrification, access to water and improved road density are significantly associated with lower levels of food insecurity. On the other hand, rising inflation rate and faster population growth have opposite effects. Thus, the results add to the growing evidence on the importance of food self-sufficiency, higher economic growth and controlled rate of aggregate inflation and population growth.

The rest of the paper is organized as follows: Section 2 discusses food security measurement and proxy indicators, data sources and data definitions. Section 3 summarizes data and emerging current and past food security progress in Africa. Section 4 introduces the equation to be estimated and the estimation method. Section 5 presents and discusses the statistical results. Section 6 concludes the paper.

2. Measuring Food Security: Data Sources and Definitions

Food and Agricultural Organization of the United Nation (FAO, IFAD and WFP, 2015) defines food insecurity or lack of food security as a situation resulting from lack of secure access to sufficient amounts of safe and nutritious food required for normal growth and development of an active and healthy life. This situation may be caused by any one or a combination/s of (i) the unavailability of sufficient food, (ii) insufficient purchasing power to obtain the quantities required, (iii) inappropriate distribution, or (iv) inadequate utilization of food at the household level. Food insecurity combined with poor conditions of health and sanitation, and inappropriate care and feeding practices are the major causes of poor nutritional status. Food insecurity may be chronic, seasonal or transitory. Thus, food insecurity is a multi-dimensional concept and, therefore, a single indicator may not capture all the aspects of food security (Barrett, 2010; Carletto *et al.*, 2013; Jones *et al.,* 2013).

In this paper, I use three proxies to capture accessibility dimensions of food insecurity classified in FAO, IFAD and WFP (2015). I proxy accessibility by the prevalence of undernourishment, the depth of food deficit and the prevalence of food inadequacy.[2] The set of variables required to analyze progress and estimation of food insecurity equations were obtained from a variety of sources. The data on food insecurity proxies and key economic and social sector data were downloaded from the website of FAO's Food Security Indicators, 2016. Data for sectoral GDP indicators were obtained from the World Bank's website on World Development Indicators, 2016.[3]

As a proxy for utilization, the FAO's prevalence of undernourishment indicator measures the probability that a randomly selected individual from the reference population is found to consume less than his/her calorie requirement for an active and healthy life. Thus, an individual with insufficient food intake needed to meet dietary energy requirements continuously is defined as undernourished or someone suffering from chronic hunger, or, hunger. FAO reports 3-year moving average prevalence of undernourishment for each country annually using the three-parameter skew-normal distribution function. This function involves three parameters: the mean level of per capita dietary energy consumption in calories, the coefficient of variation as a parameter accounting for inequality in food consumption and a coefficient of skewness to account for asymmetry in the distribution.[4]

---

[2]While there are many other measures that can proxy these aspects of food insecurity, our analysis is restricted to these measures only.

[3]The link for the FAO data is http://www.fao.org/faostat/en/#data/FS. The link for the World Bank data is http://databank.worldbank.org/data/reports.aspx?source=world-development-indicators.

[4]FAO, IFAD and WFP (2012, 2015) provide comprehensive computational methodology.

FAO defines prevalence of undernourishment as the percentage of the population with average daily caloric intake over the year less than the minimum daily requirement. Depth of food deficit measures the magnitude of the food security gap or degree to which caloric intake of the undernourished falls below minimum dietary requirements. FAO calculates depth of food deficit as 3-year averages and mean difference between intake and minimum daily caloric requirement, in kcal per person per day, among those whose intake is below the minimum daily requirement. Prevalence of food inadequacy is also in percentages and taken as a 3-year average.

The annual data are for 59 African countries over the 26-year period covering 1990–1992 to 2014–2016. Most of the proxies for food insecurity were available in the form of 3-year averages of the data. However, we assume that the annual data corresponds to middle-year. For instance, 3-year average data from 1990 to 1992 is treated as data for 1991 to simplify panel arrangements. This gives a total of 1534 observations for the study.

3. Food Security Status in Africa

3.1. *Number and Prevalence of Undernourishment*

Globally, the progress on food security has been impressive in the last three decades. With an annual reduction of about 8.5 million, the world had over 218 million fewer undernourished people in 2014–2016 than there were in 1990–1992 (Table 1).

Over 230 million decline in the Number of Undernourished (NoU) population occurred in Asia alone, and nearly 32 million in Latin America and the Caribbean. This implies a net increase of about 44 million undernourished people in the rest of the world. Within Asia the largest decline was in East Asia (150.3 million), followed by Southeastern Asia (77 million) and South Asia (9.8 million). Marked differences in PoUs across regions persist (Table 2).

Sub-Saharan Africa (SSA) remains the region with the highest prevalence of undernourishment, with modest progress in recent years. Western Asia shows no progress, while Southern Asia and Northern Africa show slow progress. Significant reductions in both the estimated number and prevalence of undernourishment have occurred in most countries of Eastern and Southeastern Asia, as well as in Latin America.

Table 1. Undernourished population (millions) and % annual change.

	Population undernourished (millions)			**% annual change between**		
Region	**1990–1992 (P1)**	**2000–2002 (P2)**	**2014–2016 (P3)**	**P1 & P2**	**P1 & P3**	**P2 & P3**
World	1010.7	929.6	792.5	−0.73	−0.86	−0.98
Africa	181.7	210.2	230.3	1.43	1.07	0.64
Eastern Africa	103.9	121.6	124.2	1.55	0.78	0.14
Middle Africa	24.2	42.4	58.9	6.84	5.74	2.59
Southern Africa	3.1	3.7	3.2	1.76	0.13	−0.90
Western Africa	44.6	35.9	31.5	−1.77	−1.17	−0.82
North Africa (exc Sudan)	6.0	6.6	4.3	0.91	−1.13	−2.32
SSA	175.7	203.6	217.8	1.44	0.96	0.46
Asia	741.9	636.6	511.7	−1.29	−1.24	−1.31
Caucasus and Central Asia	9.6	10.9	5.8	1.23	−1.58	−3.12
East Asia	295.4	221.7	145.1	−2.27	−2.04	−2.30
East Asia (exc China)	6.4	10.4	11.3	5.68	3.06	0.58
Southern Asia	291.2	272.3	281.4	−0.59	−0.13	0.22
South Asia (exc India)	81.1	86.7	86.8	0.63	0.28	0.01
Southeastern Asia	137.5	117.6	60.5	−1.32	−2.24	−3.24
West Asia	8.3	14.1	19.0	6.35	5.16	2.32
Central America	12.6	11.8	11.4	−0.58	−0.38	−0.23
South America	45.4	40.3	NA	−1.02	NA	NA
Latin America and the Caribbean	66.1	60.4	34.3	−0.78	−1.92	−2.88
Caribbean	8.1	8.2	7.5	0.11	−0.30	−0.57
Oceania	1.0	1.3	1.4	2.73	1.60	0.51

Source: FAOSTAT Website (http://www.fao.org/faostat/en/#data/FS).

Table 2. Prevalence of undernourishment, depth of food deficit and food inadequacy in Africa: 1990–1992 to 2014–2016.

Region	**Indicators**	**1990–1992 (P1)**	**2000–2002 (P2)**	**2014–2016 (P3)**	**% relative change between P1 & P3**
World	Prevalence	18.6	14.9	10.8	–41.9
	Depth	138	111	81	–41.3
	Inadequacy	25.8	21.9	16.8	–34.9
Africa	Prevalence	27.6	25.4	19.8	–28.3
	Depth	204	186	151	–26.0
	Inadequacy	34.7	32.3	25.5	–26.5
Eastern Africa	Prevalence	47.2	43.1	31.5	–33.3
	Depth	368	323	230	–37.5
	Inadequacy	55.5	52.1	40.3	–27.4
Middle Africa	Prevalence	33.5	44.2	41.3	**23.3**
	Depth	243	338	380	**56.4**
	Inadequacy	42	52.9	47.6	**13.3**
Southern Africa	Prevalence	7.2	7.1	5.2	–27.8
	Depth	46	48	37	–19.6
	Inadequacy	12.2	12.6	9.1	–25.4
Western Africa	Prevalence	24.2	15	9	–62.8
	Depth	165	101	59	–64.2
	Inadequacy	32.4	21.4	13.8	–57.4
SSA	Prevalence	33.2	30	23	–30.7
	Depth	247	221	176	–28.7
	Inadequacy	41.2	37.7	29.4	–28.6
North Africa (exc Sudan)	Prevalence	NA	NA	NA	NA
	Depth	31	32	17	–45.2
	Inadequacy	8.2	8.1	NA	NA

Data Source: FAOSTAT Website (http://www.fao.org/faostat/en/#data/FS).

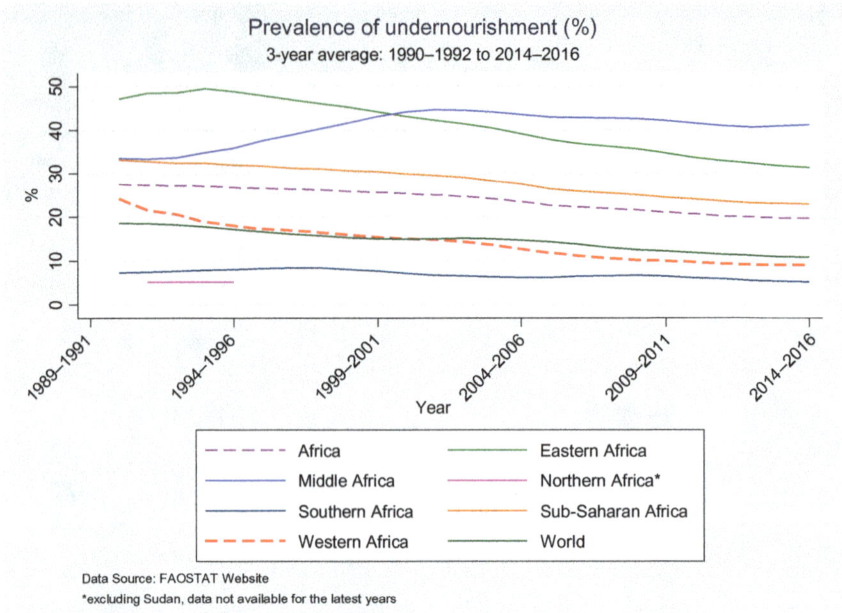

Figure 1. Regional distribution of prevalence of undernourishment between 1990–1992 and 2014–2016.

Despite the global progress, Africa has remained home for 230 million NoUs in 2014–2016 — higher from 181.7 million in 1990–1992. In terms of global share of all the NoUs, Africa has over 29% now as compared to just below 18% in 1990–1992. This implies that food security poses a serious concern for Africa and the problem is growing. The PoU has reduced from 28% in 1990–1992 to close to 20% in 2014–2016, a reduction at the rate of over 1% per annum. However, it is almost double that of the world average.

There are significant variations in the decline in PoU at the sub-regional levels (Table 2 and Figure 1). SSA added over 42 million undernourished people to the world. In 2014–2016, nearly 27% of the global and 95% of the African undernourished population were from SSA — the highest PoU for any region with nearly 218 million hungry people.

The prevalence fell from over 33% to 23% between 1990–1992 and 2014–2016. However, the pace of reduction was relatively slower since 1990s, except between 2000–2002 and 2005–2007. Overall, undernourished population count increased between 1990–1992 and 2014–2016 with an annual growth rate of 0.96 per year that resulted in addition of 42.1 million undernourished people in the region. This reflects SSA's inability to reduce its population growth rate of 2.7% per year. Other factors such as rising food prices, droughts and political instability in several countries of the region also contributed to the worrisome progress (FAO, 2015).

Eastern Africa remained the largest undernourished population in absolute terms. While the share of undernourished has fallen by over one third, with an average annual growth of 0.78%, the number of hungry people in the sub-region has risen from about 104 million in 1991 to over 124 million in 2016. In Middle Africa, the headcount of undernourished people grew under 2.5 times. The PoU also increased by 23.3%, from 33.5% in 1990–1992 to 41.3% in 2014–2016. The Southern Africa's PoU has fallen by 28% since 1990–1992. However, 3.2 million people remain undernourished. The undernourished population in Western Africa has fallen by over 13 million (29.4%) since 1990–1992. The PoU has also declined from over 24% in 1990–1992 to 9% in 2014–2016 — a decline of impressive 63%.

When compared across sub-regions within Africa, prevalence is as high as 41% in Middle Africa, and as low as 5% in Southern Africa. While in 1991, Morocco (5.3%) and Ethiopia (74.8%) were two countries with the least and the highest PoU, Gambia (5.3%) and Zambia (47.8%), respectively, replaced them in 2015.

Table 3 summarizes the distribution of improvement in terms of reduction in PoU across African countries. Sub-Saharan countries such as Angola, Benin, Cameroon, Djibouti achieved an excellent reduction of over 70% in the PoU between 1990 and 2016. In the same period, Niger, Nigeria, Togo, Gambia, Mauritania, Senegal, Ethiopia, Malawi and Mozambique performed well with reductions ranging from 50% to 70%. However, poor performances, defined as reduction of 30–50%, were recorded by Sierra Leone, Cabo Verde, Chad, Rwanda, Kenya, Congo, Guinea, Lesotho, Zimbabwe, Burkina Faso and Guinea-Bissau countries. Prevalence of undernourishment increased up to 20% in economies such as Botswana, Central African Republic, Uganda, Liberia and Namibia during the same period. Worst performers were Madagascar, Swaziland, United Republic of Tanzania and Zambia, where prevalence of undernourishment increased well over 20%.

Table 3. Progress in the prevalence of undernourishment: 1991–2015.

Progress	**Countries**
Excellent	Angola, Benin, Cameroon, Djibouti
Very Good	Niger, Nigeria, Togo, Gambia, Mauritania
Good	Senegal, Ethiopia, Malawi, Mozambique
Poor	Sierra Leone, Cabo Verde, Chad, Rwanda, Kenya
Very Poor	Congo, Guinea, Lesotho, Zimbabwe, Burkina Faso, Guinea-Bissau
Degraded	Botswana, Central African Republic, Uganda, Liberia, Namibia
Highly degraded	Madagascar, Swaziland, United Republic of Tanzania, Zambia

Note: Improvement is measured as reductions in the PoU and classified as excellent (over 70%), very good (between 60% and 70%), good (between 50% and 60%), poor (between 30% and 50%), very poor (30% but above 0), degraded (increase up to 20%), highly degraded (increase over 20%). Countries listed in this table are those for which 3-year average for 1990–1992 and 2014–2016 were available.

3.2 *Depth of Food Deficit (DoFD)*

Depth of food deficit declined globally by 57 kcal per person per day — a reduction of over 41% between 1990–1992 and 2014–2016 (Table 2 and Figure 2).

Between 1990–1992 and 2014–2016, it fell by 26% in Africa, from 204 kcal per person per day to 151 kcal per person per day, which is still much higher than the world average (81 kcal per person per day). At the sub-regional level, Western Africa is the best performing region followed by North Africa (excluding Sudan), Eastern Africa, SSA and Southern Africa. Middle Africa is the only sub-region where depth of food deficit has increased by 56.4% between 1990–1992 and 2014–2016.

3.3 *Prevalence of Food Adequacy (PoFA)*

Like prevalence of undernourishment and depth of food deficit, the decline in the PoFA continued globally, from nearly 26% in 1990–1992 to under 17% in 2014–2016 (Table 2 and Figure 3).

In the same period, African food adequacy also fell from 34.7% to 25.5% — a level of food adequacy where the world was in 1990–1992. Thus, Africa's slow progress imposes serious challenges to the progress of

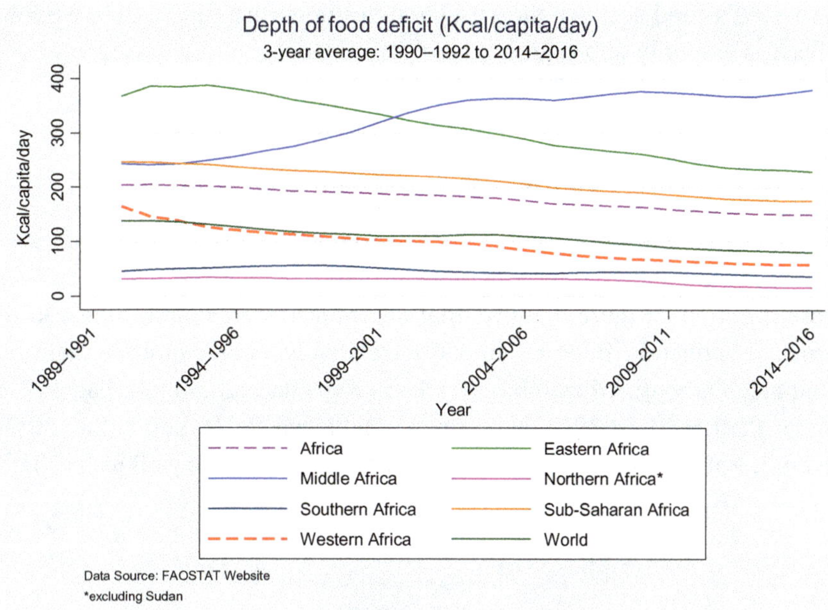

Figure 2. Regional distribution of depth of food deficit in Africa.

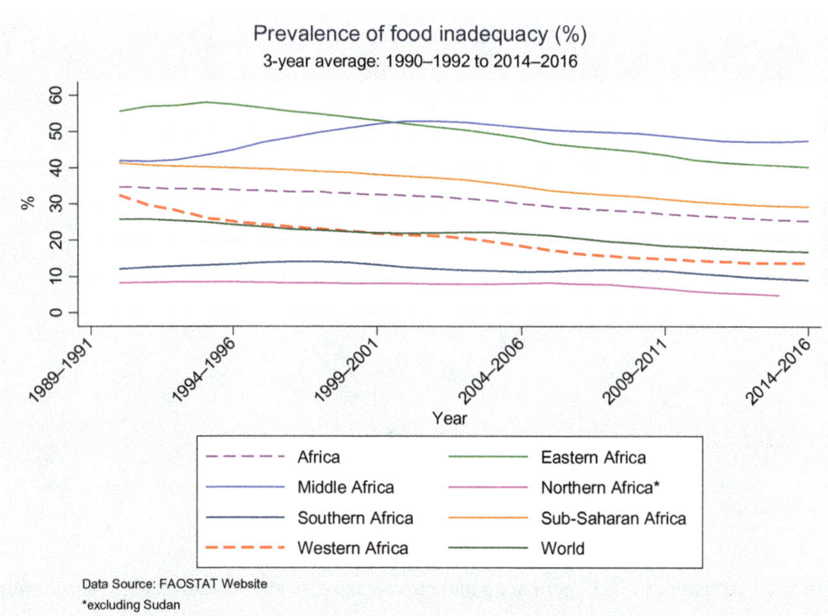

Figure 3. Regional distribution of prevalence of food inadequacy in Africa.

the world's food security targets. Though improving since 2000, Middle Africa is the only sub-region where food inadequacy increased by over 13% between 1990–1992 and 2014–2016.

3.4 *Economic Prosperity and Food Security*

Is there any association visible between GDP per capita and PoU? Are countries that increased their income also able to reduce PoU? To answer these questions, Figure 4 shows that all countries grew and improved in terms of reduction in PoU. In 1991, relatively poor countries such as Ethiopia, Dijbouti, Mozambique, Chad, Rwanda and Angola had PoUs higher than 50%. In 2015, all countries achieved PoUs well below 50%. Overall, PoU declined with per capita income in 1991 as well as in 2015,

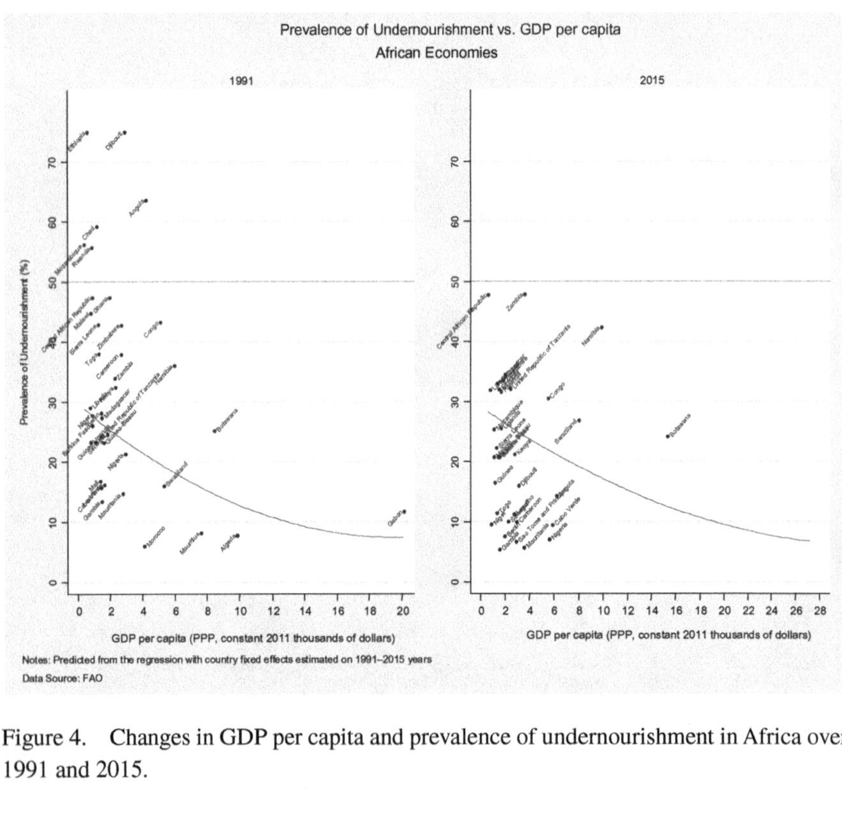

Figure 4. Changes in GDP per capita and prevalence of undernourishment in Africa over 1991 and 2015.

though the elasticity with respect to per capita GDP has been low — higher in the latest year. While some poor countries remained in the low per capita GDP and high PoU zone (e.g. Central African Republic), some with relatively large income countries — notably Botswana, Swaziland, Namibia and Congo– have higher PoUs. There is, however, a lot of variation around the regression line towards lower per capita GDP level: Liberia, Madagascar, Zimbabwe, Ethiopia and Rwanda all have slightly higher-than-expected PoUs, Siera Leone, Malawi and Kenya have slightly lower-than-expected PoUs while Mozambique and Uganda are almost on the regression line.

4. Model and Estimation Methods

To systematically assess association of African income and its components, prices, population growth, remittances, access to electricity, improved water sources and sanitation with food insecurity measures, this paper uses a panel-data regression approach with annual data from between 1990–1992 to 2014–2016 for 54 countries. The panel data approach uses variation between countries and over time.

I hypothesize that food insecurity is negatively related to income and its components, any inflow of remittance, and access to electricity, improved water sources, sanitation and road density, but positively related to prices and population growth. In this paper, I model a reduced functional form of food insecurity equation[5] as follows:

$$
\begin{aligned}
lnFIS_{i,t}^{j} &= \beta_1 lnY_{i,t-1} + \beta_2 \ln FA_{i,t-1} + \beta_3 lnP_{i,t-1} + \beta_4 lnPopgrowth_{i,t} \\
&\quad + \beta_5 X_{i,t} + \gamma_i + \tau_t + \varepsilon_{i,t}
\end{aligned}
$$

[5]Specific function form is unknown and, therefore, it is reasonable to assume a log-log functional form for this equation. As our dependent variables are 3-year averages, I have not included a lagged dependent variable as a regressor in the food insecurity equation. However, separate regressions (not shown in this paper) with lagged dependent variables. The results validate the assumption that the current level of food insecurity is influenced by past levels of food insecurity. Also, other variables such as development assistance received (*oda*), foreign direct investment inflows (*fdi*), and other forms of prices (domestic price index and its variability) were tried but not included in the final version of the model due to data unavailability and noises.

where $FIS^{j}_{i,t}$ is the food insecurity dependent variable in separate regressions for each of the *j* measures including prevalence of undernourishment, depth of food deficit, and prevalence of food inadequacy. Subscripts *i* and *t* denote an African country and time variable.

Y is income variable and enters equation as per capita gross domestic product annual % growth (*pcgdpgrowth*) or sectoral value added (*sva*) for agriculture (*sva_agr*), manufacturing (*sva_ind*) and services (*sva_ser*). *sva_agr, sva_ind, and sva_ser* are measured in constant 2010 US dollar terms.

The *FA* variable denotes food availability or supply captured through average food production (*afp*) measured as 3-year averages of constant international dollar per person. *P* is the price variable and enters equation in the form of inflation rate (*inf*) which is based on consumer prices index (CPI). *Popgrowth* variable is annual population growth in percentages.

The *X* variables include a set of other explanatory variables including personal remittances received as percentage of GDP (*remit*), access to electricity (*elec*), access to improved water sources (*water*), and road density (*roaden*). The variables *elec* and *water* are defined as percentage of population with access and *roaden* is defined as road density per 100 square kilometres of land area. *Remit* enters in log-natural form while *elec*, *water*, and *roaden* in their level. γ is country fixed effect, τ is time trend, $\varepsilon_{i,t}$ is a stochastic error term. β's are coefficients to be estimated, and all other variables are as defined above.

Pooled Cross-Sectional Ordinary Least Squares (PCOLS), Fxed Effect (FE) and the Random Effects (REs) estimators are natural approaches for estimation. However, one of the criticisms of these approaches is presence of endogeneity that potentially occurs either or through a combination of an omitted variable that is correlated with some regressors or the dependent variable and at least one of the independent variables are determined simultaneously in a system, or the presence of measurement error in at least one of the regressors. In the presence of potential endogeneity, estimates may not be efficient or consistent.[6] Some

[6]In the presence of endogeneity, an Instrumental Variable (IV) or General Method of Moments (GMMs) regression approach is used to consistently estimate the coefficients. However, applications of such techniques require additional variables and longer data series. I note that despite the large coverage of countries and years, some of the variables

explanatory variables such as *pcgdpgrowth* in the food insecurity equation might be endogenous. However, the aim of this paper is to establish association and not causal effects. For the sake of simplicity, I assume that there is no reverse causality running from explanatory variables to dependent variables, and to reduce the risk of endogeneity from reverse causation, I use the lagged values of suspected variables. Thus, the estimation strategy adopted in this paper is use all the three approaches and test for their suitability.

For all the three dependent variables, four model specifications were run. I use *pcgdpgrowth* and *sva* variables in separate specifications. This is done to avoid highly collinear variables in the same model. Specification 1 includes only *pcgdpgrowth,* but excludes sva variables, with all other variables remaining the same. Specification 2 adds *elec* variable in Specification 1. Specification 3 includes three *sva*-related variables (*sva_agr, sva_ind and sva_ser*), *but* excludes *pcgdpgrowth* from Specification 2. Assuming that the access to electricity, improved water sources, and road density are strongly correlated with the *pcgdpgrowth*, Specification 4 does not include any income variables but only *elec*, *water* and *roaden*.

The results from PCOLS, FE and RE approaches were similar — though not the same.[7] Two tests of suitability choice between PCOLS vs FE, and FE vs RE were conducted. Based on the evidence, use of fixed effects regression approach was finalized and reported in Tables 4–6 of Section 5. The results for other approaches can be obtained upon request.

5. Results

Tables 4–6 show results for the factors associated with prevalence of undernourishment, depth of food deficit, and prevalence of food inadequacy, respectively.

---

have large numbers of observations missing making it hard to use sophisticated techniques.

[7]One of the departures in the result was that agricultural along with industry and service sector shares of output were not significant in the random effects.

5.1. *Economic Growth*

Consistent across all the specifications, a higher per capita GDP growth is significantly associated with reduction in the prevalence of undernourishment, depth of food deficit, prevalence of food inadequacy, and thus, with improved food security. While statistically significant at 1% level of significance, the degree of association captured through elasticity is quite low. For instance, *ceteris paribus*, a 10% increase in the per capita GDP growth is associated with reductions in the PoU, DoFD and PoFA, respectively, at 0.05%, 0.04% and 0.03%. This suggests that the extent to which economic growth should improve food security situation is very low.

Next, I consider major sectoral components of GDP. The negative and significant coefficient for agricultural value added to GDP means that after controlling for other variables in Specification 3 of Tables 4–6, higher growth of agricultural output is associated with larger reductions in PoU, DoFD and PoFA. The statistical as well as economic importance of agricultural output is very significant. A 1% higher agricultural output is associated with reductions in PoU and PoFA by 0.23%, and in DoFD by 0.29%. The other two sectors, industry and services, are not significant in any of the equations. This implies that while contribution of industry and service sector outputs are important for the economy to grow, it does not significantly contribute to food security in Africa.

5.2. *Food Production*

Highly significant and large negative coefficients of average food production show that higher food supply is essential for food security. The result is consistent across all specifications and all the indicators. The elasticity of supply w.r.t. food security indicators of access varies from –0.34% for PoFA to −1.32% for DoFD.

5.3. *Inflation Rate*

On average, higher inflation rates[8] mean significantly higher levels of PoU, DoFD and PoFA — the degree of association is weak though

---

[8] In other specifications (not reported here, but can be obtained from author upon request), I also used domestic price index and its variability in place of inflation rate. The results

Table 4. Panel data fixed effects regression results for prevalence of undernourishment.

Explanatory variables	**Spec 1**	**Spec 2**	**Spec 3**	**Spec 4**
Ln(Afp(t–1))	−1.163***	−0.931***	−0.429**	−1.048***
	(0.217)	(0.196)	(0.179)	(0.207)
Ln(pcgdpgrowth (t–1))	−0.005***	−0.002		
	(0.001)	(0.002)		
Ln(sav_agr (t–1))			*−0.233***	
			(0.114)	
Ln(sav_ind (t–1))			−0.010	
			(0.128)	
Ln(sav_ser (t–1))			−0.102	
			(0.122)	
Ln(inf (t–1))	0.0001**	0.0002***	0.000	0.000
	(0.0001)	(0.0001)	(0.001)	(0.001)
Ln(popgrowth (t))	0.150***	0.057	0.049	0.028
	(0.051)	(0.073)	(0.069)	(0.047)
Ln(remit (t))	−0.042**	−0.045*	−0.043*	0.002
	(0.021)	(0.023)	(0.023)	(0.012)
Elect (t)		−0.012**	−0.005	−0.000
		(0.004)	(0.004)	(0.005)
Roadden(t)				−0.015***
				(0.003)
Water(t)				−0.021***
				(0.006)
Constant	8.634***	7.931***	12.575***	9.727***
	(1.051)	(0.913)	(2.140)	(1.017)
Observations (*N**T*)	656	638	571	309
R-squared	0.405	0.533	0.527	0.742
Number of country	41	41	38	35

Note: Dependent variable prevalence of undernourishment is in log-natural form. Number of observations vary across specifications due to missing values in the variables. Country specific fixed effects are adjusted for robust variance-covariance matrix of the estimators (VCE) after model fitting. Robust standard errors in parentheses. $^{***}p < 0.01$, $^{**}p < 0.05$, $^{*}p < 0.1$.

Table 5. Panel data fixed effects regression results for depth of food deficit.

Explanatory variables	**Spec 1**	**Spec 2**	**Spec 3**	**Spec 4**
Ln(Afp(t–1))	−1.315***	−1.058***	−0.483**	−1.033***
	(0.249)	(0.222)	(0.219)	(0.232)
Ln(pcgdpgrowth (t–1))	−0.004*	−0.001		
	(0.002)	(0.002)		
Ln(sav_agr (t–1))			−0.288**	
			(0.140)	
Ln(sav_ind (t–1))			−0.027	
			(0.144)	
Ln(sav_ser (t–1))			−0.090	
			(0.142)	
Ln(inf (t–1))	0.0002**	0.0003***	0.000	0.000
	(0.000)	(0.000)	(0.001)	(0.001)
Ln(popgrowth (t))	0.142**	0.049	0.032	0.016
	(0.064)	(0.092)	(0.079)	(0.051)
Ln(remit (t))	−0.053**	−0.052*	−0.050*	−0.003
	(0.025)	(0.028)	(0.026)	(0.014)
Elect (t)		−0.012**	−0.004	0.002
		(0.005)	(0.005)	(0.006)
Roadden(t)				−0.017***
				(0.003)
Water(t)				−0.025***
				(0.006)
Constant	11.170***	10.413***	15.911***	11.696***
	(1.229)	(1.062)	(2.619)	(1.128)
Observations ($N*T$)	736	718	651	335
R-squared	0.393	0.492	0.469	0.673
Number of country	43	43	40	37

Note: Dependent variable depth of food deficit is in log-natural form. Number of observations vary across specifications due to missing values in the variables. Country specific fixed effects are adjusted for robust variance-covariance matrix of the estimators (VCE) after model fitting. Robust standard errors in parentheses. $***p < 0.01$, $**p < 0.05$, $*p < 0.1$.

Table 6. Panel data fixed effects regression results for prevalence of food inadequacy.

Explanatory variables	**Spec 1**	**Spec 2**	**Spec 3**	**Spec 4**
Ln(Afp(t–1))	−1.029***	−0.817***	−0.359**	−0.817***
	(0.202)	(0.177)	(0.162)	(0.176)
Ln(pcgdpgrowth (t–1))	−0.003*	−0.001		
	(0.002)	(0.002)		
Ln(sav_agr (t–1))			−0.229**	
			(0.092)	
Ln(sav_ind (t–1))			−0.016	
			(0.108)	
Ln(sav_ser (t–1))			−0.083	
			(0.108)	
Ln(inf (t–1))	0.0001**	0.0002***	0.000	0.000
	(0.0001)	(0.0001)	(0.001)	(0.001)
Ln(popgrowth (t))	0.126**	0.050	0.035	0.024
	(0.049)	(0.070)	(0.058)	(0.039)
Ln(remit (t))	−0.038**	−0.036*	−0.034*	0.000
	(0.019)	(0.020)	(0.018)	(0.009)
Elect (t)		−0.010**	−0.003	0.001
		(0.004)	(0.004)	(0.004)
Roadden(t)				−0.012***
				(0.003)
Water(t)				−0.020***
				(0.005)
Constant	8.263***	7.620***	12.139***	8.719***
	(0.989)	(0.842)	(1.753)	(0.872)
Observations (*N*T*)	711	693	626	320
R-squared	0.402	0.518	0.508	0.713
Number of country	42	42	39	36

Note: Dependent variable prevalence of food inadequacy is in log-natural form. Number of observations vary across specifications due to missing values in the variables. Country specific fixed effects are adjusted for robust variance-covariance matrix of the estimators (VCE) after model fitting. Robust standard errors in parentheses. $^{***}p < 0.01$, $^{**}p < 0.05$, $^{*}p < 0.1$.

(Specifications 1 and 2 only). However, result is not consistent across all specifications. When controlling for sectoral output, population growth, remittances received, access to electricity or improved water and road density, inflation rate does not show significant associations (Specifications 3 and 4).

5.4. *Population Growth*

Population growth is significant and has positive coefficient with reasonably higher magnitude (Specification 1). This means that accelerated population growth is associated with a deterioration in food security situations.

5.5. *Remittances*

The results establish that higher share of received personal remittances in the GDP is significantly associated with the lower level of food insecurity. A 1% increase in the received personal remittances as % of GDP is associated with reduction of over 0.04% PoU, 0.05% DoFD and over 0.03% PoFA. This result complements the literature on the productive uses of remittances[9] and their positive role in reducing the risks of households' food insecurity directly by increasing food consumption or indirectly by reducing food price shocks (Nguyen and Winters, 2011; Mango *et al.*, 2014; Combes *et al.*, 2014).

---

show that price index is not significantly associated with the food security measures. However, variability in the domestic food index is significantly associated with higher depth of food deficit, and higher prevalence of food inadequacy.

[9]In other specifications (not reported here, but can be obtained from author upon request), I also used foreign direct investment net inflows as % of GDP and Net Official Development Assistance (ODA) received (% of GNI) to supplement remittances. However, both the variables were not significant in any of the specifications. Considering data availability issues and its indirect effect on per capita GDP and its composition, I decided not to include them in the results presented in this paper.

5.6. *Access to Electricity, Improved Water Sources and Road Density*

Access to electricity (Specification 2), access to water sources and road density (Specification 4) have significantly negative association with food insecurity measures. This means that better electrification, improvements in the access to water and better road infrastructure coverage might help to improve food security, possibly through improvement in health, reductions in the population growth and transport connectivity.

6. Conclusions

The main finding of this chapter is that increase in food availability through increased food production, agricultural output share, aggregate per capita income growth, personal remittances received and better infrastructure are key factors to contribute in reducing food insecurity in Africa. Faster population growth and rising prices can deteriorate food security situation.

This paper uses three indicators, prevalence of undernourishment, depth of food deficit and prevalence of food inadequacy to measure access dimension of food insecurity. The data for up to 59 African countries from 1990 to 2016 was studied. The evidence indicates that aggregate economic growth is not sufficient to deliver improved food security, but a sustained improvement in the agricultural output and productivity through investments in infrastructure and technological innovations are required. In this way, agricultural output can be increased without impacting on high inflation rate, particularly food inflation.

This study is not free from limitations related to data issues, soundness of methodologies and choice of exhaustive sets of regressors. First, the series of variables have a number of missing observations that reduce number of observations included in the regression by more than half in some of the specifications. Second, the assumption of no endogeneity is strong and effects nature of the causal relationship. Third, several potential regressors are not included in the model due to data limitations. This might affect the analysis by imputing omitted variable bias.

Despite outlined limitations, this paper contributes to the literature on United Nations' SDG goal 2 "end hunger, achieve food security and improved nutrition, and promote sustainable agriculture" by providing empirical evidence on factors associated with undernourishment and food inadequacy in Africa. The results, that agricultural productivity and sustainable food production are necessary to improve food security, complement United Nations' SDGs' targets.

References

Barrett, C. (2010) "Measuring Food Insecurity", *Science*, Vol. 327, pp. 825–828.

Carletto, C., Zezza, A. and R. Banerjee (2013) "Towards Better Measurement of Household Food Security: Harmonizing Indicators and the Role of Household Surveys", *Global Food Security*, Vol. 2, pp. 30–40.

Combes, J. L., Ebeke, C. H., Etoundi, S. M. N. and T. U. Yogo (2014) "Are Remittances and Foreign Aid a Hedge Against Food Price Shocks in Developing Countries?" *World Development*, Vol. 54, pp. 81–98.

FAO, IFAD and WFP (2012) *The State of Food Insecurity in the World 2012: Economic Growth is Necessary but not Sucient to Accelerate Reduction of Hunger and Malnutrition*. Rome: Food and Agriculture Organization of the United Nations.

FAO, IFAD and WFP (2013) *The State of Food Insecurity in the World 2013: The Multiple Dimensions of Food Security*. Rome: Food and Agriculture Organization of the United Nations.

FAO, IFAD and WFP (2015) *The State of Food Insecurity in the World 2015: Meeting the 2015 International Hunger Targets: Taking Stock of Uneven Progress*. Rome: Food and Agriculture Organization of the United Nations.

Jones, A. D., Ngure, F. M., Pelto, G. and S. L. Young (2013) "What are We Assessing When We Measure Food Security? A Compendium and Review of Current Metrics", *Advanced Nutrition*, Vol. 4, pp. 481–505.

Mango, N., Zamasiya, B., Makate, C., Nyikahadzoi, K. and S. Siziba (2014) "Factors Influencing Household Food Security Among Smallholder Farmers in the Mudzi District of Zimbabwe", *Development Southern Africa*, Vol. 31, No. 4, pp. 625–640.

Nguyen, M. C. and P. Winters (2011) "The Impact of Migration on Food Consumption Patterns: The Case of Vietnam", *Food Policy*, Vol. 36, No. 1, pp. 71–87.

Chapter 10

Agricultural Research, Technology and Nutrition in Sub-Saharan Africa

Raghav Gaiha[*,‡] **and Shantanu Mathur**[†,§]

[*]*University of Manchester, UK*
[†]*International Fund for Agricultural Development, Italy*
[‡]*raghavdasgaiha@gmail.com*
[§]*s.mathur@ifad.org*

Abstract

The objective of this study is to examine the relationships between agricultural research, technology and nutrition in Sub-Saharan Africa (SSA), drawing upon a rich and insightful literature. African agriculture has the lowest productivity compared with other regions of the world. Agricultural development has enormous potential to make a significant contribution to reducing malnutrition and associated ill health. An assessment is carried out through a review of a large number of studies. These examined the factors determining adoption of innovative agricultural technology; their benefits and the underlying mechanisms; sustainability of the benefits; empowerment of women farmers and child nutrition; and the prospects of youth employment in agriculture and elsewhere. A case is then made for greater investment in agricultural research.

Keywords: Agricultural research, technology, production and diet diversity, nutrition, Sub-Saharan Africa.

1. Introduction

African agriculture has the lowest productivity (output per hectare) when compared to other regions of the world. The Green Revolution observed in Asia did not occur in Africa for reasons such as the different institutional context, greater diversity in cropping patterns (requiring higher investments in research), limited physical infrastructure, particularly irrigation, and defective rural financial systems (Mellor, 2014). Today, the consensus on agricultural development in Africa concerns the adoption of the Green Revolution package and the "classical" pathway of modernization — intensification based on modern inputs (improved seeds and inorganic fertilizers). This development option was supported by international research agencies and adopted by governments. There is, however, growing evidence of difficulties in ensuring the sustainability of such a model (Jayne *et al.*, 2014). It relies on non-renewable fossil fuels and the efficiency of costly fertilizers is reduced by soil degradation in many regions of the continent. This soil degradation is a consequence of continuous cultivation and the lack of crop rotation where high population densities exist, resulting in soil acidification and deficiencies in soil organic carbon and micronutrients.

Agricultural research has generated several kinds of technology with high potentials for impact, but the expected impact on farmers' productivity, livelihood and quality of life has not been fully realized. Institutional innovations are needed to improve productivity and make public agricultural institutions more responsive to markets, more accountable to the communities they serve and better recognized as an important tool for achieving economic growth. Other studies have shown that huge productivity gains are possible and accrue where governments allocate the necessary resources to agricultural research and development. In Sub-Saharan Africa (SSA), however, public investment in agriculture is still far below what is needed, despite commitments by African governments to allocate 10% of their public spending on it. The challenge is to develop technology that is relevant to small farmers and to enable them to transform their farms into viable small businesses that make a vital contribution to local and national economies. This calls for client-oriented agricultural research.

FAO defines prevalence of undernourishment as the percentage of the population with average daily caloric intake over the year less than the minimum daily requirement. Depth of undernourishment measures the degree to which caloric intake of the undernourished falls below minimum dietary requirements. In a recent contribution, Pande (2018) draws attention to the slow progress in reducing undernourishment in Africa and its sub-region, SSA. Using 3-year averages of FAO estimates, the total Number of Undernourished (NoU) declined from 1010.7 million in 1990–1992 to 792.5 million in 2014–2016. Thus, the world had over 218.2 million fewer undernourished persons in 2014–2016 than in 1990–1992. The Proportion of Undernourished (PoU) declined from 18.6 to 10.8%, as also the Depth of Undernourishment (DoU) from 138 kcal per capita per day to 81 kcal. In contrast to the global progress, Africa remained home to 230 million NoUs in 2014–2016 — much higher than the 181.7 million in 1990–1992. In terms of global share of all the NoUs, Africa has over 29% now as compared to just below 18% in 1990–1992. The PoU, however, recorded a slow reduction from 27.6% to 19.8%, as also DoU from 204 to 151 kcal. Thus, undernourishment remains a serious concern for Africa.

Although difficult to ascertain whether it is a trend reversal, two recent FAO reports (2017a, 2017b) show a rise in hunger globally as well as in Africa. The NoU in the world suffering from chronic food deprivation began to rise in 2014 — going from 775 million people to 777 million in 2015 — and is now estimated to have increased further, to 815 million in 2016. The stagnation of the global average of the PoU from 2013 to 2015 is the result of two offsetting changes at the regional level: in SSA, the share of undernourished people increased, while there was a continued decline in Asia in the same period. However, in 2016, the PoU increased in most regions except Northern Africa, Southern Asia, Eastern Asia, Central America and the Caribbean. The deterioration was most severe in SSA and South-Eastern Asia (FAO, 2017a, 2017b).[1]

---

[1] As noted in *The Economist* (November 11–17, 2017), "too many economies depend on commodity exports. In 2016, weak commodity prices were partly responsible for a slowdown in

Undernutrition is widespread and a key reason for poor child health in many developing countries. In SSA, around 40% of children under the age of five suffer from stunted growth, that is, severely reduced height-for-age relative to their growth potential. Stunting is a result of periods of undernutrition in early childhood, and it has been found to have a series of adverse long-term effects in those who survive childhood. It is negatively associated with mental development, with human capital accumulation, with adult health, and with economic productivity and income levels in adulthood (Larsen and Lilleør, 2017).

Vitamin A deficiency is associated with higher risk of morbidity and mortality, and ocular disorders such as night blindness, xerophthalmia and blindness, affecting infants, children and women during pregnancy and lactation. African regions account for the greatest number of preschool children with night blindness and for more than one quarter of all children with sub-clinical vitamin A deficiency (Hotz *et al.*, 2012; WHO, 2016).

The central premise is that agricultural development has enormous potential to make significant contribution in reducing malnutrition and the associated ill health. With its close links to both the immediate causes of undernutrition (diets, feeding practices and health) and its underlying determinants (such as income, education, access to Water, Sanitation and Hygiene (WASH) and health services and gender equity), the agriculture sector can play a strong role in improving nutrition outcomes (Gillespie and van den Bold, 2017).[2]

Several different pathways between agriculture and nutrition are identified with some overlap.[3] Agriculture generates income that can be spent on nutrition-enhancing goods and services, although agriculture is generally a more important source of income for the poor and undernourished, both directly, and through the so-called "multiplier effects" on other sectors. Because of various market failures, however, farmers may choose to grow food that they consume, thus rendering agriculture a special sector for nutrition, but also opening up complex dynamic policy trade-offs.

economic growth across SSA to 1.4%, its most sluggish pace in more than two decades. With the population growing by about 3% a year, people on average got poorer last year", p. 4.

[2]For a cogent and comprehensive but somewhat sceptical assessment, see Timmer (2015).

[3]Six pathways are identified in Gillespie and van den Bold (2017).

The macroeconomic linkages between agricultural production conditions and food prices drive consumption decisions. Few linkages go beyond price and income to focus on the linkages between child undernutrition and maternal socio-economic and nutritional status. Agricultural production conditions can affect women's decision-making power and control of nutrition-relevant resources, as well as their ability to manage the care of young children, which is of huge importance for nutrition (Gillespie and van den Bold, 2017).

Food systems are changing rapidly. Globalization, trade liberalization and rapid urbanization have led to major shifts in the availability, affordability and acceptability of different types of food, which has driven a nutrition transition in many countries in the developing world. Food production has become more capital-intensive and supply chains have grown longer as basic ingredients undergo multiple transformations. Expansion of fast food outlets and supermarkets has resulted in dietary shifts. The consumption of low nutritional quality, energy-dense, ultra-processed food and drinks, and fried snacks and sweets has risen dramatically in the past decade. Combined with increasingly sedentary lifestyles, rates of overweight and obesity and associated diet-related chronic diseases have spiked (Carletto *et al.*, 2015).

The concomitant shift to the more market-oriented nature of agricultural policies means that agricultural technology and markets play a more important role in determining food prices and rural incomes, and more food is consumed from the marketplace rather than from own production. The greater market orientation of food production and consumption has increased the bidirectional links between agriculture and nutrition: agriculture still affects nutrition, but food and nutritional demands increasingly affect agriculture. Increasing demands for energy-intensive products exacerbate environmental impacts of food value chains: for example, excessive use of agricultural chemicals to extract more dietary energy from every hectare while contaminating the very food it produces, along with the groundwater and soil; and the greenhouse gas emissions from livestock industries to feed the ever-increasing demand for meat and dairy products. Weather related shocks could result in greater crop failures and higher food prices (Carletto *et al.*, 2015).

Evidence also points to improved impacts on nutrition if agricultural interventions are targeted to women and when specific work is done around women's empowerment (Gillespie and van den Bold, 2017).

Agriculture has a substantial role in meeting the youth employment challenge facing Africa, given the inability of the urban economy to absorb the young entrants to the labour force in rural areas. There will be vast opportunities for the innovative young people in agricultural systems as they adapt to a range of challenges in the near future. These challenges relate to raising productivity in a sustainable way, integration into emerging high value chains and healthy diets (Suttie, 2015).

The focus of the study is therefore on whether agricultural research through improved technology directly or indirectly will help improve nutrition in SSA (or more broadly in Africa). A thorough review of recent evidence is carried out and a case is made for greater investment in agricultural research and complementary measures. Other related themes explored here are potential of innovative women and young farmers for greater productivity and better nutritional outcomes. An assessment is given of how diversified food production, value chains and food preferences determine nutritional outcomes. Attention is given to sustainability of agricultural technologies. A thorough review of returns from agricultural research serves as the basis for greater investment in it. This chapter ends with a summary of the major findings from a broad policy perspective.

2. Determinants of Technology Adoption

The extant literature has focused on determinants of technology adoption such as relaxation of credit, input and infrastructural constraints as well as building awareness of and providing easier access to information on new technologies. In particular, the evidence identifies empirically formal and informal channels that affect the decision process of technology adoption. Formal channels include extension services, information campaigns, demonstration trials by extension agents, membership of agricultural associations and participation in research programme activities (Hasan *et al.*, 2015). Informal channels refer to all social networks of smallholder farmers, learning from neighbours' experiences, learning-by-doing and spill-over effects (Garbero *et al.*, 2016).

Adoption follows a progressive decision path. Lindner *et al.* (1982) were the first to analyze the time lag from availability of new technology to definite adoption decision. They identify three constituents of the entire time lag: the first is the awareness lag, when farmers discover the existence of new technology; the second is the evaluation lag, when farmers try out the innovation; and the third and last lag is the ultimate decision of adoption or dis-adoption of the new technology. Because of lack of data, these authors evaluate the impact of distance from source of information and education on the first two lags. They find that the lower the distance from source of information, the higher is the probability of being aware and trying out technologies and that education partly offsets the effect of distance, implying that more educated farmers can have access to information despite the distance. Subsequent studies examine awareness and adoption rates (Diagne and Demont, 2007; Asuming-Brempong *et al.*, 2011; Simtowe *et al.*, 2012), others (e.g. Moser and Barrett, 2006) focus on the try-out and adoption rates, while Lambrecht *et al.* (2014) examine the determining factors of all the three lags.

Diagne and Demont (2007), in their analysis of both the determinants and impact of adoption, recognize the existence of two main sources of bias, namely *non-exposure bias* and *positive selection bias*. The former is due to the fact that, given the limited initial diffusion of a new technology, farmers who have not been exposed to it cannot adopt it, but they might have adopted it had they been exposed to it. Non-exposure bias may thus underestimate the true adoption rate of the entire population, given the limited diffusion of new technology. Positive selection bias is instead due to the fact that farmers voluntarily get in touch with extension services and participate in the overall exposure to information diffusion of new technology. Hence, farmers who decide to get involved in the information accumulation process of new technologies are more likely to adopt them and are thus systematically different from those who do not self-select in the exposure. Moreover, some farmers or communities are targeted by research programmes and extension services, whereas others are not, and targeted populations have higher probability to adopt new technologies. Positive selection bias is therefore likely to overestimate the true adoption rate of the entire population. The authors use the Average Treatment Effect (ATE) method.[4]

---

[4]In order to control for these two sources of bias, the authors implement the Average Treatment Effect (ATE) method, which allows for the estimation of the population mean

Studies based on measurement of ATE show a population adoption gap, meaning that the estimated demand for new technology is quite high, but its diffusion does not cover the entire population and does not satisfy the potential demand. Diagne and Demont (2007) estimate the adoption gap of NERICA in Cote d'Ivoire equal to 18%, where only 4% of farmers are jointly exposed and have adopted NERICA. The adoption gap of NERICA in Ghana, estimated by Asuming-Brempong *et al.* (2011), is instead equal to 44% and that of improved groundnut in Malawi, estimated by Simtowe *et al.* (2012), is 12%.

Specifically, the main factors that determine the awareness of a new technology include social characteristics of farmers and agro-ecological conditions in a targeted area. In particular, farmers who are more aware of a technology have higher education (Simtowe *et al.,* 2012), live in proximity to research institutions and universities (Asuming-Brempong *et al.*, 2011) and have more social capital, which includes participation in collective actions, membership of non-agricultural organizations and network of credit channels (Lambrecht *et al.*, 2014; Yokouchi and Saito, 2016).[5]

Both social characteristics and economic constraints determine the try-out step. This is positively influenced by factors such as learning from others, higher liquidity (Moser and Barrett, 2006), and access to information and extension services (Lambrecht *et al.*, 2014; Bezu *et al.*, 2014; Kikulwe *et al.*, 2012). In particular, younger farmers living near the market, with social capital and labour endowments, are more likely to experiment with a new technology (Lambrecht *et al.*, 2014). The continued adoption step is largely influenced by economic constraints, demographic actors and dissemination mechanisms, such as extension (Asuming-Brempong *et al.*, 2011). Following Moser and Barrett (2006), in addition to liquidity, social capital (learning from others) and peer effects (attitude of conformity to neighbouring farmers' behaviour) play an important role in determining continued adoption. A third study (Lambrecht *et al.*, 2014),

---

adoption outcome and the Average Treatment Effect on the Treated (ATT). The difference between these two components gives the population non-exposure bias, also called the population adoption gap, which provides useful information on what would have been the adoption rate if the diffusion of technology had been complete. For a more detailed exposition, see Garbero *et al.* (2016).

[5]For a review of the econometric methods used, see Garbero *et al.* (2016).

however, reports that the continued adoption decision is mainly determined by credit and liquidity constraint, and by the quality of extension services.[6] The latter facilitates the adoption decision process allowing farmers to continue with the new technology, after the trial period. Economic and financial constraints hamper continued adoption.

While the decision process is essentially dynamic, and requires a dynamic framework, the majority of studies have relied on cross-sectional datasets, which do not allow for an analysis of a dynamic learning process. Also, the ones that do employ panel data, do not examine the dynamic decision making process. For example, Kikulwe *et al.* (2012) simply determine the factors of adoption at the baseline year. Garbero *et al.* (2016) fill this gap. It adds to existing knowledge, by first analyzing the determinants of technology adoption with a special focus on the dynamics of the adoption decision process. The role of path or state dependence is assessed, namely, the role of past experience in the adoption decision process. This aspect has not been sufficiently analyzed in the agricultural technology adoption literature with the exception of Cowan and Gunby (1996). Moreover, the impact of agricultural technology on farmers' welfare and agricultural productivity is estimated, using observational data and non-experimental methods in a dynamic framework and 3 years' panel data from Uganda. The endogeneity of the adoption decision is taken into account along with selection on both observables and unobservables. Following Doss (2006), Garbero *et al.* (2016) examine the drivers of technology adoption and its impact in a broader context. For the estimation of technology adoption, in addition to the most common socio-economic explanatory variables, it controls for the technology adoption decision realized in the previous year in order to examine preferences of households towards technology adoption in a dynamic setting. For the impact assessment, the authors estimate the effects of technology on poverty, and other welfare indicators by taking into account households' adoption decision histories.[7]

State dependence is defined as the direct effect of technology adoption status in the previous period on the current or contemporary technology adoption status. The measure of technology used is improved seeds. A key

---

[6]For an insightful study of effectiveness of different providers of extension services in Uganada, see Hasan *et al.* (2015).

[7]For two related studies, see Asfaw *et al.* (2012a, 2012b).

question that this study seeks to answer is whether state dependence is spurious or real. In the former case, state dependence is due to observed or unobserved households' heterogeneity; whereas in the latter, state dependence actually drives the technology adoption process.

Characteristics included in different specifications are: household size, sex and age of household head, number of dependents in the household, parcel size in hectares, household distance to village centre, distance from village centre to agricultural extension centre, household distance to a major road, whether the household head attended secondary school, asset index, occurrence of irregular rains, occurrence of erosion on arable land, source of technical agricultural information by district, agro-ecologic zone of the household, season and region of the household. State-of-the-art econometric methods are used to examine state dependence of technology adoption.[8]

The state dependence of technology adoption is confirmed. The presence of state dependence means that previous choice in the type of technology used affects current choice. A household that adopted improved seeds in the period t-1 has a 4.79 percentage points higher probability of adopting improved seeds again in the period t compared to another which did not adopt improved seeds in the period t-1. Moreover, the initial technology adoption decision significantly influences current technology adoption decision, even more than the lagged adoption (7.8%).

Among household characteristics, the probability of technology adoption increases if the household's head is male and better educated, and household size is larger; parcel size does not have any impact. Somewhat surprisingly, distances from the village centre to the market and household distance to a major road have no effect on adoption while distance from village centre to agricultural extension services lowered adoption. Extension plays a key role in facilitating adoption of new technology. Among all sources of extension advice, only extension services provided by National Agricultural Advisory Services (NAADS) have a positive effect on adoption. Regions characterized by tropic-cool/sub-humid agro-ecological zone are negatively associated with adoption of new technology.

---

[8]For technical details, see Garbero *et al.* (2016).

3. Impact

Several studies have sought to analyze the determinants of uptake and the reasons why farmers adopt technologies (Doss, 2006) and their causal effects on agricultural productivity. These studies have focused mostly on the impact of yield-increasing and cost-reducing technologies. Nevertheless, some of the yield-increasing technologies are also associated with quality-improving technologies (Kabunga *et al.*, 2014), which consist of new seeds varieties that not only increase productivity and reduce cost per unit of output, but also allow for a better quality of agricultural output in terms of nutritional characteristics and taste.

The relevant literature has also documented the pathways through which agricultural research enhances standard of living conditions and welfare outcomes in developing countries, namely, higher agricultural productivity, lower production cost, reduction of food prices, higher wages and employment, and lower losses due to diseases or unfavourable climatic conditions. Hence, both producers and consumers are likely to benefit. A selection of these studies is reviewed below, drawing upon Garbero *et al.* (2016) and other research.

A recent meta-analysis by Stewart *et al.* (2015), examining the impact of agricultural technology, emphasizes that the majority of the studies reviewed are plagued by methodological challenges and mostly analyse the role of agricultural research using observational data and non-experimental designs. In the absence of randomized experiments where farmers are randomly distributed to two groups, namely, adopters and non-adopters, farmers choose to adopt agricultural technologies on a voluntary basis, or are systematically selected by project implementers or development institutions based on their propensity to participate in the technology adoption decision. This implies that adopters and non-adopters can be systematically different, due to *self-selection* or generally selection based on observable or unobservable characteristics, which renders any assessment of the impact of adoption on welfare outcomes with *ex-post* observational data problematic.

Bezu *et al.* (2014) account for the endogeneity of input subsidy and area under improved maize to estimate the impact of households' decision to use improved maize varieties on household welfare, using a 3-year panel dataset.[9] Another notable study by Donstop-Nguezet *et al.* (2011) seeks to capture the effects of adoption of New Rice for Africa (NERICA) on productivity, income and poverty of Nigerian rice farmers.[10]

Turning to the actual magnitude of the impact of the concerned technologies, the overall effect from the reviewed studies is positive, but these impact magnitudes vary by outcome variable and are sensitive to the choice of the estimator employed. For instance, improved chick pea and pigeon pea in Tanzania lead to increases in the average expected consumption per adult equivalent by 24.6% and to 103%, respectively (Asfaw *et al.*, 2012b). However, these authors, using the same dataset but adopting a different econometric method (Asfaw *et al.*, 2012a), found that adoption of improved pigeon pea increases consumption expenditure by 31% for adopters on average and reduces the Foster-Greer-Thorbecke poverty indices, namely, the head-count index, the poverty gap and the severity of poverty index by a range of 12–13%; 8–10% and 4.4–8.1%, respectively. Some other studies assess impact of technology adoption on income of farmers and households. Bezu *et al.* (2014) found that a 1% increase in improved maize area in Malawi is associated with a 0.48% increase in income of adopters, a 0.34% increase in own maize consumption and a 0.24% increase in assets. Positive impacts on welfare are due also to size of land, while there is a negative impact of family size once the labour force is taken into account.

Tissue culture banana technology adoption in Kenya increases annual farm and household income by $500 and $662, respectively, an increase by a factor of 2 in farm income and of 89% in household income (Kabunga *et al.*, 2014). The increase in total household income represents a positive spill-over from adopters to non-adopters. Larger household sizes

---

[9]They use the control function approach and instrumental variables to correct for the endogeneity of input subsidy and improved maize variety.

[10]They use two instrumental variable-based estimators: the first is the non-parametric Wald estimator proposed by Imbens and Angrist (1994) which requires only the observed outcome variable y, the treatment status variable d, and an instrument z. The second IV-based estimator is Abadie's (2003) generalization of the LATE estimator of Imbens and Angrist (1994) to cases where the instrument z is not totally independent of the potential outcomes but will become so, conditional on x, a vector of covariates that determine the observed outcome y. However, these methods do not seem to lead to an unbiased estimate of impact given the presence of weak instruments (Garbero *et al.*, 2016).

negatively affect both per capita farm income and total household income while land size and off-farm activities exhibit a protective effect on household income only; in addition, credit constraints were found to have a negative effect on household income. Last, adoption of tissue culture banana was also found to reduce food insecurity and severe food insecurity by 0.44 and 0.32 index points, respectively.

Adoption of NERICA was also found to positively increase household income, along with other variables characterizing household demographic structure, such as gender, age and education of household head and household size in Nigeria (Dontsop-Nguezet *et al.*, 2011).

Several studies confirm that poorer and more educated households benefit more from technology adoption. This could be because the poor start from a low base and the more educated are able to use new technology more effectively. Specifically, the empirical evidence highlights the positive impact of improved seeds varieties on consumption expenditure and poverty (Asfaw *et al.*, 2012a, 2012b). Also, Bezu *et al.* (2014) find that poorer households benefit more, while differences by gender are not significant. By contrast, the impact of NERICA adoption in Nigeria is larger for educated, elderly, males in rainfed upland and lowland and in the irrigated technology areas (Donstop-Nguezet *et al.*, 2011) in addition to the poorest farmers who benefited most.

Using state-of-the-art econometric methods to account for endogeneity of technology adoption, Garbero *et al.* (2016), estimated the impact of agricultural technology adoption on per capita expenditure, poverty and maize yields in Uganda.[11] Daily per adult expenditure expressed in US$ PPP increased by 5% due to improved agricultural technology. It also led to a reduction in the likelihood of being poor by 11%. Other measures of poverty (poverty gap and poverty severity) also reduced. The impact on maize yields ranged between 21% and 28% by season. An important insight is that, with state dependence, the value of adoption for farmers increases with the level of adoption. Adequate extension services could create positive feedbacks leading to much higher adoption rates and significant welfare improvements. Yet another study that breaks new ground is Mekonnen *et al.* (2017).

[11]These methods include propensity score matching, Heckman selection model and endogenous switching regression model (ESRM). For details, see Garbero *et al.* (2016).

The major determinants of technology adoption in Ethiopia have been identified as risk aversion, perceptions about new technologies, access to extension and advisory services, and access to credit, with human capital, livestock holdings, land size, and tenure security being other socio-economic factors. However, little attention has been given to the role social networks and especially social learning play in technology adoption. Mekonnen *et al.* (2017) enrich the sparse literature by offering a fresh perspective and robust empirical evidence, based on a state-of-the-art econometric methodology. The novelty of this analysis lies in an assessment of the relative importance of networks of male and female members of the same households for social learning in technology adoption and for improved farm productivity.

Specifically, this study investigates whether individuals belonging to the same group tend to behave similarly in terms of adopting row-planting, a recent innovation in Ethiopian agriculture due to: (1) endogenous or peer effects, (2) exogenous or contextual effects and (3) correlated effects. Besides, it tests for effects of social networks on farm productivity. To overcome some of the problems related to identification, this study uses a random assignment of matches within the sample, employs non-linear as well as dynamic empirical specifications, and controls for exogenous characteristics of peers.[12]

The analysis is based on a household survey conducted by the authors between January and March 2014. The baseline survey used a mix of purposive and random sampling to select 390 households from three study sites in Oromia region in Ethiopia: Bakko-Sibu Siree, Lume-Adaa, and Hettosa-Tiyyo.

The results show that belonging to certain groups such as *iddirs* (funeral groups), maintaining relationship with network members in terms of kinship or informal forms of insurance, or a high frequency of meetings with a network member all appear to increase the probability of a network connection being an information link. Moreover, there is robust evidence of network externalities in the adoption of row-planting, especially in the case of female networks and for farm productivity. Finally, extension services and other programmes that promote agricultural innovations and

[12]For further details, see Mekonnen *et al.* (2017).

their diffusion need to identify the "right" networks to be most efficient, such as female networks in the case of row-planting. The results thus imply that investment in the formation of groups, rather than simply using existing networks, may also be worthwhile.

Agricultural growth in Ethiopia as a major contributor to overall economic growth was a remarkable occurrence for Africa, which lags in agricultural performance globally and is increasingly dependent on imported staple foods to feed its population. An understanding of the Ethiopian experience offers important lessons for the rest of Africa.

From this perspective, Bachewe *et al.* (2017) make an important contribution in two ways. (i) They identify the sources of this growth using an adjusted Solow decomposition model, which allows measurement of the extent to which modern inputs contributed to this growth. (ii) Using a set of comprehensive datasets, they offer new (and update existing) evidence on changes in modern input adoption over the 2004–2014 period. An upshot of this analysis is that, under certain conditions, significant agricultural growth can be achieved in Africa in a relatively short period. An influential view that the preconditions for fast, intensification-driven output growth might not be present in Africa is rejected. Indeed, it is argued that this situation is rapidly changing — partly driven by rapid population growth, increasing land scarcity, urbanization, better transport and communication infrastructure, higher incomes, and an emerging middle class — at least in parts of Africa. These changing incentives combined with an enabling environment might then lead to improved agricultural performance across the continent.

A methodological innovation is the modelling of simultaneous use of more than one modern input. A multinomial probit model is used to assess factors associated with adoption of only chemical fertilizer, only improved seeds, or both chemical fertilizers and improved seeds, in contrast to the reference category of adoption of neither input.[13]

Agricultural output more than doubled, due to area expansion, but, more importantly, due to significant yield increases. The increased productivity is partly explained by rapid uptake of several improved agricultural technologies. However, some of this agricultural growth cannot be

[13]For further details, see Mekonnen *et al.* (2017).

explained by increased adoption of modern inputs and other production factors. Significant growth in TFP, 2.3% per year on average, also contributed to this growth. Further, the adoption of modern technologies was rapid and their contribution to agricultural growth was especially higher in the second half of the last decade. In the first half, agricultural growth was largely driven by area expansion and TFP growth.

Major drivers for the increasing adoption of modern inputs seem to be multiple, and enabled by significantly higher expenditures in the agriculture sector. First, Ethiopia expanded agricultural extension system in the last decade, with one of the highest extension agent-to-farmer ratios in the world. Second, access to markets rose substantially. Third, improved access to education led to a significant decrease in illiteracy in rural areas. Fourth, high international prices of export products as well as improved modern input–output ratios for local crops provided better incentives for the agriculture sector over the last decade. These factors together accelerated adoption of improved technologies, and consequently agricultural productivity. However, other factors played a role as well, including good weather, better access to MFIs in rural areas, improved tenure security and a well-functioning safety net (Mekonnen *et al.*, 2017).

Gillespie and van den Bold (2017) assess welfare impacts for developing countries, based on a recent review of agriculture and nutrition links in six countries (three in South Asia, and three in SSA), as part of the Leveraging Agriculture for Nutrition in South Asia (LANSA) and Leveraging Agriculture for Nutrition in East Africa (LANEA) initiatives. Here, we confine ourselves to the latter.

LANEA illuminates agriculture–nutrition pathways in East Africa, in Kenya, Ethiopia and Uganda, countries where agriculture retains an important role. In all three countries and East Africa, research focused on agriculture as a source of food, with particularly limited research and evidence on women's participation in agriculture and their own nutrition and health status. In Ethiopia, it was difficult for households to achieve food security solely through household production. Land ownership had a positive impact on food security, with women's land tenure security particularly important in rural areas. Female-headed households were more likely to experience a decrease in asset holdings due to volatility in food prices, putting pressure on women's time. Besides, net purchasers of food were more vulnerable to food price increases, particularly the urban poor, and that, lastly, adolescent boys were favoured over adolescent girls in allocation of household resources. In Kenya, interventions to improve vegetable, Animal Source Foods (ASF), and fruit production produced mixed results, but ownership of livestock and milk consumption was associated with better nutrition outcomes. Poorer households, however, faced challenges with intensive dairy production due to high input costs. Although income from on- and off-farm employment and food-for-work was associated with better food security and variety and quantity of foods consumed, it did not always lead to improvements in nutritional status, particularly if health and child care practices were suboptimal. Taking into account the role of food prices, especially households without access to food produced locally struggled to achieve adequate food consumption, and it was difficult for them to meet nutritional requirements with their own food production, particularly when production was influenced by seasonality. Women's employment in agriculture was found to have positive impacts on nutrition in the household when women had decision-making power over resource allocation. In Uganda, evidence from randomized controlled trials showed positive impacts from biofortified crops, including orange-fleshed sweet potato, on vitamin A status among women and children. Ownership of livestock was associated with better household food security in Kampala. Evidence also showed mixed impacts on the links between women's empowerment, intrahousehold decision-making, and better nutrition outcomes.[14]

Larsen and Lilleør (2017) presented one of a few rigorous assessments of the impact on early childhood nutrition, measured as height-for-age, of an agricultural intervention that improved food security in the lean season among smallholder farmers in Northern Tanzania by providing them with a "basket" of new technology options.

The agricultural intervention is called Rural Initiatives for Participatory Agricultural Transformation (RIPAT). The specific instance of this intervention evaluated was the first RIPAT programme (RIPAT I), implemented by a local NGO, RECODA, in eight villages in Arumeru District in the Arusha Region of Northern Tanzania between 2006 and 2009. The stated overall development goal of RIPAT is to reduce poverty and improve food security among smallholder farmers by facilitating high and sustainable

[14]For a list of important contributions, see Gillespie and van den Bold (2017). More on women's empowerment, and livestock as a source of nutrition later.

levels of adoption of improved agricultural and livestock technologies disseminated.

The technology options comprise new banana cultivation techniques; new improved banana and other perennial and annual crop varieties; conservation agriculture for improved land utilization (such as minimum soil disturbance, cover crops, intercropping, rotation, and diversification of crops); post-harvesting technologies; improved animal husbandry; multipurpose trees for fodder, fruit, or firewood; soil and water conservation, including rain water harvesting; and savings groups. Each farmer was free to choose which technologies to adopt on his/her own farm according to his/her own needs, constraints and resources.

Height-for-age is a strong biological marker of the nutritional status of children during the first 1,000 days of their lives, from conception to 2 years of age. During this period, children have very high growth rates; and consequently, when subject to spells of growth faltering, children quickly fall behind the height-for-age growth curves of their peers, with limited chances of catching up subsequently.

This study, using post-treatment data, analyses whether the three-and-a-half-year-long agricultural intervention led to an improvement in the height-for-age measures among such young children. A rigorous methodology is used to determine the impact of the basket of technologies on stunting.[15] The agricultural intervention, RIPAT, improved drought resilience among the participating "children".

While investment in agriculture has a (relatively) high return on investment, in many cases, increases in food production and consumption have not contributed significantly to improvement in nutrition and health. This is in part because of lack of hygiene and sanitation and poor medical

[15]Larsen and Lilleør (2017) follow the identification strategy in Duflo (2003) and exploit the fact that height-for-age captures early-life undernutrition in the first 1,000 days, from conception to 2 years of age. A difference-in-differences comparison of cohorts conceived before and after the phase-in of the project is carried out, where only the latter cohort lived all of their first 1,000 days under full project implementation. Under the assumption of a common growth profile for all children in absence of treatment, the height-for-age measures allows the authors to control for systematic differences in nutritional levels between older children in treatment and comparison households prior to the onset of intervention activities.

services. Considering specifically agricultural interventions — mainly related to home gardening and animal/dairy production — evidence is mixed in terms of their impacts on nutrition. While there is evidence of positive impacts on intermediary nutrition outcomes, such as dietary diversity, household production and consumption, and child and maternal intake of "target" foods and micronutrients, impact on nutrition outcomes — particularly child anthropometry and micronutrient status — was much more limited, except in relation to vitamin A intake and status.

3.1. *Production Diversity, Dietary Diversity and Nutrition*

Lack of dietary diversity is viewed as the major cause of micronutrient malnutrition in Sub-Saharan Africa. Imbalanced diets resulting from consumption of mainly high carbohydrate based-diets also contribute to productivity losses and reduced educational attainment and income. Consequently, micronutrient malnutrition is currently the most critical for food and nutritional security problem as most diets are often deficient in essential vitamins and minerals. In Tanzania, for example, most rural and urban households consume mainly staples as their main food, which are high in carbohydrates, but low in micronutrients and vitamins. Staple food items increase energy availability but do not improve nutritional outcomes if not consumed together with micro-nutrient rich foods (Kennedy *et al.*, 2007).

Recent studies have attempted to establish the linkage between land use or cropping pattern and dietary diversity of households. Herforth (2010) and Jones *et al.* (2014), for example, examined the relationship between farm diversity and dietary diversity among households in African countries and conclude that there is a strong relationship between dietary and farm diversity. However, there are a few limitations. Consider the Jones *et al.* (2014) study. They used a multiple linear regression model to analyze the interlinks between farm production diversity and household dietary diversity. Although the authors found a positive relationship between the two constructs, many of the relevant covariates (education, age, location) were omitted, biasing the effect of production diversity.

Second, the data used for analysis do not account for the proportion of consumption of own household produced food and associated seasonal effects. Most importantly, production diversity cannot be treated as exogenous as it is a household choice variable.

Some of these gaps are sought to be filled by Rajendran *et al.* (2014). They hypothesize: (i) large-scale farmers have more diverse dietary patterns; (ii) higher level of education of farmers leads to positive and significant association with dietary diversity: (iii) increased diversity of crops in farmers' fields leads to more diverse diets of the households, and (iv) decision making and control of income by female headed households leads to greater dietary diversity. These hypotheses were tested using multiple linear regression models by controlling for other covariates in the model, based on Tanzanian data. The farmers were categorized into "vegetable cum maize-based households" and "only maize-based households." Farmers designated as vegetable cum maize-based households grew vegetables, maize and other staples, whereas only maize-based households were those that cultivated maize and other staple crops with no vegetables. To correct for the bias among these two groups, the authors randomly selected an equal proportion from each group — 15 farm households from each category, making a total of 30 farm households per village. Overall, 300 farm households that cultivated maize and vegetables in each of the 10 villages, selected from Babati, Kongwa and Kieto districts in Tanzania, were surveyed from July to August, 2013, using a structured questionnaire. A dietary diversity score, based on FAO guidelines (FAO, 2011), was used. The dietary diversity scores described in these guidelines consist of a simple count of food groups that a household or an individual has consumed over the preceding 24 hours recall period. 16 food groups were constructed based on local food consumption. Individual dietary diversity scores aim to reflect nutrient adequacy, whereas the Household Dietary Diversity Score (HDDS) is a snapshot of the economic ability of a household to access a variety of foods (FAO, 2011). This study used two different measurements of variables such as crop count and Simpson's Index to measure farm diversity in agricultural seasons (both dry and rainy seasons). The crop count sums the total number of different crop species cultivated by the households in a crop year (i.e. March 2012 to February 2013), whereas Simpson's Index describes evenness of distributed area under cultivation for different crop species in cropping pattern.[16] It seeks to examine the effect of crop diversity on dietary diversity of farm households.[17] Both crop count and Simpson's index were not significantly associated with dietary diversity after controlling for other covariates in both models. Covariates such as number of people in household, monthly per capita expenditure on food, net cultivated area under irrigation for all crops, proportion of total vegetables consumed from own production and decision-making and control of income by female headed households exhibited strong influences on dietary diversity. These variables positively and significantly influenced dietary diversity in both cases. Briefly, crop diversity does not influence dietary diversity after controlling for other covariates.

There are a few factors, however, that undermine the robustness of the results. These limitations are similar to the ones encountered earlier. One is the use of farm diversity as an exogenous variable. In fact, farm diversity is a response to weather and price risks (a more diversified crop portfolio protects the farmer better against such risks), and relative profitability of different crops and animal husbandry. A more refined methodology that adjusts for the endogeneity of these and other variables (the split between food and non-food expenditure) is thus needed. Another major limitation is that the analysis of nutritional impact has to go beyond groups of food commodities consumed. There is an important linking role of food value chains that encompass the preferences of vendors (including supermarkets and other retailers) and consumers. What recent literature has shown is that even the poor respond to changes in relative food prices as well as express a preference for variety in food.

A positive relationship between farm production diversity and dietary diversity is plausible, because smallholder farmers consume at home much of what they produce (Muller, 2009). However, this is more

[16] Simpson's diversity index is commonly used to measure biodiversity. High scores (close to 1) indicate high diversity, and low scores (close to 0) indicate low diversity.

[17] It used multiple linear regression models employing cross-section data collected through a primary survey. This model is designed to control for the effects of other covariates (i.e. individual and household characteristics, land ownership, irrigation, regional effects, non-farm income, expenditure on food and non-food items) in order to capture the net effect of farm diversity on dietary diversity.

plausible for a subsistence economy than one in which market transactions are prominent. Instead of producing everything at home, households can buy a variety of food in the market when they generate sufficient income. Farm diversification may contribute to income growth and stability. Besides, as the majority of smallholder households in developing countries also have off-farm income sources, the link between production diversity and diet diversity is further undermined. Finally, when relying on markets, nutrition effects in farm households will also depend on how well the markets function and who decides how farm and off-farm incomes will be allocated to food. It is well known that income in the hands of women frequently results in more nourishing food — especially for children.

Sibhatu *et al.* (2014) analyze the relationship between production and consumption diversity in smallholder farm households with data from four developing countries: Indonesia, Kenya, Ethiopia, and Malawi. These four countries were selected mainly because of availability of suitable and recent household data. The results are classified under (i) association between production and diet diversity, (ii) role of market access, and (iii) role of selling and buying food.[18] Farm production diversity is positively associated with dietary diversity, but the effect is relatively small. In the pooled sample, producing one additional crop or livestock species leads to a 0.9% increase in the number of food groups consumed. This effect, however, varies across the countries in question. In Kenya and Ethiopia, the coefficient estimates are very small and not statistically significant. In these two countries, average production diversity is quite high; further increasing farm diversity would hardly contribute to higher dietary diversity. One indicator of market access is the geographic distance from the farm household to the closest market where food can be sold or bought. The estimated coefficients are negative in all models, implying that households in remoter regions have lower dietary diversity. Better market access through reduced distances could therefore contribute to higher dietary diversity. Comparing the magnitude of the estimated coefficients in the pooled model reveals that reducing market distance by

[18] A Poisson regression model is used.

10 km has the same effect on dietary diversity as increasing farm production diversity by one additional crop or livestock species.[19]

A more pertinent question is whether this also leads to more healthy diets. Depending on the type of food outlets available in a particular context, buying food may possibly be associated with rather unhealthy dietary diversification, for instance, through increased consumption of fats, sweets, or sugary beverages. This is examined by using alternative dietary diversity scores as dependent variables, including only more healthy food groups. The finding that better market access tends to increase dietary diversity also holds with this alternative specification. However, it is not self-evident that this specification is clearly superior for two reasons: (i) one is the failure to distinguish between processed and unprocessed foods, say, vegetables (e.g. eating French fries and eating boiled potato) with vastly different nutritional implications; and (ii) at best, dietary diversity (restricted or unrestricted) is an approximation to nutrients' intake as there are substitutions both within and between food groups in response to income and price changes (a case in point is different grades of rice).[20]

Another approach is to measure what households sell and buy. This information is only available for the samples from Ethiopia and Malawi. A dummy, used as an additional explanatory variable, takes the value of one if the household sells at least parts of its farm produce to the market, zero otherwise. The estimated coefficient is positive and significant. It is also much larger than the production diversity coefficient. This comparison suggests that facilitating the commercialization of smallholder farms may be a better strategy to improve nutrition than promoting more diversified subsistence production. Furthermore, the negative and significant interaction term confirms that market participation reduces the role of production diversity for dietary quality.

---

[19]The interaction term between production diversity and market distance is not significant in most cases. The positive and significant interaction coefficient in the Malawi case suggests that the role of production diversity is more important in remoter regions where farms tend to be more subsistence-oriented. This seems plausible except that endogeneity of production diversity is an issue, as discussed later.

[20]See, for example, Timmer (1981), Behrman and Deolalikar (1989), Jha *et al.* (2009) and Gaiha *et al.* (2014).

Accordingly, dietary diversity is measured in terms of the food purchased in the market. The farm production diversity coefficient is significantly negative, meaning that more diversified farms tend to buy less diversified foods in the market. This is perhaps not surprising: if the farm produces diverse foods itself, diversity from the market may not be needed to the same extent. However, diversified own production can substitute for diversity from the market only partially, because more than half of all of the food consumed in sample households is purchased.

Better market access in terms of shorter distance and more off-farm income opportunities increase the level of purchased food diversity. If off-farm income opportunities are greater in rural areas with short distances to market, the market access effect can't be disentangled from the income effect. The interaction between level of farm income and participation in off-farm activities is often complex as small farmers tend to work as labourers in the latter while relatively affluent dominate as owners in more remunerative enterprises.[21] The two important inferences are: (i) increasing on-farm diversity among smallholders is not always the most effective way to improve dietary diversity and should not be considered a goal in itself; and (ii) in many situations, facilitating market access through improved infrastructure and other policies to reduce transaction costs and price distortions seems to be more promising than promoting further production diversification as such. There are three caveats, however. One is the endogeneity of production diversity. Unless this is corrected, the coefficients are likely to be biased or suspect. The second is lack of uniformity of food baskets across countries/sub-regions (Masset *et al.*, 2012). The third is that regardless of how diet diversity is measured, it cannot on its own capture nutritional effects. A direct test may

[21]To test for such bias, the authors re-estimated the regression models, this time including socioeconomic and demographic characteristics — such as farm and household size, as well as age, education, and gender of the household head — as additional explanatory variables. Some of these other factors are significant, but the estimated coefficients for farm production diversity and market access do not change much. The authors interpret this as evidence that the main results do not suffer from omitted variable bias. These additional variables, however, do not resolve the endogeneity of production diversity. For example, farm diversity could be a risk-averse response to crop price uncertainty and expansion of high value chains (e.g. tomato for making ketchup, coffee for upgrade to export quality).

yield more reliable estimates of nutritional outcomes in which the dependent variables are calories, proteins, fats and micronutrients (Gaiha *et al.*, 2014).

Another estimation strategy that allows for *simultaneity* in production and consumption decisions is intuitively more appealing (Dillon *et al.*, 2015). An appropriate procedure is to induce an exogenous change in production and assess its subsequent effects on diet. This study investigated the *quasi-exogenous* increase in on-farm diversity among Africa RISING beneficiary households in Malawi to examine the link between production and dietary diversity. Three groups of households were recruited into this research study: all households who were testing innovations as of June 2013 ("beneficiary" group), randomly sampled households in project villages who did not participate in the project ("non-beneficiary" group), and randomly sampled households from non-project villages representing similar development domains as Africa RISING villages ("control" group). The main findings obtained are as follows.

Beneficiary households had more diverse farms, on average and across quartiles, relative to non-beneficiary and control group households. No statistically significant differences were found between beneficiary households and the other two groups in terms of the household dietary diversity index which is measured by the count of food items consumed within the household. No statistically significant differences were found between beneficiary households and households in the other two groups in terms of the value of foods consumed during the reference week.

In brief, improvements in product diversity did not translate into better diets, measured by the diversity and value of foods consumed within the household.

Two caveats are in order: (i) the Herfindahl index as a measure of diet diversity is better as it allows for shares of different food commodities in household food expenditure[22]; and (ii) because of higher and rising shares of oily and processed foods, the correspondence between diet diversity and nutritional intake needs careful verification.

[22]For an application, see Gaiha *et al.* (2014).

4. Livestock and Nutrition

ASF are nutritionally dense sources of energy, protein, and other essential micronutrients. Thus ASF enable children and pregnant and breastfeeding women to obtain calories in adequate quantities as well as high quality proteins, micronutrients and overall better nutrition. Since ASF also are a major source of iron, zinc, calcium, riboflavin, vitamin A, vitamin B-12 and retinol, and increasing the intake of ASF and the micronutrients they contain has numerous positive benefits including linear growth, improved educational attainment and health status, leading to long-term improvements in income and productivity.

Using nationally representative data for Uganda, Azzarri *et al.* (2015) examines such linkages between livestock ownership, consumption and nutrition. Uganda offers a promising environment for this analysis due to a combination of high prevalence of livestock ownership, recent growth in the livestock sector, and high levels of malnutrition — 33% of stunting and 50% of anaemia prevalence in children under five. They use household survey data from the 2005/2006 Uganda National Household Survey (UNHS) and the 2009/10 Uganda National Panel Survey (UNPS). Three livestock categories — large ruminants (bulls, cows, calves), small ruminants (goats and sheep), and poultry (chickens, turkeys, and ducks) are considered. The empirical analysis of child nutritional outcomes uses standardized anthropometric indicators. *Z*-scores for height-for-age (HA), weight-for-age (WA), weight-for-height (WH) are computed based on the 2006 World Health Organization's new Child Growth Standards. An innovative econometric methodology is used.[23]

The analysis confirms significant differences in the consumption patterns of ASF between livestock owners and non-owners: the number of large ruminants owned or managed has a positive effect on dairy consumption but not on beef consumption. While the number of small ruminants does not have a significant effect on consumption of goat and sheep

[23]The authors examine in the first stage whether the consumption of ASF depends on ownership of the three livestock categories using a tobit specification with random effects; and, in the second, the effect of ownership of livestock categories on child anthropometric outcomes using a probit.

meat, ownership of poultry affects chicken consumption positively. In particular, there is a positive effect of the number of poultry on chicken consumption and of the number of large ruminants on dairy consumption above and beyond the indirect effect of these livestock types through livestock income, controlling for welfare level (proxied by total per-capita consumption expenditure tercile). There is, however, a weak association between livestock ownership and child nutritional status, specifically on the probability of being underweight and wasted (limited to children between 2–5 years of age), but no association with stunting. Also, while ownership of small ruminants reduces the probability of children of age 2–5 years being underweight, ownership of large ruminants partly counters that effect.

Yet another study (Kassa *et al.*, 2015) assesses the impact of animal source food interventions on nutrition-related outcomes in Ethiopia (in the Horn of Africa). The analysis examines the impact of a women-focused goat development project expanded to include interventions to promote vitamin A intake, nutrition and health education, training in gardening and food preparation, and distribution of vegetable seeds. Goat owning households consumed all produced milk; 87% by the adults as *hoja*; children in the participating households had slightly more diversified diets; they were also more likely to consume milk more than 4 times a day. A methodological limitation is that no correction is made for self-selection bias.

So if we go by the findings of Azzarri *et al.* (2015) for Uganda, from a policy perspective, promoting (small) livestock ownership has the potential for affecting human nutrition in Sub-Saharan African countries, but the direction and size of the effect is still controversial. In contexts where markets are imperfect, supporting livestock ownership may be conducive to improving diets by a direct access channel, as well as providing further livelihood opportunities and increased income.

5. Biofortification

Soil micronutrient deficiencies are thought to be severe in SSA, where 75% of the total arable land has serious soil fertility problems. Insufficient micronutrient availability in soils in these regions not only causes low crop productivity, but also poor nutritional quality of the crops that contributes to malnutrition in the human population.

Diets in SSA (especially among resource poor households) are often low in diversity and dominated by staple crops such as maize, rice, cassava, sorghum, millet, banana and sweet potato. Such diets are poor in micronutrients (minerals and vitamins) and consequently micronutrient deficiencies are widespread (FAO, 2015). The chronic lack of micronutrients causes severe but often invisible health problems, especially among women and young children: hence "hidden hunger".

In SSA, micronutrient deficiencies contribute 1.5–12% of the total Disability Adjusted Life Years (DALYs). Alarming numbers suffer from iron-deficiency anaemia, which affects more than half of the female population in countries such as DR Congo, Ghana, Mali, Senegal and Togo. Selenium contributes to the human diet through uptake by crops from the soil. Even mild to moderate deficiencies of micronutrients can lead to severe human health problems, generally related to sub-optimal metabolic functioning, decreased immunity and consequently increased susceptibility to infections, growth failure, cognitive impairment and, finally, reduced productivity (de Valenca *et al.*, 2017). Direct interventions comprise dietary diversification, micronutrient supplementation, modification of food choices and fortification. Biofortification increases the content and/or bioavailability of essential nutrients in crops during plant growth through genetic and agronomic pathways (Garcia-Bauellos *et al.*, 2014; Gibson, 2007).

Vitamin A deficiency is associated with the higher risk of morbidity and mortality, and ocular disorders such as night blindness, xerophthalmia and blindness, affecting infants, children and women during pregnancy and lactation. Among populations at risk, vitamin A deficiency is estimated to affect more than 200 million women and children. African regions account for the greatest number of preschool children with night blindness and for more than one-quarter of all children with sub-clinical vitamin A deficiency (Hotz *et al.*, 2012).

Although the primary cause of vitamin A deficiency is its inadequate consumption, there have been relatively few large-scale, agricultural, food-based interventions implemented to address the problem, and fewer still have been adequately evaluated. For example, homestead and/or community garden production of vitamin A-rich fruits and vegetables has been promoted in a few populations with some success.

Sweet potato varieties most commonly cultivated in Africa are white or pale yellow having no or little provitamin A, and have a relatively high DM content. However, provitamin A-rich varieties, known as Orange Sweet Potato (OSP), have been bred through the process of biofortification or have been introduced and evaluated, and are suitable for Africa in terms of preferred agronomic and consumer traits. Due to the high content of β-carotene in some African-grown OSP varieties, the relatively high seasonal consumption of sweet potato can contribute substantially to increased vitamin A intake adequacy.

Mozambique is a country with modest use of sweet potato as a staple food. However, the prevalence of vitamin A deficiency is very high, and the coverage of vitamin A supplementation varies. Zambézia Province in Central Mozambique is more reliant on roots and tubers than on maize, has among the highest rates of stunting and underweight in the country and the lowest rates of vitamin A supplementation.

A nearly 3-year long, large-scale intervention to introduce several OSP varieties using agricultural extension and market development activities, product development, combined with demand creation and nutrition education, was implemented in rural communities of Zambézia Province, Mozambique. The study implemented two models of intervention to compare the effect of different durations of inputs on outcomes. In the detailed and meticulous scrutiny of this intervention, Hotz *et al.* (2012) hypothesized that intakes of OSP and vitamin A would be greater when exposure to key intervention components was extended to 3 years compared with 1 year. A prospective randomized, controlled effectiveness evaluation of both models was carried out.[24]

This large-scale intervention had a substantial impact on the dietary intake of OSP among women and preschool children. The increase in OSP

---

[24]An intervention to introduce household-level cultivation of OSP was implemented between 2006 and 2009 in 144 selected villages from four districts, combined in three strata (Milange, Gurue and Mopeia/Nicoadala) of Zambézia Province, Mozambique. This was a large-scale intervention reaching more than 12000 farm households and was designed to learn lessons about scaling up the dissemination of OSP.

intake in the intervention groups was largely attributed to a direct substitution of white and yellow sweet potato varieties. The incorporation of OSP in the diet translated to a large, significant increase in vitamin A intakes by these subgroups and hence reduced the prevalence of inadequate vitamin A intakes. There were no major differences in the impact on OSP or vitamin A intakes between the model 1 and model 2 groups, indicating that the magnitude of impact observed in the present study was not diluted by the less intensive intervention in model 2. Similar substitution rates across age groups suggest that OSP was equitably shared among the women and children of different ages.

The wide acceptance of OSP in populations where white or yellow sweet potatoes are usually consumed has been observed elsewhere in SSA, and can thus be plausibly generalized.

The increases in OSP intake were similar between the two intervention models. This implies that additional project inputs to supervise and support the village-level promoters in repeating agriculture and nutrition education sessions through the 2nd and 3rd years of the intervention did not translate into additional impact in the amount of OSP consumed, vitamin A intake or the prevalence of inadequate vitamin A intake. This is an important policy finding as the additional cost of maintaining direct, community-level contact by project staff beyond the 1st year of intervention is not justified in these sweet potato-producing areas and the maintenance of district-level activities and mass media may be sufficient to maintain behaviour change after the 1st year.

Some constraints to implementing agronomic biofortification are briefly noted. Development of the biophysical, economic, social and political environment is necessary to facilitate proper technologies, allocation of resources and food processing systems. A key issue is the commercialization of smallholder agriculture to create markets for extra production, because otherwise investments in (extra) mineral fertilizer are not economically feasible. Mapping of micronutrient deficiencies in order to provide field-specific fertilization recommendations remains a challenge. Furthermore, knowledge and tools should be accessible and affordable for farmers in rural African regions. Finally, new fertilizer products and management practices need to be matched with local socio-cultural environments in order to enhance adoption (Saltzman *et al.*, 2013). It is important to raise awareness about proper food processing and consumption that stimulate micronutrient uptake into the human body.[25]

6. Home Gardens

Over the recent years there has been growing interest to strengthen and intensify local food production in order to mitigate the adverse effect of global food shocks and food price volatilities. Consequently, home gardens are being viewed as a strategy to enhance household food security and nutrition. Home gardens are an integral part of local food systems and the agricultural landscape of developing countries all over the world and have endured the test of time.

Studies of homestead food production programmes have found improvements in production of targeted nutrient- rich foods within households, but have not found impact on child nutrition. A critical intermediate step requiring assessment is whether production of these more diverse foods leads to their actually being eaten, improving the diversity and quality of children's diets in those households.[26] Reviews of interventions aiming to increase the diversity of agricultural production and assess impact on diet and nutrition have found in general that the specific foods or food groups targeted by an intervention go into the diets of target beneficiaries, but have not demonstrated impact on nutritional status (anthropometry) — mainly because the original evaluations were not properly designed to capture such an effect (e.g. Abebe *et al.*, 2006).

The household garden is a small-scale production system supplying plant and animal consumption and utilitarian items either not obtainable, affordable, or readily available through retail markets, field cultivation,

[25] As some of the discussion overlaps with sustainable technology discussion, some details are omitted here to avoid repetition.

[26] Homestead gardens are found in backyards, farmyards, kitchens, small patches of available land, vacant lots, and along roadsides and the edges of fields. They are generally close to a house and source of water and are managed by family members using low-cost inputs. Their products include fruits, vegetables, herbs, condiments, and sometimes secondary staples such as legumes and sweet potatoes, most of which are grown for household consumption. The nutrition impacts of homestead gardens have been relatively well documented.

hunting, gathering, fishing, and wage earning. Featuring ecologically adapted and complementary species, household gardens are marked by low capital input and simple technology. Home gardens can be described as a mixed cropping system that encompasses vegetables, fruits, plantation crops, spices, herbs, ornamental and medicinal plants as well as livestock that can serve as a supplementary source of food and income.

The most fundamental social benefit of home gardens stems from their direct contributions to household food security by increasing availability, accessibility, and utilization of food products. Home gardens are maintained for easy access to fresh plant and animal food sources in both rural and urban locales. Food items from home gardens add substantially to the family energy and nutritive requirements on a continuous basis. Resource-poor families often depend more on home gardens for their food staples and secondary staples than those endowed with a fair amount of assets and resources such as land and capital. For poor and marginalized families unable to afford expensive animal products to fulfil their nutritional needs, home gardens offer a cheap source of nutritive foods.

Various studies conclude that, while adding to the caloric quantity, home gardens supplement staple-based diet with a significant portion of proteins, vitamins, and minerals, leading to an enriched and balanced diet particularly for growing children and mothers. Additionally, plants from the gardens — especially spices and herbs — are used as flavour enhancers, teas, and condiments. Furthermore, the integration of livestock and poultry activities into home gardening reinforces food and nutritional security for the families as milk, eggs, and meat from home-raised animals provide the main and, in many instances, the only source of animal protein. In some places, home gardeners are also engaged in mushroom cultivation and beekeeping and even small fresh water fish ponds are incorporated into the garden space adding to the share of proteins and other nutrients available for the family.

Even though there are only a few published narratives, home gardens have been proposed as an option for food and nutritional security in disaster, conflict, and other post-crisis situations. Home gardens based on enset and coffee are an integrated farming system that not only provide subsistence and complementary food products for Ethiopian families, especially during famines, but also provide the primary means of employment for the household.

In a post-conflict setting, assistance and reconciliation mechanisms work best and result in environmental, social and economic benefits when there is a cultural or traditional linkage between the target population and the intervention. Hence, home garden projects offer a realistic solution, as in most countries home gardening is a regular day-to-day activity amongst the households, especially for women. In addition, home gardens when properly managed provide a four-in-one solution to the food and nutrition problem by increasing household food availability, enabling greater physical, economic and social access, providing an array of nutrients, and protecting and buffering the household against food shortages (Galhena *et al.*, 2013).

A generous portion of the plants found in home gardens have some medicinal value and they can be used to treat many common health problems in a cost-effective manner. For instance, home gardens in Bukoba district of Tanzania contained plant species grown entirely for medicinal purposes. Based on a study conducted by Brun *et al.* (1989) in Senegal, evaluating the food and nutritional impact of home gardening, it was found that, although the gardens did not make a major contribution to food consumption and nutrition, they were instrumental in improving the women's income and social status as well as their awareness of evolving food habits in urban areas.

Evidence from Southeastern Nigeria shows that tree crops and livestock produced in home gardens accounted for more than 60% of household income. In many cases the sale of produce from home gardens improves the financial status of the family providing additional income, while contributing social and cultural amelioration. The fact that home production requires fewer inputs and investment is extremely important for resource-poor families that have limited access to production inputs. Yet moderately rigorous crop and livestock production in home gardens can generate as much revenue per unit area as field crop production.

Home gardens provide multiple environmental and ecological benefits. They serve as the primary unit that initiates and utilizes ecologically friendly approaches for food production while conserving biodiversity and natural resources. Home gardens are usually diverse and contain a rich composition of plant and animal species. A study of home gardens in Southern Ethiopia identifies a significant concentration of plants used as vegetables, fruits, herbs, medicines, yams, and spices.

Kumar *et al.* (2015) point out that evidence is needed on the direct links between food production within a household, ingestion of that food by individual household members, and subsequent effects on nutritional status. The motivation for this study is to address the gap in our understanding of how diversity of agricultural production affects the dietary diversity and nutritional status of children living in farming communities in SSA, using household survey data from a rural district in central Zambia. An innovative econometric methodology is used that allows for the endogeneity of dietary diversity and anthropometric outcomes but treats production diversity as exogenous. In a more refined methodology, endogeneity of production diversity has also to be taken into account. To examine whether greater household production diversity trickles down to dietary diversity among young children, they examine the relation between household production diversity and dietary intake among children aged 6–23 months. And finally, they examine the link between production diversity and nutritional status of children aged 6–23 months and children aged 24–59 months.

The three production diversity variables assessed are significantly associated with individual dietary diversity outcomes in young children aged 6–23 months.[27] These results suggest that the diversity of diets consumed by infants and young children is directly related to diversity in agricultural production in these semi-subsistence households. Production diversity is not associated with nutritional status (as measured through anthropometry) in younger children, but in children over the age of 24 months there is a more consistent pattern between agricultural production diversity and linear growth. In older children, agricultural production diversity is positively associated with HAZ scores and

[27]Production diversity is measured in terms of: (i) total number of crops (including field crops and fruits and vegetables) cultivated; (ii) total number of agricultural activities engaged in (production of field crops, production of fruits and fruits/vegetables, rearing animals and production of animal source foods); and (iii) production of seven different food groups that correspond to those groups used in the child dietary diversity index.

inversely associated with stunting. These associations, while small, are consistent, and are in line with what is known about biological processes affecting children of different ages. Diversity of agricultural production thus has an important impact on dietary diversity in young children in subsistence households, and subsequently on nutritional status as these children age.

Another study (Gillespie and van den Bold, 2017) reports mixed evidence on the impact of home gardening and animal/dairy production on nutrition. While there is evidence of positive impacts on intermediary nutrition outcomes, such as dietary diversity, household production and consumption, and child and maternal intake of "target" foods and micronutrients, impact on nutrition outcomes — particularly child anthropometry and micronutrient status — was much more limited, except in relation to vitamin A intake and status.

A third detailed study (Kidala *et al.*, 2000) focuses on Tanzania. It assesses the impacts of promotion of home production, consumption and storage of vitamin A-rich foods, health and nutrition education. They observed lower serum vitamin A and higher helminths in the treatment areas. Overall, after the treatment, higher intakes of vitamin A-rich foods were associated with higher serum vitamin A. There was a significantly higher percentage of households with homestead gardens and production of vitamin A-rich vegetables in treatment areas. Besides, the authors observed better knowledge, attitudes, practices about use of vitamin A, and higher shares using solar driers for vitamin A foods, and higher 7-day frequency of intake of vitamin A foods. A limitation is that there is no correction for self-selection bias.

Masset *et al.* (2012) carry out a meta review with a strong methodological flavour and cautious interpretation of results. In a broad brush but rigorous review of 23 studies of impact of agricultural interventions on child nutrition, they make several insightful comments for policy design and implementation.

Central to the review are examples of interventions (such as home gardens and the production of bio-fortified crops) with the explicit goal of improving the nutritional status of children. One limitation is that it is a distillation of the studies reviewed without going into contextual specificities.

A large majority of the studies are of home gardens (n = 15), and much smaller numbers of biofortification (2), small-scale fisheries and aquaculture (3), dairy development (1), and animal husbandry and poultry development (1). Rigorous evaluations of the effect of dairy development, animal husbandry, and fisheries projects are extremely rare. In the case of biofortification programmes, the lack of evidence is largely due to the novelty of the interventions.

In most cases, home garden programmes increased the consumption of fruit and vegetables, aquaculture and small fisheries interventions increased the consumption of fish, and dairy development projects increased the consumption of milk. A difficulty is that an increase in the consumption of the food item targeted by the intervention does not imply an improvement in the overall diet, because substitution effects in consumption occur. For example, in one case, although the consumption of vegetables, rice, and fish increased after the intervention, the consumption of pulses decreased. This suggests that indicators of the diversity of the diet or analysis of the full consumption basket are better indicators than is consumption of the specific food promoted by an intervention.

Two studies assessed the effect on iron intake of children and found no statistically significant differences in the average haemoglobin concentrations between children in the project and control groups. Another study assessed the effect of fish consumption on iron intake at the household level and found a modest effect by using food as per micronutrients conversion tables. The observed effect would have been even smaller after consideration of the actual body absorption of the iron ingested.[28]

Nine studies reported effects on concentration of serum retinol from blood samples. However, only four of these studies reported means and standard deviations of observations on children in project and control areas. The difference between the mean serum retinol concentration in the project and control group for each study is reported with a 95% confidence interval. Overall, the effect of the interventions is a difference of 2.4 μg/dL in serum retinol between project and control areas (z test of significance 6.35; $P < 0.001$). This summary effect is the weighted mean of the effects found by the individual studies. This meta-analysis provides

[28]For details of the studies cited, see Masset *et al.* (2012).

some support to the hypothesis that agricultural home garden interventions improve vitamin A intake among children under the age of 5.

Anthropometric data were collected by 13 of the 23 studies included in the review, but only eight studies used these data to calculate prevalence of stunting, underweight, and wasting. Only one study found a statistically significant effect on prevalence of stunting, whereas three studies found a positive effect on prevalence of underweight and two found a positive effect on wasting.

Overall, these results provide little support for the hypothesis that agricultural interventions help to reduce undernutrition. However, they should not be interpreted as evidence of the absence of an effect.

In sum, the interventions reviewed had a positive effect on the production of agricultural goods promoted, but there was no effect on households' total income. The interventions were successful in promoting the consumption of specific foods, but not in dietary changes. There was no effect on the absorption of iron and some on absorption of vitamin A. The effects on the prevalence of stunting, wasting, and underweight among children under 5 years of age were limited and mixed.

7. Women's Empowerment, Agriculture and Nutrition

Women are vitally important agents, both in their roles as producers and as custodians of household welfare. Their importance, moreover, is generally greater in the lowest-income settings and among households with high dependency ratios — in which a large proportion of household members are nonearning and often nutritionally vulnerable dependents.

The resources and income flows that women control often have positive impacts on household health and nutrition. In some countries, women tend to lack access to economic opportunities outside the domestic sphere to which traditional customs often confine them, especially in rural areas. They are also very often severely constrained by time and the multiple — often simultaneous — roles they play as producers and caregivers. Agricultural programmes and policies that empower and enable women and that involve them in decisions and activities throughout the life of the programme achieve greater nutritional impacts (World Bank, 2007).

We now review the evidence for selected African countries.

Although women comprise more than 50% of the agricultural workforce in most of the Eastern and Southern Africa (ESA) region, the productivity gap between men and women farmers persists. To illustrate how wide the gap is, in Tanzania, Malawi, Uganda narrowing the gender gap in agricultural productivity has the potential of raising the gross domestic product by US$105 million, US$100 million, and US$65 million, respectively (IFAD, FAO and WFP, 2015). Women farmers typically use lower levels of purchased technological inputs, such as fertilizers and high-yielding seed varieties. That women lack access to these key technological inputs explains a significant portion of the productivity gap. They are often hesitant to adopt these technologies if they do not control the benefits that accrue from adopting. Moreover, women also face unique challenges, due to their lifecycle and reproductive roles, which further influence their participation on- and off-farm.

In Kenya, new varieties of sweet potatoes rich in beta-carotene were introduced to women farmers with an end goal of improving vitamin A intake of young children, thereby preventing vitamin A deficiency. The Kenyan study showed a significant increase in the intake of vitamin A-rich foods, among children whose mothers received both the production-focused intervention of planting materials and access to agricultural extension services, and the consumption-focused intervention of nutrition education and training in food processing and preparation. By contrast, there was a decrease in vitamin A food intake (30%, but not statistically significant) for children whose mothers received only the production-focused inputs. This example suggests that: (a) women's farm production offers an entry point for interventions that can improve nutrition; and (b) interventions that increase women's agricultural productivity and increase their health and nutrition knowledge may yield more benefits than ones that target only productivity or only knowledge.

Once food is produced and enters the household, women are principally responsible for processing it. Food processing can often improve the nutritional quality of foods and increase dietary diversification. Women process oilseeds, such as sunflower or sesame seeds, to produce cooking oil; transform cassava into *gari*; smoke and dry fish and meat; and process and preserve fruits and vegetables. Thus, women's roles in food processing offer yet another entry point for interventions that can enhance family nutrition (Kurz and Johnson-Welch, 2000).

A few case studies, however, reveal some unexpected outcomes (World Bank, 2007). Although this study draws upon a rich literature from different regions, we focus more on African evidence. Failure to understand cultural norms and the gender dynamics within the household can result in unanticipated outcomes. In the Gambia, for example, a project geared to increasing women's rice production was so successful that the land it was grown on was reclassified internally within the household (von Braun *et al.*, 1994). This resulted in output from that land being sold by men as opposed to women. Women therefore lost their original income stream, but did retain an increased labour commitment. Vegetables and legumes are often regarded as women's crops. Recognizing this, a project in Togo was successful because it promoted the introduction of soybeans as a legume rather than as a cash crop. Promotion as a cash crop would have resulted in the crop switching to male control. Interventions promoting the production of animal source foods also assessed their impact on maternal income or women's control over income. The results were quite mixed. For example, an intervention involving intensified dairy farming in Kenya showed that an important share of the additional income was controlled by women, whereas in Ethiopia men's incomes benefited significantly more from intensified dairying than did women's. Whether women's income is likely to increase depends on the livestock or aquaculture production system, the nature of the intervention, and cultural beliefs and practices relating to gender. Even if the intervention is targeted to women's livestock and aquaculture activities, women lose control over the income generated by those activities.

Successful interventions are more likely to take into account the range of factors that differentially enable or constrain men and women in terms of access to resources like land and services like credit. These constraints often limit their roles as decision makers in the household or community. The significance of gender equity is particularly critical because women's status and decision-making power directly affect the nutritional status of their children.

Poor levels of human capital, health, and nutrition significantly constrain women's ability to work as efficient agricultural producers. Low levels of human capital may influence women's productivity in two ways. First, they may take longer to perform the same agricultural task. Second, they may not use certain technologies if they lack the information and knowledge required to use it. In fact, a significant portion of the on-farm productivity gap in Malawi is explained by the labour productivity gap, which is larger than the land productivity gap. Women are found to spend more time working on the farm, which diminishes the size of the overall productivity gap, but increases the labour productivity gender gap because women take longer to perform the same task as compared to men (Palacios-López and Lopez, 2014).

Evidence further suggests that, on average, women have lower access to extension as compared to their male counterparts (Quisumbing *et al.*, 2014), which compounds the problem of lower education levels of women. When they do have access to extension, they are more likely to adopt new technologies.

Rural women are less likely to have land under their control than rural men. Improving tenure security and access to land has direct consequences for bolstering investments in long-term financial capital demanding technologies. Tenure security in nine West African countries led to improved tree planting and investments in land significantly, but did not affect short-term investments such as use of purchased, productive inputs. The influence that women have on agricultural decision-making is, however, higher when women own land individually.

Several factors, such as collateral requirements, mobility restrictions, significant transaction costs, and cultural barriers, impede women from accessing financial products and credit. Moreover, they may also have less demand for credit if seeking financial products in formal systems and being entrepreneurial implies stepping outside the boundaries of prevalent social and cultural norms. In such contexts, interventions that provide access to financial products to women farmers through familiar structures, such as rural savings and credit cooperative organizations, may induce women to seek credit due to the prevalence of strong peer effects.

A useful way of shortening the link between technology innovation and adoption by women is to make them centre stage in the technology innovation and product design process. In Tanzania, for example, a solar powered irrigation pump has been developed that irrigates approximately one acre of land in 6–12 hours. The pump is portable and can be easily transported between fields, offering an opportunity for developing custom hiring irrigation service businesses for women entrepreneurs and women-led cooperatives. Besides, policy should take into account not just cultural appropriateness but also the fact that women have multiple objectives while working on the farm and more likely to adopt technologies that prioritize their household food and nutrition security.

In Mozambique, an experimental evaluation of the fertilizer subsidy programme reveals a relatively low uptake of fertilizer and improved seed varieties by farmers, potentially due to other credit or information limitations. Indeed, adoption of new technologies by women farmers requires a set of complementary policies such as innovative financing mechanisms along with providing actual knowledge about technologies and bringing the technologies to the door-step. When simultaneously implemented, such complementary policies are more likely to enhance technology adoption by women.

In Western Kenya, farmers were encouraged to use fertilizers by providing them with time-limited fertilizer discounts in the form of free delivery, right after the harvest season. An evaluation suggests that such small nudges were much more effective in encouraging fertilizer use instead of much larger price subsidies during the planting season.

Encouragement and nudges through social networks of women induce adoption as women rely more on their informal social networks than men. Strengthening women's land rights, starting from shifts in inheritance laws to land rental laws, is essential to women trusting that their investments in agricultural technologies will support their long-term personal, household, and community level goals. Evaluation of South Africa's Land Redistribution for Agricultural Development programme, for example, suggests that beneficiaries experienced a 25% increase in their consumption expenditures. Moreover, while their living standards initially dropped, after over 3 years, the beneficiaries experienced benefits of the order of 150% in their living standards.

There are improved impacts on nutrition if agricultural interventions are targeted to women and when specific work is done around women's empowerment (for example, through behaviour change communication), mediated through women's time use, women's own health and nutrition status, and women's access to and control over resources as well as intra-household decision-making power (Gillespie and van den Bold, 2017).

8. Value Chain Analysis and Nutrition

Recent reviews of the contribution of agriculture in improving nutrition show that although agricultural programmes have immense potential to improve nutrition, this potential is yet to be realized. Limitations in the design and implementation of agriculture interventions, as well as a lack of clarity in terms of nutrition goals and interventions, are partly responsible for the paltry evidence. Even more important, the lack of rigour in most of the existing impact evaluations prevents any clear conclusions regarding the contribution of agriculture in improving nutrition (Ruel and Alderman, 2013).

Value chain concepts are useful in designing strategies to achieve nutrition goals. Central to this approach is identifying opportunities where chain actors benefit from the marketing of agricultural products with higher nutritional value. However, value chain development focuses on efficiency and economic returns among value chain transactions, and the nutritional content of commodities is often overlooked.

A food value chain is a form of food supply chain, or the series of processes and actors that take a food from its production to consumption and disposal as waste. In a *value chain*, the emphasis is on the value (usually economic) accrued (and lost) for chain actors at different steps in the chain, and the value produced through the functioning of the whole chain as an interactive unit. A value chain is commodity specific, and thus involves only one particular food that is relevant within a diet.

Improved chain relations and overall chain performance could yield tangible benefits in terms of economic returns and, potentially, poverty reduction (Gelli *et al.*, 2015). As value chains are crucial in determining food availability, affordability, quality, and acceptability, they have potential to improve nutrition. What is required is to identify opportunities where value chain actors benefit from supplying the market with agricultural products of higher nutritional value. Value chain development, however, has rarely focused attention on consumers — consumers are simply considered as purchasers driving the ultimate source of demand. In this light, the value chain strategy is likely to be enriched by a stronger consumer focus, and, in particular, a focus on consumer nutrition and health. The empirical evidence on the role of value chains in improving nutrition is, however, scanty and mixed.

Basically, nutrition results from the quality of the overall diet, not just from the nutrient content of an individual food. In value chains, the focus is generally commodity specific, rather than on how to integrate multiple chains to contribute to an enhanced quality of diet. There may be offsetting impacts such that, if one value chain works better and consumption of the associated food increases, consumption of other foods may decline.

Another major concern is the lack of clarity in terms of the pathways linking value chain activities to nutrition. This includes understanding the requirements that need to be achieved in order for value chains to bring about increased consumption of nutritious food. In turn, it is necessary to understand what constraints prevent these requirements from being met and the interventions that are likely to be most effective in overcoming these constraints.

The availability (quantity available on the market), affordability (price), and quality (including nutrition content and food safety) influence consumption at the interface between the value chain and the food environment. The intake of nutritious food complements the consumption of other foods in the diet, which may be self-produced or purchased on the market. The nutritious food may be shared within the household or consumed by only a few household members. Increasing the demand for nutritious foods would also lead to expanding marketing opportunities for producers. This increased demand stimulates agricultural production, particularly for smallholders who face market access constraints, especially as increased demand may be a relatively stable revenue channel and a low-risk venture for producers.

When the supply of nutritious foods is limited, interventions could expand supply through advanced production technologies, or mechanisms to reduce input costs so production of those crops is relatively more profitable. Other supporting measures include the provision of insurance, access to credit, and land titling. Examples of relevant interventions that enhance nutritional value include fortification, enrichment, processing multiple foods into more nutritious products, food safety and detoxification, labelling, and sensitization.

In sum, on the demand side, the central issue is how to promote consumption of nutritious foods by target populations that may not be able to afford a healthy diet. Similarly, on the supply side, an important concern is the feasibility of targeting the poorest smallholders and informal enterprises along the value chain, particularly, involving women.

A few examples are discussed below to elucidate the potential of value chains for enhancement of nutritional value and the constraints that must be addressed. Chronic undernutrition is pervasive in Nigeria, with rates of stunting and underweight alarmingly high and with little progress over the last decade. There are major disparities in nutrition outcomes between the wealthy and poor, between the north and south, and between urban and rural areas. Micronutrient deficiencies are widespread across social groups. Vitamin A deficiency, for example, is associated with 25% of child and maternal deaths. Together with direct nutrition interventions, it is necessary to improve the functioning of food value chains and provide access to nutrient-dense foods to the urban and rural poor.

Robinson *et al.* (2014) maps current value chains for two products, cowpeas and soyabeans, and complementary products, focusing on whether they meet a set of key criteria: availability, affordability, acceptability and nutritional quality. It examines in detail each stage of the value chains for these products: production and supply, wholesale, processing, distribution/retail and consumer groups, and identifies the constraints facing them. For the present study, we confine ourselves to cowpeas. Cowpeas make a substantial contribution to the nutrition of poor populations in Nigeria.[29] Markets for cowpea products are mainly informal, and the majority of products are produced by small-scale businesses and sold

[29]Cowpea grains contain an average of 24% protein and 62% soluble carbohydrates. They are rich in thiamine, folates and iron, and also contain zinc, potassium, magnesium, riboflavin, vitamin B6 and calcium, as well as the amino acids lysine and tryptophan. Nutrient-density varies among cowpea varieties in Nigeria, and some varieties have been highlighted as especially good sources of micronutrients (Robinson *et al.*, 2014).

locally. Few formal sector businesses have invested in cowpea products, and there is limited innovation in value-added products. A merit of cowpea foods is that they are readily acceptable to diverse populations, widely available across the country and can be distinguished from less nutritious alternatives. However, affordability and availability of cowpeas is constrained by major supply-side problems. Cowpea prices fluctuate between seasons, due to the susceptibility of grains to degradation and low use of improved storage technologies. Although simple, safe and low-cost technologies are available in the form of improved storage bags, these are not prominent in wholesale and transport stages of the value chain. Besides, existing preservation techniques make use of pesticides that create risks of toxic contamination.

There is substantial involvement from businesses across Nigeria in producing cowpea products. The vast majority of these businesses operate in the informal economy, often at a very local scale. In addition to processors, businesses are also involved in agricultural inputs and storing, transporting and wholesaling cowpeas. Processors of cowpea products use four standard distribution models to reach consumers: street food vendors, restaurants and fast food companies, institutional providers (such as schools or hospitals) and supermarkets.

In order to overcome supply-side constraints, Robinson *et al.* (2014) make a few specific recommendations. These include (i) raising of yields of cowpeas. Factors underlying poor yields comprise the high cost of inputs for cowpea production, limited use of improved seeds, infestation by pests, drought and irregular rainfall and inconsistent government policies, especially on input subsidies and incentives. (ii) The price of cowpeas during the high season can be as much as double that during the low season. Although cowpeas are overall the most affordable protein source in most of Nigeria, during the high season they are not affordable to poor populations. Improving use of storage technologies along the value chain, including on-farm facilities, transportation and storage facilities in markets would help alleviate this constraint. (iii) Value chain actors use pesticides to reduce weevil damage, but these chemicals persist throughout the value chain and have caused poisoning and even death in people eating cowpea. There are safe and effective storage solutions in Nigeria (i.e. PICS bags).

9. Sustainable Technologies

Two aspects are of prime importance: scaling up successful agricultural practices, and prioritizing sustainable intensification approaches and integrating them into agricultural technology in the local context. Less-favoured areas need to receive attention in policy matters, especially in the context of the threat to agriculture from climate change and/or globalization of agricultural trade.

Two specific concerns are: restoration of soil fertility and judicious use of water. Both conservation technologies can also be pursued in some low-productivity areas. However, they have not caught the attention of policymakers. Extension of both these measures would help raise productivity and save resources in these areas.

A few examples illustrate the potential and constraints. The Ethiopian economy relies on its agricultural sector as a fundamental instrument for poverty alleviation, food security and economic growth. However, this sector is prone to land degradation — depletion of soil organic matter, soil erosion and lack of adequate plant nutrient supply. These problems are getting worse in many parts of the country, particularly in the highlands. Furthermore, climate change is likely to accelerate land degradation in Ethiopia. Although there is substantial evidence on the adoption and productivity impacts of soil and water conservation measures in Ethiopia, the evidence on adoption and productivity impacts of other land management practices, including Minimum Tillage (MT) and Commercial Fertilizer (CF) use, is scanty. Specifically, evidence is lacking on the relative contribution of these practices to agricultural productivity in low vs. high agricultural potential areas.

Kassie *et al.* (2011) fills this gap by examining the productivity gains associated with adoption of MT and CF use in the high and low agricultural potential areas of the Ethiopian highlands. To do this, the authors use household- and plot-level data from the Tigray and Amhara administrative regions.[30] They employ both semi-parametric and parametric methods. The parametric analysis is based on matched samples of

[30]The Tigray region is typical of the low moisture and generally low agricultural potential areas. The dataset of the Amhara region allows an intraregional comparison of the

adopters and non-adopters, obtained from the Propensity Score Matching (PSM) process.[31]

The results provide evidence of a strong impact of MT on agricultural productivity, compared with the impact of CF, in the low agricultural potential areas. In the high agricultural potential region, however, CF has a very significant and positive impact on crop productivity, whereas MT has no significant impact.

From a policy perspective, these findings stress the need for moisture-conserving technologies in semi-arid environments. Specifically, the productivity advantages of MT in the low-potential areas come from its ability to conserve soil moisture in dry environments. Further, the findings suggest that CF is less profitable in this area owing to inadequate soil moisture. In addition, the non-profitability of CF in low-potential areas indicates that investing in CF in these environments is a financial risk, which has considerable relevance for resource-constrained areas, such as rural Ethiopia.

More importantly, the analysis suggests that different strategies are needed for different environments. For instance, in the low agricultural potential areas, government and non-governmental organizations should focus more on promoting MT as a yield-augmenting technology. Relying on external inputs (such as chemicals and fertilizers) in low-potential areas, which has been the strategy in the past, is not likely to be beneficial unless moisture availability is enhanced.

Good soil conditions that enhance micronutrient availability for crop uptake are essential for the success of agronomic biofortification. It is often recommended to optimize soil conditions through Integrated Soil Fertility Management, which is defined as "a set of soil fertility management practices that necessarily include the use of mineral fertilizer, organic inputs and improved germplasm". The combination of mineral fertilizers and organic inputs is beneficial, because they have complementary functions and enhance mutual effectiveness. Animal manures, for example, are a good source of many micronutrients. Manzeke *et al.* (2014)

---

performance of SLM practices because the dataset covers both low and high agricultural potential areas.

[31] For further details, see Kassie *et al.* (2011).

report that when Zn-enriched fertilizer was applied together with cattle manure and forest leaf litter, there were larger increases in maize grain yield and Zn concentration in the grain. Long-term application of organic matter to the soil not only increases total Zn content of the soil but also the proportion of labile Zn, which is the readily available form for plant uptake.

Agronomic biofortification has so far been most effective with Zn and Se. Many African soils suffer from multiple micronutrient deficiencies, as a result of their inherent soil properties and continuous cropping without nutrient replenishment. Current fertilization programmes in African countries primarily focus on NPK fertilizers, but many soils are non-responsive to NPK due to (multiple) micronutrient deficiencies. Soil modification with small amounts of (multiple) micronutrients is a sustainable strategy to increase yields and nutritional quality of crops (Vanlauwe *et al.*, 2015). A review of experiments from 10 African countries on the impact of Zn-enriched fertilizers showed that soil Zn application increased the Zn concentration in maize, rice and wheat grains by, respectively, 23%, 7% and 19% and by 30%, 25% and 63% through foliar application (Joy, 2015). Moreover, another agronomic benefit is that seedlings from seeds with high Zn concentration have better growth performance and resilience against environmental stress, so positive impacts on productivity may be seen in the next cropping generation.

Application of micronutrient-enriched fertilizers has minimal negative environmental impact. Most micronutrients are not susceptible to leaching because they are strongly bound in the soil. When micronutrient demand and supply are well-matched, negative environmental effects are unlikely. In fact, crop health improves when micronutrient deficiencies in the crop are alleviated. The improved general crop health enhances growth and nutrient uptake efficiency, as well as resilience against pests and diseases, thus reducing the need for pesticides and herbicides.

An important question is whether agronomic biofortification is an effective, feasible and sustainable approach to alleviate micronutrient deficiencies; especially in comparison with other intervention strategies such as genetic biofortification, food fortification, supplementation and dietary diversification? An unequivocal answer is difficult as the literature is sparse.

A particularly interesting example is of legumes in Malawi as a potentially important source of nutrition and restoration of soil fertility. Legumes are good sources of a range of macro- and micronutrients, and they substantially improve the quality of grain/root/tuber-based diets, for both young children and other family members. The use of legume plant residues can improve soil fertility and potentially contribute to future harvests. Among the few studies, a notable one is the Soils, Food, and Health Communities Study (SFHC) in northern Malawi's Soils Food and Health Communities Project. The SFHC study explored whether a legume system intervention could improve soil fertility, food security, and child nutrition (Kerr and Chirwa, 2004). However, there is no update on its outcomes.

10. Youth Employment in Rural Areas

There is no agreed definition of youth. The 15–24-year-old age range is commonly used, notably by the UN agencies, but the African Union defines youth as those in the 15–35-year-old age group.

The 15–24-year-old age group represents 20% of SSA's population today and, unlike in other regions, this youth share will remain high and stable (19% in 2050). In absolute terms, SSA's youth will grow from nearly 200 million in 2015 to nearly 400 million in 2050, and its share in the labour force will remain the highest in the world, even if following a declining trend. Representing 37% today — in comparison with 30% in India, 25% in China and 20% in Europe — it should still account for 30% in 2050 (ILO, 2016).

Agriculture has a substantial role in meeting the youth employment challenge facing Africa. Even in a most optimistic scenario, non-farm and urban sectors are not likely to absorb more than two thirds of young labour market entrants over the next decade. But there will be vast opportunities for the innovative young people in agricultural systems as they adapt to a range of challenges in the near future. These challenges relate to raising productivity in a sustainable way, integration into emerging high value chains, and healthy diets (Sumberg *et al.*, 2012).

While the challenges are daunting, the potential benefits of addressing them are enormous. Higher prices, more integrated value chains, widening connectivity to markets in some areas, and greater private and public engagement in the sector are creating new opportunities (Suttie, 2015). A major barrier is, however, strong negative preferences/attitudes of the youth towards agriculture.

Tadele and Gella (2012) make an attempt to capture attitudes and aspirations of rural in- and out-of-school young people towards agriculture, based on field-work in two regions in Ethiopia: Amhara Region, East Gojjam Zone — Gozamin Woreda (Chertekel Kebele); and Southern Nations, Nationalities and Peoples Region (SNNPR), Alaba Tembaro Zone, Qedida Gamella Woreda (Geshgolla Kebele). Focus Group Discussions (FGDs) were carried out with older farmers (men and women), young farmers (men and women), school students in grades 7 and 8 (aged around 16–18 years) (boys and girls), and young people who have left school but are not farming (boys/men and girls/women, in some cases college students, aged around 20–25 years). We will confine ourselves mostly to the views of the young.

The farmer was described variously as 'someone who labours to feed others'; tied to his land; and lacking, participants perceived, any other option than simply being a farmer. Life as a farmer was tied to life in a village which most respondents saw as hard and demanding. Yet there was considerable heterogeneity in the views of the young. Participants in both sites agreed that agriculture has changed significantly over the last decade. The introduction and adoption of agricultural inputs such as improved seeds, fertilizers and better farming methods (such as slash ploughing, sowing seeds in rows, water pumps, modern beehives) have produced significant increases in productivity and earnings.

There were competing narratives on whether agriculture was becoming more desirable to young people as a result. On the one hand, participants felt that these developments were making agriculture more and more profitable and therefore more appealing. However, they felt that there was a huge obstacle in engaging in it — scarcity of land. Although the dominant view was that young people are disinterested in agriculture, some participants pointed out that this was not always the case.

Disaggregation of farming preferences by age, gender, in- and out-of-school offers interesting contrasts. Young boys and girls currently attending school mostly viewed agriculture as a dead end: an option they were either unwilling to consider at all or only as a last resort. Specifically, the life of the farmer was perceived as tiring and hard, a life of endless toil with little gain. Girls attending school were more negatively inclined towards farming. They described the lives of their parents as traditional and backward and wished for a better life which they sought to attain through their education. Besides, shortage of land discouraged them more. A slightly more positive attitude towards agriculture was evident among young people who had left school, either failing to complete high school for various reasons or to qualify for higher level education. Although this group of respondents were equally aware of the grimness of traditional agriculture and the life of the common farmer, many were not dismissive of agriculture as a possible future livelihood, while a few even saw it as a preferred livelihood option, under improved conditions. Negative attitudes towards agriculture were not confined to the young. Although older farmers and officials acknowledged that agriculture can be a very lucrative livelihood, none wanted their children to follow in their footsteps. This was the case even for those whose lives had improved and even though agriculture was now as good a livelihood as any other, if not better. Given negative attitudes of family and society about agriculture, informal work in urban areas is preferred by young people who have attended school even if it is low paying and as back-breaking as agriculture.[32]

Apart from the inability of the urban economy to accommodate a huge influx of labour from the rural agricultural sector, the government considers rural educated youth as instrumental in bringing about a transformation in agricultural skills, knowledge and productivity. However, there is a sense of injustice and deprivation among young people, especially those who are already in agriculture and struggling to find plots and

[32]Rural youth rarely consider farming to be a "best job" or even a "good job" when one takes into account the very low returns provided by agriculture and the harsh conditions of work with hand tools. In fact, agriculture is probably one of the most difficult ways to make a living and, above all, it does not offer a desirable social status. Recognizing agriculture as a viable employment option is even more challenging when economic and social restrictions related to access to productive resources are taken into account. All these limitations are exacerbated for young women who, in general, have no prospect of land access due to rules of inheritance, and who know that they will mainly have to work for their husbands (ILO, 2016).

those willing to go into agriculture but unable to do so with no means of accessing farmland. Thus, the government has not effectively addressed either the attitude of many young people towards agriculture or the obstacles preventing their entry into the sector.

Access to land was the top concern for young people in both sites studied, and the government needs to consider how to facilitate land acquisition for young people interested in agriculture. Moreover, and no less important, is the imperative to address infrastructural needs of rural people and catalysing the social and economic transformation of rural areas which would, in the long run, make agriculture more attractive. Despite such negativity, it is argued that agriculture has a substantial role in meeting the youth employment challenge facing Africa. While the challenges are daunting, the potential benefits of addressing them are enormous. Higher prices, more integrated value chains, widening connectivity to markets in some areas, and greater private and public engagement in the sector are creating new opportunities (Suttie, 2015).

Africa's complex agro-ecologies and highly diverse production systems demand a level of agricultural research that is only feasible with reversal of decades of underinvestment in it. For now, growth in agricultural productivity will have to come from wider use of superior technologies that have worked elsewhere — improved seeds, breeds, cropping methods, conservation practices, and equipment. Over the past decade, more farmers across Africa have started to adopt such technologies, but at a slow pace.

As demand for food rises, growth in total factor productivity checks rise in real food prices and helps create jobs. Without sustaining productivity growth through agricultural research, the development of farming skills, and the adoption of new and better varieties, growth in output will come through increased use of purchased inputs such as fertilizer and agro-chemicals. Short-term gains in productivity, however, will be costly, increasing the real price of food, and eroding potential gains to producers, consumers, and society at large.

Africa offers ample opportunities for *simultaneous* increases in average farm size and in employment. Declining average farm size in Africa suggests that constraints on land markets are already hindering the prospects for young people and becoming stronger (World Bank, 2015).

Broadly, there are four options for young farmers: continue on the family plot but with a different mix of enterprises; establish their own operations on new land; combine farming with part-time other work; or wage employment on large or mid-size commercial holdings. These options/pathways vary in their requirements for land, capital, and skills. The first two — full-time employment on the family farm and full-time farming on a new holding — are the most prevalent.[33]

In this pathway, the skills and labour of multiple young adults in the household could enable specialization. Given demand for their labour, those capable of earning off-farm wages could do so, thus adding to the household's capital. Superior technologies, such as conservation tillage, require high investment of labour at peak periods, and a household with several young adults could undertake the required work. A combination of pooled off-farm earnings, a shift in farming technology to higher-value and more commercial products, and aggregation of household labour at peak periods, would enable small farms to absorb young adults constructively.

The second pathway involves a group of young people leaving the farm of their childhood and establishing a new and separate holding, ideally larger than the parcel they left. Those more likely to succeed in such an undertaking would probably be relatively experienced in farming and hence on the older end of the age range for "youth." These farmers would require land, start-up capital, and advisory services or training to handle technical and managerial responsibilities.

In the third pathway, young people may be independent part-time farmers, either managing their own holdings or contributing to family operations described under pathway 1, with enough capital to establish themselves as sellers of services, a trader, or an occasional wage worker. Higher-value agriculture will use services more intensively and create employment for those who can provide them. Demand for transport, plant protection, veterinary services, mechanized field operations, and advice

[33]A household survey in nine African countries in 2008 showed that 51% reported that inheriting land already under cultivation was the most common means for young people to obtain land, while 16% would be allocated land not previously cultivated, 9% would rent or borrow land, and 12% would buy land (Proctor and Lucchesi, 2012).

can be met by young men and women with the capital and skills to start a small business.

In the fourth pathway, young people take wage work, whether formal or informal, on large commercial farms or in the processing and service sectors. These young people need skills to handle a range of tasks and equipment. At a minimum, for the most basic low-skilled work, they need good health to perform in gruelling working conditions. Such wage work could be combined with other activities, or it could be a temporary option until better opportunities appear.

To create opportunities commensurate with the number of young people who will need employment, constraints on the acquisition of capital, land, and skills must be removed or relaxed.

A few selected initiatives are delineated below. Allowing alternative forms of collateral, such as chattel mortgages, warehouse receipts, and the future harvest, can ease the credit constraints — especially for young farmers. The OHADA7 Uniform Act on Secured Transactions, in effect in 17 SSA countries, was amended at the end of 2010 to allow borrowers to use a wide range of assets as collateral, including warehouse receipts and movable property such as machinery, equipment, and receivables that remain in the hands of the debtor. Leasing also offers young farmers some relief, as it requires either no or less collateral than typically required by loans. A case in point is DFCU Leasing in Uganda, which gave more than US$4 million in farm equipment leases in 2002 for items such as rice hullers, dairy processing equipment, and maize milling equipment. Despite leasing's potential to relieve constraints on access to mechanical technology, few firms have entered this business. Some outgrower arrangements prefinance inputs and assure marketing channels. In Mozambique, Rwanda, Tanzania, and Zambia, Rabo Development (a subsidiary of Rabobank) offers management services and technical assistance to financial institutions, which, in turn, finance supply chains with a range of agricultural clients. Participants include commercial farmers, farmers with little commercial presence, and an intermediate group of farmers with ambitions to grow commercially.

Microinsurance in Africa almost doubled between 2006 and 2009 from a very small base. Microinsurance differs from traditional insurance by being available through well-trusted yet innovative channels and by offering low premiums, products with simple designs, flexible payments for premiums, and prompt settlement of claims. For example, more than 11,000 Kenyan maize farmers, some with barely 1 acre, have obtained insurance policies that cover significant losses when drought or excess rain destroys their harvest.

None of these innovations in rural finance is relevant exclusively to young people. Nor should young people be segregated as a group and offered financial services designed specifically for them. The risks of working with the young are high, and separating them from a larger pool for sharing risks would make them even less attractive to financial institutions. Indeed, any and all innovations in finance that facilitate sustainable outreach to small farmers and rural entrepreneurs should be supported. When necessary, additional features should be added to enable these programmes to serve young people.

The two aspects of land administration that matter most to young entrants to the labour force are the need to improve security of tenure and the need to relax controls on rental. Land redistribution will also enhance young people's access to land. In general, policies and measures that help the poor to gain access to land will also help young people.

Young Africans must be equipped with basic reading, writing, and numeracy skills, and the ability to use digital technology to access and interpret information. Beyond these basics, the skills required for individuals in pathways 1 and 2 may differ from the skills required in pathways 3 and 4. The majority of farmers, who will have little more than a primary school education, will need access to effective agricultural extension services to sharpen their skills. It is anticipated that a growing and diversifying agricultural sector will create jobs that demand increasingly advanced technical and professional skills, from processing and marketing to agricultural research.

Returns to schooling in rural areas rise with the pace of technological innovation in farming. More educated farmers are often the first to adopt new seed, tillage practices, fertilizer, and animal breeds. Besides, it is necessary to improve both basic education and agricultural vocational education for women and to enhance rural women's access to extension services. Essentially, the agriculture that will attract the young will have to be profitable, competitive, and dynamic. These same characteristics are needed for agriculture to deliver growth, to improve food security, and to preserve a fragile natural environment (World Bank, 2015).

The development of agro-food businesses represents a significant opportunity for youth employment and for local development, due to powerful growth linkages to the rest of the economy. The growing food demand in Africa is a major avenue for agro-processing, which can easily be developed using Small and Medium-sized Entities (SMEs) and with intermediate technology. This option requires less capital, is more labour intensive and facilitates the proliferation of units in rural boroughs and small towns, offering employment and entrepreneurial opportunities, local value added and new incomes. Agro-processing SMEs can also facilitate the resolution of post-harvest problems, which are a significant issue in SSA resulting in a loss of revenue for farmers.

In addition, agro-industrial enterprises can provide inputs and services to the farm sector, stimulate market-induced innovation through farmers' participation in value chains and networks, and motivate other enterprises in the production of goods and services. They can be effective contributors to the local economy, the diversification of which will open new opportunity spaces for youth with more diversified and attractive jobs (ILO, 2016).

In the Niger Delta, for instance, the IFAD-supported Community Based Natural Resource Management Programme is promoting a new category of entrepreneur-cum-mentor called the "N-Agripreneur". These N-Agripreneurs are energetic university graduates who own and run medium-scale enterprises at different stages of food value chains. They deliver business development services to producers, especially young people, who are interested in agro-based activities, such as farming as a business, small-scale processing, input supply and marketing. Their success is reflected in more interconnected, stable and prosperous communities and local food systems, as well as jobs for the (mostly young) entrepreneurs (Suttie, 2015).

In order to enable young people to respond to the environmental, economic and nutrition challenges of the future, they must develop suitable capacities. A case in point is Information and Communications Technologies (ICTs) which can develop young people's capacities, while improving communication and easing access to information and decision-making processes. Investing in extending these technologies to rural areas, in particular targeting young people — who are generally more adaptable to their use — has allowed them to keep themselves up-to-date with market information and new opportunities.[34]

11. Returns on Agricultural Research and Technology

Agricultural research has generated several kinds of technology with high potentials for impact, but the expected impact on farmers' productivity, livelihood and quality of life has not been fully realized. Institutional innovations are needed to improve productivity and make public agricultural institutions more responsive to markets, more accountable to the communities they serve, and better recognized as an important tool for achieving economic growth. Other studies have shown that huge productivity gains are possible and accrue where governments allocate the necessary resources to agricultural research and development. In SSA, however, public investment in agriculture is still far below what is needed, despite commitments by African governments to allocate 10% of their public spending to it. The challenge is to develop technology that is relevant to small farmers and to enable them to transform their farms into viable small businesses that make a vital contribution to local and national economies. This calls for client-oriented agricultural research.

An aggregate investment of $7,120 million (1990 US dollars) produced benefit/cost ratios higher than 1, indicating efficient investments. The study also showed that research projects have generated more than 90% of the total CGIAR benefits (Raitzer, 2003). Over 80% out of this is attributed to plant genetic improvement, and the remainder to cassava mealy bug biological control. A negligible proportion is attributed to policy research. Similarly, the average internal profitability rate for investments made on research and dissemination of Sahel varieties of rice in the

[34]A survey in *The Economist* (November 11–17, 2017) draws attention to the enormous potential of ICT in Africa, "every 10% increase in mobile phone penetration in poor countries speeds up GDP growth per person by 0.8–1.2 percentage points a year. And when people get mobile internet, the rate of growth bumps up again", p. 6.

Senegal River Valley is estimated at over 221%, which is considerably higher than the cost of access to capital valued at 18% for the period 1995–2004.[35]

A thematic review of the rates of return is illuminating.

11.1 *Impact of Crop and Livestock Commodity Research on Economic Growth*

Maize improvement in West and Central Africa (1971–2005) — improved varieties were derived from the CGIAR and their National Agricultural Research Systems (NARS) partners' research — saw increase in adoption of improved varieties from less than 5% in the 1970s to about 60% in 2005 and with annual economic benefits estimated at $2.9 billion, an increasing trend over time, and an overall rate of return to research investment (CGIAR and national) of 43%.

Improved varieties of cowpeas, which provide both food and livestock feed, are being widely adopted in the dry savannah of West Africa, with estimated benefits of $299 million to $1.1 billion which are likely to accrue during 2000–2020.

Eastern and Southern Africa have also registered impressive gains, where improved varieties of common bean, developed with farmer participation, have been adopted on about 50% of the total bean area over 15 years. A study conducted in 2008 estimates that the new varieties are strengthening food security and raising incomes in 5.3 million rural households. The benefits of bean improvement research for Africa are estimated to have a current value of roughly $200 million, compared to costs of about $16 million (CGIAR, 2011).

New Rice for Africa, or NERICA, which combines the high yields of Asian rice with African rice's resistance to local pests and diseases, has spread to about 250,000 hectares in upland areas, helping to reduce national rice import bills and generating higher incomes in rural communities.

[35]For sources, see Seck *et al.* (2013).

In Mozambique, the introduction of new orange-fleshed sweet potato significantly increased the intake of vitamin A among young children. In Kenya, Farm Concern International undertook a women targeted work on commercialization of traditional leafy vegetables, which was later shown to be effective in increasing consumption of the micronutrient-rich vegetables. Millet also was found to be very beneficial because of its high content of the minerals phosphorus, manganese and magnesium.

The development of a vaccine against an "orphan" livestock disease in Africa has huge potential benefits. The production and delivery of this vaccine for East Coast fever — a tick-transmitted disease that threatens some 25 million cattle in 11 countries of eastern, central and southern Africa — is now in the hands of private sector partners. It is expected to save more than a million cattle, with benefits worth up to US$270 million a year in the countries where the disease is now endemic.

11.2. *Impact of Natural Resource Management Research on Economic Growth*

A set of case studies published in 2007 indicates that such research is giving highly positive returns on investment, based partially on the benefits for agricultural productivity. If methodologies were available for gauging the environmental benefits as well, the returns would no doubt be much higher. By 2002, more than 66,000 farmers in Zambia had adopted an agro-forestry system called "fertilizer tree fallows", which renews soil fertility using on-farm resources. The system has been shown to boost maize production while reducing production risks and soil erosion, with benefits of up to $20 million, compared with an investment of about $3.5 million.[36]

11.3. *Impact of Agricultural Research on Nutrition*

Berti *et al.* (2004) reported that most agriculture interventions increased food production, but did not necessarily improve nutrition or health.

[36]For further details, see Seck *et al.* (2013).

Furthermore, in the last few years, there has been an increase of interest in how to shape agriculture for more impacts on nutrition, particularly among mothers and children. Several reviews concluded that the current state of empirical evidence for impacts on nutrition ascribed to defined agricultural interventions is weak and mixed.[37] The statistical significance of impacts has been documented in a few cases, mainly in terms of micronutrient status (usually vitamin A). However, net effects across all nutrients have not been documented and there is apparent lack of sound, empirical evidence on the efficacy, effectiveness at scale, and cost-effectiveness of all kinds of agricultural intervention on nutrition. This remains a barrier to policy advocacy.

11.4. *Impact of Agricultural Research on Poverty Reduction and Food Security*

Thirtle *et al.* (2003) explored the relationship between agricultural productivity and poverty in 48 developing countries between 1985 and 1993. They found that a 1% improvement in crop yields reduced the proportion of people living on less than US$1 per day by 0.6%. Rice varietal improvement research has contributed tremendously to increase rice production in several countries. In each country, the benefits from rice research are, on average, 10 times higher than the total agricultural research investment. Research has also helped to uplift large numbers of the rural poor above the poverty line. According to more recent impact assessment studies in SSA, national and international organizations are making a big impact in reinforcing food security and alleviating poverty through rice research. Rice varietal improvement contributed, on average, US$375 million per year to the region's economy. Overall, improved varieties have increased net revenues by $93 per hectare, with the highest gains in irrigated and rainfed lowland ecologies. The annual returns to investment in rice research now exceed 20%.

There are many reports of NERICA's positive impact on farmers' livelihood across SSA, from Guinea in West Africa to Uganda in East

[37] For further details, see Seck *et al.* (2013).

Africa. Impact studies also reveal that rice research contributes effectively to the realization of almost all the Millennium Development Goals, including halving levels of poverty and hunger, promoting education, improving health, reducing child mortality, empowering women and ensuring environmental sustainability (Seck *et al.*, 2013).

Another important staple is maize. Maize improvement research had a benefit-cost ratio of 21 in the region. This means that every dollar invested in maize research generated additional food worth $21. Estimates for country-level benefit-cost ratio ranged from 11 (Mali) to 84 (Nigeria), with an average rate of return of 43% in West and Central Africa. Since maize and rice are major staples in large regions of Africa, it is clear that investment in agricultural research is yielding perceptible impacts on food security and poverty reduction.

In general, however, agricultural research has had mixed impact on well-being in this region. For example, there is no emphasis on research by the NARS on reducing undernutrition. Thus there are cases of malnutrition in the face of abundant food supply because of the lack of integrating researches on crop production, nutrition and health. Also, research on the processing of farm produce in SSA is missing in the agenda of all the programmes. The absence of programmes for attracting increased participation of the private sector in African agricultural research is compounded by insufficient investment in university education for science and technology (Mokwunye, 2010).

Nevertheless, the rates of return are high on agricultural research. As several impacts are inter-related, for example, women's empowerment, nutrition, poverty and sustainability, the rates of return may imply that these can be neatly separated thematically. This would be an oversimplification and misleading. However, if social valuation of these benefits differ, the social rates of return on agricultural research are likely to be substantially higher. Another refinement will be to assign probabilities to these outcomes so that their certainty equivalent values could be computed.[38]

[38]For an integrated analytical framework for impact assessment of agricultural research combining the main themes/pathways, see Mathur and Gaiha (2003).

12. Discussion

African agriculture has the lowest productivity when compared to other regions of the world. The Green Revolution observed in Asia did not occur in Africa for many reasons relating to the different institutional context, greater diversity in cropping patterns (requiring higher investments in research), limited physical infrastructure, particularly irrigation, and defective rural financial systems.

Agricultural research has generated several kinds of technology with high potentials for impact, but the expected impact on farmers' productivity, livelihood and quality of life has not been fully realized. Huge productivity gains are possible and accrue where governments allocate the necessary resources to agricultural research and development. In SSA, however, public investment in agriculture is still far below what is needed, despite commitments by African governments to allocate 10% of their public spending to it.

Although difficult to ascertain whether it is a trend reversal, recent FAO reports (2017a, 2017b) show a rise in hunger globally as well as in Africa. The NOU in the world suffering from chronic food deprivation began to rise in 2014 — going from 775 million people to 777 million in 2015 — and is now estimated to have increased further, to 815 million in 2016. The deterioration was most severe in Sub-Saharan Africa and Southeastern Asia (FAO, 2017a, 2017b).

In SSA, micronutrient deficiencies contribute 1.5–12% of the total Disability Adjusted Life Years (DALYs). Alarming numbers suffer from iron-deficiency anaemia, which affects more than half of the female population in countries such as DR Congo, Ghana, Mali, Senegal and Togo. Selenium contributes to the human diet through uptake by crops from the soil. Even mild to moderate deficiencies of micronutrients can lead to severe human health problems, generally related to sub-optimal metabolic functioning, decreased immunity and, consequently, increased susceptibility to infections, growth failure, cognitive impairment and, finally, reduced productivity (WHO, 2016; de Valenca *et al.*, 2017).

Besides, around 40% of children under the age of five suffer from stunted growth, that is, severely reduced height-for-age relative to their growth potential. Stunting is a result of periods of undernutrition in early childhood, and it has been found to have a series of adverse long-term effects in those who survive childhood. It is negatively associated with mental development, with human capital accumulation, with adult health, and with economic productivity and income levels in adulthood (Larsen and Lilleør, 2017).

It was argued that agricultural development has enormous potential to make significant contributions to reducing malnutrition and associated ill health. With its close links to both the immediate causes of undernutrition (diets, feeding practices, and health) and its underlying determinants (such as income, food security, education, access to WASH — water, sanitation and hygiene — and health services, and gender equity), the agriculture sector can play a much stronger role than in the past in improving nutrition outcomes.

An assessment was carried out through a review of a large number of studies that examined the factors determining adoption of innovative agricultural technology, their benefits and the underlying mechanisms, sustainability of the benefits, empowerment of women farmers and child nutrition, and prospects of youth employment in agriculture and elsewhere. A case was then made out for greater investment in agricultural research.

The main factors that determine the awareness of a new technology include social characteristics of farmers, and agro-ecological conditions in a targeted area. In particular, farmers that are more aware of a technology have higher education, live in proximity to research institutions and universities, and have more social capital, which includes participation in collective actions, membership of non-agricultural organization and network of credit channels.

Both social characteristics and economic constraints determine the tryout step. This is positively influenced by factors such as learning from others, higher liquidity, and access to information and extension services. In particular, younger farmers living near the market, with social capital and human capital endowments are more likely to experiment with a new technology.

The continued adoption step is largely influenced by economic and demographic factors, and dissemination mechanisms, such as extension. The role of path or state dependence is assessed, namely, the role of past experience in the adoption decision process. Moreover, the initial technology adoption decision significantly influences current technology adoption decision, even more than the lagged adoption (Garbero *et al.*, 2016).

A rich shelf of innovative technologies by itself is not enough. Agricultural extension is expected to play a key role in facilitating adoption of new technology. However, there are few examples of successful extension. There is growing evidence that the private sector is taking over some of the functions which were formerly performed by governments — especially in African countries facing severe budget constraints. Two policy concerns are: (i) reform in extension services, and (ii) creation of enabling conditions for the private sector to have a more influential role in targeting marginal and women farmers for better nutritional outcomes.

The pathways through which agricultural research enhances standard of living conditions and welfare outcomes comprise higher agricultural productivity, lower production cost, reduction of food prices, higher wages and employment, and lower losses due to diseases or unfavourable climatic conditions. Hence, both producers and consumers are likely to benefit. However, many of the studies reviewed lack analytical rigour, casting serious doubts about their inferences (Masset *et al.*, 2012). Subject to this caveat, some of the principal findings are reviewed below.

Improved chick pea and pigeon pea in Tanzania lead to more than moderate increases in the average expected consumption per adult equivalent; increase in improved maize area in Malawi is associated with increase in income of adopters, in own maize consumption and increase in assets; tissue culture banana technology adoption in Kenya increases annual farm and household income substantially as well as reduces food insecurity; adoption of NERICA positively increases household income, along with other variables characterizing household demographic structure, such as gender, age and education of household head and household size in Nigeria; the impacts of improved seeds on per capita expenditure, poverty and maize yields in Uganda were significant; evidence from randomized controlled trials showed positive impacts from biofortified crops, including orange-fleshed sweet potato, on vitamin A status among women and children; there were mixed impacts on the links between women's empowerment, intra-household decision-making, and better nutrition outcomes; in Kenya, interventions to improve vegetable, ASF and fruit production produced mixed results, but ownership of livestock and milk consumption were associated with better nutrition outcomes. In contexts where markets are imperfect, supporting livestock ownership is conducive to improving diets by a direct access channel, as well as providing further livelihood opportunities and increased income.

Height-for-age is a strong biological marker of the nutritional status of children during the first 1,000 days of their lives, from conception to 2 years of age. During this period, children have very high growth rates; and consequently, when subject to spells of growth faltering, children quickly fall behind the height-for-age growth curves of their peers, with limited chances of catching up subsequently.

An assessment of impact of the basket of technologies, offered under RIPAT, on stunting in northern Tanzania is insightful. The technology options comprise new banana cultivation techniques; new improved banana and other perennial and annual crop varieties; conservation agriculture for improved land utilization (such as minimum soil disturbance, cover crops, intercropping, rotation, and diversification of crops); post-harvesting technologies; improved animal husbandry; multipurpose trees for fodder, fruit, or firewood; soil and water conservation, including rain water harvesting; and savings groups. A key to RIPAT's success was that each farmer was free to choose which technologies to adopt on his/her own farm according to his/her own needs, constraints, and resources.

Drought resilience improved among the participating farmers in northern Tanzania. Besides, there was a significant positive impact on the height-for-age *z*-scores of young children who had been fully exposed to the project in their early life. Similarly, there was a substantial reduction in stunting prevalence among the young group of RIPAT children of around 18 percentage points.

An important policy insight that emerges is that, since the impacts were measured almost 5 years after the start of the project, which lasted three and a half years, these are sustainable impacts, but not necessarily quick impacts. There is thus potential for agricultural interventions in alleviating undernutrition and that they can indeed be very effective.

Lack of dietary diversity is viewed as the major cause of micronutrient malnutrition in SSA. Imbalanced diets resulting from consumption of mainly high carbohydrate based-diets also contribute to productivity losses and reduced educational attainment and income. Consequently, micronutrient malnutrition is currently the most critical for food and nutritional security problem as most diets are often deficient in essential vitamins and minerals.

In some cases, crop diversity does not influence dietary diversity after controlling for other covariates. However, the methodology is suspect, since there is little recognition of the fact that farm diversity is a response to weather and price risks (a more diversified crop portfolio protects the farmer better against such risks), and relative profitability of different crops and animal husbandry. Another major limitation is that the analysis of nutritional impact has to go beyond groups of food commodities consumed. Even among small holders a positive relationship between farm production diversity and dietary diversity is found to be weak (Kenya, Malawi and Ethiopia). If market transactions are prominent, instead of producing everything at home, households can buy a variety of food in the market when they generate sufficient income.

An assessment of the implications of buy and sell decisions of smallholders is thus useful. If a household sells part of its production, it results in greater dietary diversity (Ethiopia and Malawi). On the other hand, if farm production is more diverse, the household tends to buy less diverse food from the market. However, diversified own production can substitute for diversity from the market only partially, because more than half of all of the food consumed in sample households is purchased.

Two inferences follow: (i) increasing on-farm diversity among smallholders is not always the most effective way to improve dietary diversity and should not be considered a goal in itself; and (ii) in many situations, facilitating market access through improved infrastructure and other policies to reduce transaction costs and price distortions seems to be more promising than promoting further production diversification as such.

In SSA, micronutrient deficiencies contribute 1.5–12% of the total Disability Adjusted Life Years (DALYs). Alarming numbers suffer from iron-deficiency anaemia, which affects more than half of the female population in countries such as DR Congo, Ghana, Mali, Senegal, Togo. Direct interventions comprise dietary diversification, micronutrient supplementation, modification of food choices and fortification. Biofortification increases the content and/or bioavailability of essential nutrients in crops during plant growth through genetic and agronomic pathways.

Vitamin A deficiency is associated with the higher risk of morbidity and mortality, and ocular disorders such as night blindness, xerophthalmia and blindness, affecting infants, children and women during pregnancy and lactation. African regions account for the greatest number of preschool children with night blindness and for more than one-quarter of all children with sub-clinical vitamin A deficiency.

Even though currently food fortification and supplementation are the most commonly used strategies to alleviate micronutrient deficiencies among humans, biofortification (agronomic and/or genetic) is considered to have more potential in the long-term because it seems more cost-effective, and practical.

Sweet potato varieties most commonly cultivated in Africa are white or pale yellow having no or little provitamin A, and have a relatively high DM content. However, provitamin A-rich varieties, known as OSP, have been bred through the process of biofortification or have been introduced and evaluated, and are suitable for Africa in terms of preferred agronomic and consumer traits. Due to the high content of β-carotene in some African-grown OSP varieties, the relatively high seasonal consumption of sweet potato can contribute substantially to increased vitamin A intake adequacy.

A nearly 3-year long, large-scale intervention to introduce several OSP varieties using agricultural extension and market development activities, product development, combined with demand creation and nutrition education, was implemented in rural communities of Zambézia Province, Mozambique. A detailed and rigorous evaluation of this intervention shows a substantial impact on the dietary intake of OSP among women and preschool children. The increase in OSP intake in the intervention groups was largely attributed to a direct substitution of white and yellow sweet potato varieties. The incorporation of OSP in the diet translated to a large, significant increase in vitamin A intakes by these subgroups and hence reduced the prevalence of inadequate vitamin A intakes.

There were no major differences in the impact on OSP or vitamin A intakes between the groups exposed for 3 years or one. The cost saving in the less intensive version is enormous and of considerable policy significance.

The similar substitution rates across age groups suggest that OSP was equitably shared among the women and children of different ages.

The wide acceptance of OSP in populations where white or yellow sweet potatoes are usually consumed has been observed elsewhere in Sub-Saharan Africa, and can thus be plausibly generalized.

Focusing on home gardening and animal/dairy production, evidence is mixed in terms of their impacts on nutrition. While there is evidence of positive impacts on intermediary nutrition outcomes, such as dietary diversity, household production and consumption, and child and maternal intake of "target" foods and micronutrients, impact on nutrition outcomes — particularly child anthropometry and micronutrient status — was much more limited, except in relation to vitamin A intake and status. The fact that home production requires fewer inputs and investment is extremely important for resource-poor families that have limited access to production inputs. Yet moderately rigorous crop and livestock production in home gardens can generate as much revenue per unit area as field crop production. Home gardens provide multiple environmental and ecological benefits.

A useful policy insight emerges from a review of studies of home gardens selected on certain criteria. In many cases, home garden programmes increased the consumption of fruits and vegetables, aquaculture and small fisheries interventions increased the consumption of fish, and dairy development projects increased the consumption of milk. A difficulty is that an increase in the consumption of the food item targeted by the intervention does not imply an improvement in the overall diet, because substitution effects in consumption occur. For example, in one case, although the consumption of vegetables, rice, and fish increased after the intervention, the consumption of pulses decreased. This suggests that indicators of the diversity of the diet or analysis of the full consumption basket are better indicators than is consumption of the specific food promoted by an intervention. Indeed, as argued here, there is a strong case for going beyond food basket to their nutritional content.

Women are vitally important agents, both in their roles as producers and as custodians of household welfare. The resources and income flows that women control often have positive impacts on household health and nutrition. Agricultural programmes and policies that empower and enable women and that involve them in decisions and activities throughout the life of the programme achieve greater nutritional impacts. However, failure to understand cultural norms and the gender dynamics within the household can result in unanticipated outcomes. In the Gambia, for example, a project geared to increasing women's rice production was so successful that the land it was grown on was reclassified internally within the household. This resulted in output from that land being sold by men as opposed to women. Women therefore lost their original income stream, but remained committed to working long hours.

There are improved impacts on nutrition if agricultural interventions are targeted to women and when specific work is done around women's empowerment (for example, through behaviour change communication), mediated through women's time use, their own health and nutrition status, and their access to and control over resources as well as intra-household decision-making power. Further, encouragement and nudges through social networks of women induce adoption as they rely more on their informal social networks than men.

The link between production and dietary diversity is incomplete without acknowledging the important role of value chains in nutritional outcomes. An important fact, however, is that a value chain is commodity specific, and thus involves only one particular food that is relevant within a diet. What is thus required is to identify opportunities where value chain actors benefit from supplying the market with agricultural products of higher nutritional value. But value chain development has rarely focused attention on consumers — consumers are simply considered as purchasers driving the ultimate source of demand. In this light, the value chain strategy is likely to be enriched by a stronger consumer focus, and, in particular, a focus on consumer nutrition and health. The empirical evidence on the role of value chains in improving nutrition is, however, scanty and mixed.

Briefly, on the demand side, the central issue is how to promote consumption of nutritious foods by target populations that may not be able to afford a healthy diet. Similarly, on the supply side, an important concern is the feasibility of targeting the poorest smallholders and informal enterprises along the value chain, particularly, involving women.

From the perspective of sustainable development, two major concerns are: scaling up successful agricultural practices, and prioritizing sustainable intensification approaches and integrating them into agricultural technology in the local context. Less-favoured areas need to receive attention in policy matters, especially in the context of the threat to agriculture from climate change and/or globalization of agricultural trade.

Focusing on conservation technologies, attention needs to be given to restoration of soil fertility and judicious use of water. Both conservation technologies can also be pursued in some low-productivity areas. However, they have not caught the attention of policymakers. Extension of both these measures would help raise productivity and save resources in these areas.

Although there is substantial evidence on the adoption and productivity impacts of soil and water conservation measures in Ethiopia, the evidence on adoption and productivity impacts of other land management practices, including MT and CF use, is scanty. But a few insights emerge from a detailed assessment. There is a strong impact of MT on agricultural productivity, compared with the impact of CF, in the low agricultural potential areas. In the high agricultural potential region, however, CF has a very significant and positive impact on crop productivity, whereas MT has no significant impact. Hence different strategies are needed for different environments. For instance, in the low agricultural potential areas, government and non-governmental organizations should focus more on promoting MT as a yield-augmenting technology. Relying on external inputs (such as chemicals and fertilizers) in low-potential areas, which has been the strategy in the past, is not likely to be beneficial unless moisture availability is enhanced.

Many African soils suffer from multiple micronutrient deficiencies, as a result of their inherent soil properties and continuous cropping without nutrient replenishment. Current fertilization programmes in African countries primarily focus on NPK fertilizers, but many soils are non-responsive to NPK due to (multiple) micronutrient deficiencies. Soil modification with small amounts of (multiple) micronutrients is a sustainable strategy to increase yields and nutritional quality of crops. A review of experiments from ten African countries on the impact of

Zn-enriched fertilizers showed that soil Zn application increased the Zn concentration in maize, rice and wheat grains. Moreover, another agronomic benefit is that seedlings from seeds with high Zn concentration have better growth performance and resilience against environmental stress, so positive impacts on productivity may be seen in the next cropping generation.

Application of micronutrient-enriched fertilizers has minimal negative environmental impact. Most micronutrients are not susceptible to leaching because they are strongly bound in the soil.

An important question is whether agronomic biofortification is an effective, feasible and sustainable approach to alleviate micronutrient deficiencies; especially in comparison with other intervention strategies such as genetic biofortification, food fortification, supplementation and dietary diversification. An unequivocal answer is difficult as the literature is sparse. Nevertheless, a few observations are in order.

A key issue is the commercialization of smallholder agriculture to create markets for the extra production, because otherwise investments in (extra) mineral fertilizer are not economically feasible. Mapping of micronutrient deficiencies in order to provide field-specific fertilization recommendations remains a challenge. Furthermore, knowledge and tools should be accessible and affordable for farmers in rural African regions. Finally, new fertilizer products and management practices need to be matched with local socio-cultural environments in order to enhance adoption. It is important to raise awareness about proper food processing and consumption that stimulates micronutrient uptake into the human body.

The 15–24-year-old age group represents 20% of SSA's population today and, unlike in other regions, this youth share will remain high and stable. Agriculture has a substantial role in meeting the youth employment challenge facing Africa, given the inability of the urban economy to absorb fully the young entrants to the rural labour force. It is argued that there will be vast opportunities for the innovative young people in agricultural systems as they adapt to a range of challenges in the near future. These challenges relate to raising productivity in a sustainable way, integration into emerging high value chains, and healthy diets. A major barrier is, however, strong negative preferences/attitudes of the youth towards agriculture. Unfortunately, the governments have not effectively addressed either the attitude of many young people towards agriculture or the obstacles preventing their entry into the sector. To create opportunities commensurate with the number of young people who will need employment, constraints on the acquisition of capital, land, and skills must be removed or relaxed.

Some options that may help the young as well as others include allowing alternative forms of collateral, such as chattel mortgages, warehouse receipts, and the future harvest; leasing also offers young farmers some relief, as it requires either no or less collateral than typically required by loans; outgrower arrangements that pre-finance inputs and assure marketing channels; microinsurance offering low premiums, flexible payments, and prompt settlement of claims. However, an exclusive focus of the young in these innovative financial arrangements may add to the risks of financial institutions and undermine their attractiveness to the latter. Indeed, any and all innovations in finance that facilitate sustainable outreach to small farmers and rural entrepreneurs should be supported. When necessary, additional features should be added to enable these programmes to serve young people.

The two aspects of land administration that matter most to young entrants to the labour force are the need to improve security of tenure and the need to relax controls on rental. Land redistribution will also enhance young people's access to land.

Young Africans must be equipped with basic reading, writing, and numeracy skills, and the ability to use digital technology to access and interpret information. A growing and diversifying agricultural sector will create jobs that demand increasingly advanced technical and professional skills, from processing and marketing to agricultural research. Development of agro-food businesses represents a significant opportunity for youth employment and for local development, due to powerful growth linkages to the rest of the economy.

A case can be made for higher investment in agricultural research. A few examples illustrate the high returns. (i) Maize improvement in West and Central Africa gave a return of 43%. (ii) In SSA, national and international organizations are making a big impact in reinforcing food security and alleviating poverty through rice research. Overall, improved varieties have increased net revenues by $93 per hectare, with the highest gains in irrigated and rainfed lowland ecologies. The annual returns to investment in rice research now exceed 20%.

Impact studies also reveal that rice research contributes effectively to the realization of almost all the Millennium Development Goals, including halving levels of poverty and hunger, promoting education, improving health, reducing child mortality, empowering women and ensuring environmental sustainability.

Yet agricultural research has had mixed impact on well-being in this region. Specifically, there is no emphasis on research by the NARS on reducing undernutrition. Thus there are cases of malnutrition in the face of abundant food supply because of the lack of integrating researches on crop production, nutrition and health.

13. Concluding Observations

To conclude, institutional innovations are needed to improve productivity and make public agricultural institutions more responsive to markets, more accountable to the communities they serve, and better recognized as an important tool for achieving economic growth. Huge productivity gains are possible and accrue where governments allocate the necessary resources to agricultural research and development. In SSA, however, public investment in agriculture is still far below what is needed. The challenge is to develop technology that is relevant to small farmers and to enable them to transform their farms into viable small businesses that make a vital contribution to local and national economies and improve nutrition. But better nutritional outcomes are contingent on clear research priorities established through an integrated and empirically valid analytical framework that encompasses the pathways identified and assessed here.

Although the effects of agricultural interventions on nutrition are largely limited or missing, it would be a mistake to infer that the absence of a significant effect implies that there is no effect. Few in number, their use of rigorous methodologies nevertheless yields significant effects on nutrition.

Acknowledgements

We are grateful to the editor, Raghbendra Jha, for meticulous editorial advice, and P. Winters, A. Garbero, R. Omar, Manoj K. Pandey, Katsushi S. Imai and Nidhi Kaicker for valuable suggestions. The views expressed are personal and not necessarily of the organizations the authors are affiliated to.

References

Abadie, A. (2003) "Semiparametric Instrumental Variable Estimation of Treatment Response Models", *Journal of Econometrics*, Vol. 113, pp. 231–263.

Abebe, T., Wiersum, K., Bongers, F. and F. Sterck (2006) "Diversity and Dynamics in Homegardens of Southern Ethiopia," in *Tropical Homegardens: A Time-tested Example of Sustainable Agroforestry*, ed. Nair BMKPKR. Dordrecht, The Netherlands: Springer Science.

Asfaw, S., Kassie, M., Simtowe, F. and L. Lipper (2012a) "Poverty Reduction Effects of Agricultural Technology Adoption: A Micro-evidence from Rural Tanzania", *Journal of Development Studies*, Vol. 48, pp. 1288–1305.

Asfaw, S., Shiferaw, B., Simtowe, F. and L. Lipper (2012b) "Impact of Modern Agricultural Technologies on Smallholder Welfare: Evidence from Tanzania and Ethiopia", *Food Policy*, Vol. 37, pp. 283–295.

Asuming-Brempong, S., Gyasi, K. O., Marfo, K. A., Diagne, A., Wiredu, A. N. and A. Asuming-Boakye (2011) "The Exposure and Adoption of New Rice for Africa (NERICAs) Among Ghanaian Rice Farmers: What is the Evidence?" *African Journal of Agricultural Research*, Vol. 6, No. 27, pp. 5911–5917.

Azzarri, C., Zezza, A., Haile, B. and E. Cross (2015) "Does Livestock Ownership Affect Animal Source Foods Consumption and Child Nutritional Status? Evidence from Rural Uganda", *The Journal of Development Studies*, Vol. 51, No. 8, pp. 1034–1059. DOI: 0.1080/00220388.2015.1018905.

Bachewe, F. N., Berhane, G., Minten, B. and A. S. Taffesse (2017) "Agricultural Transformation in Africa? Assessing the Evidence in Ethiopia", *World Development*, Articles in Press.

Behrman, J. R. and A. Deolalikar (1989) "Is Variety the Spice of Life? Implications for Calorie Intake", *The Review of Economics and Statistics*, Vol. 71, No. 4, pp. 666–672.

Berti, P. R., Krasevec, J. and S. FitzGerald (2004) "A Review of the Effectiveness of Agriculture Interventions in Improving Nutrition Outcomes", *Public Health Nutrition*, Vol. 7, No. 5, pp. 599–609.

Bezu, S., Kassie, G. T., Shiferaw, B. and J. Ricker-Gilbert (2014) "Impact of Improved Maize Adoption on Welfare of Farm Households in Malawi: A Panel Data Analysis", *World Development*, Vol. 59, pp. 120–131.

Blanken, J., von Braun, J. and H. de Haen (1994) "The Triple Role of Potatoes as a Source of Cash, Food, and Employment: Effects on Nutritional Improvement in Rwanda", in *Agricultural Commercialization, Economic Development, and Nutrition,* eds. J. von Braun and E. Kennedy (pp. 276–294). Baltimore, MD: Johns Hopkins University Press.

Brun, T., Reynaud, J. and S. Chevaussus-Agnes (1989) "Food and Nutrition Impact of One Home Garden Project in Senegal", *Ecology of Food and Nutrition*, Vol. 23, pp. 91–108.

Carletto, G., Ruel, M., Winters, P. and A. Zezza (2015) "Farm-level Pathways to Improved Nutritional Status: Introduction to the Special Issue", *The Journal of Development Studies*, Vol. 51, No. 8, pp. 945–957.

CGIAR (2011) 40 Findings on the Impacts of CGIA R Research, CGIAR.

Cowan, R. and P. Gunby (1996) "Sprayed to Death: Path Dependence, Lock-in and Pest Control Strategies", *The Economic Journal*, Vol. 106, No. 436, pp. 521–542.

de Valençaa, A. W., Bakeb, A., Brouwerb, I. D. and K. E. Gillera (2017) "Agronomic Biofortification of Crops to Fight Hidden Hunger in Sub-Saharan Africa", *Global Food Security*, Vol. 12, pp. 8–14.

Diagne, A. and M. Demont (2007) "Taking a New Look at Empirical Models of Adoption: Average Treatment Effect Estimation of Adoption Rates and their Determinants", *Agricultural Economics*, Vol. 37, Nos. 2–3, pp. 201–210.

Dillon, A., Mcgee, K. and Oseni, G. (2015) "Agricultural Production, Dietary Diversity and Climate Variability", *The Journal of Development Studies*, Vol. 51, No. 8, pp. 976–995.

Donstop-Nguezet P. M., Diagne, A. and V. O. Okoruwa Ojehomon (2011) "Impact of Improved Rice Technology (Nerica Varieties) on Income and Poverty Among Rice Farming Households in Nigeria: A Local Average Treatment Effect (Late) Approach", *Quarterly Journal of International Agriculture*, Vol. 50, No. 3, pp. 267–291.

Doss, C. R. (2006) "Analyzing Technology Adoption Using Microstudies: Limitations, Challenges, and Opportunities for Improvement", *Agricultural Economics*, Vol. 34, No. 3, pp. 207–219.

Duflo, E. (2003) "Grandmothers and Granddaughters: Old-age Pensions and Intrahousehold Allocation in South Africa", *World Bank Economic Review*, Vol. 17, No. 1, pp. 1–25.

FAO (2011) *Guidelines for Measuring Household and Individual Dietary Diversity*. Rome.

FAO (2015) *The State of Food Insecurity in the World – Meeting the 2015 International Hunger Targets: Taking Stock of Uneven Progress*. Food and Agriculture Organization of the United Nations, Rome.

FAO, IFAD and WFP (2017a) Global Report on Food Crises 2017. Rome.

FAO, IFAD, UNICEF, WFP and WHO (2017b) *The State of Food Security and Nutrition in the World 2017. Building Resilience for Peace and Food Security*. Rome: FAO.

Gaiha, R., Jha, R. and V. S. Kulkarni (2014) *Diets, Malnutrition, and Disease: The Indian Experience*. New Delhi: Oxford University Press.

Galhena, D. H., Freed, R. and K. M. Maredia (2013) "Home Gardens: A Promising Approach to Enhance Household Food Security and Wellbeing", *Agriculture & Food Security*, Vol. 2, p. 8.

Garbero, A., Gaiha, R., Marionand, P. and E. Porreca (2016) *Agricultural Research and Welfare in Uganda*. SKD, IFAD, Rome.

Garcia-Banuelos, M. L., Sida-Arreola, J. P. and E. Sanches (2014) "Biofortification — Promising Approach to Increasing the Content of Iron and Zinc in Staple Food Crops", *Journal of Elementology*, Vol. 19, No. 3, pp. 865–888.

Gelli, A., Hawkes, C., Donovan, J., Harris, J., Summer, A., de Brauw, A., Spencer, H., Johnson, N., Garrett, J. and D. Ryckembusch (2015) "Value Chains and Nutrition: A Framework to Support the Identification, Design, and Evaluation of Interventions", IFPRI Discussion Paper 01413.

Gibson, R. S. (2007) "The Role of Diet- and Host-Related Factors in Nutrient Bioavailability and thus in Nutrient-Based Dietary Requirement Estimates", *Food and Nutrition Bulletin*, Vol. 28, No. 1 (Suppl International), pp. S77–S100.

Gillespie, S. and M. van den Bold (2017) "Agriculture, Food Systems, and Nutrition: Meeting the Challenge", *Global Challenges*, Vol. 1, pp. 1–12.

Hasan, M. F., Imai, K. S. and T. Sato (2015) "Impacts of Agricultural Extension on Crop Productivity in Uganda", DP2012-34, Kobe University.

Herforth, A. (2010) "Promotion of Traditional African Vegetables in Kenya and Tanzania: A Case Study of an Intervention Representing Emerging Imperatives in Global Nutrition", Ph.D thesis, Cornell University, Ithaca, NY.

Hotz, C., Loechl, C., de Brauw, A., Eozenou, P., Gilligan, D., Moursi, M., Munhaua, B., van Jaarsveld, P., Carriquiry, A. and J. V. Meenakshi (2012) "A Large-scale Intervention to Introduce Orange Sweet Potato in Rural

Mozambique Increases Vitamin A Intakes Among Children and Women", *British Journal of Nutrition*, Vol. 108, pp. 163–176.

ILO (2016) "World Employment and Social Outlook: Trends 2016", Geneva, Switzerland.

Imbens, G. and J. Angrist (1994) "Identification and Estimation of Local Average Treatment Effects", *Econometrica,* Vol. 61, pp. 467–476.

Jayne, T. S., Chamberlin, J. and D. Headey (2014) "Land Pressures, the Evolution of Farming Systems, and Development Strategies in Africa: A Synthesis", Food Policy, Vol. 48, pp. 1–17.

Jha, R., Gaiha, R. and A. Sharma (2009) "Modelling Variety in Consumption Expenditure on Food in India", *International Review of Applied Economics*, Vol. 23, No. 4, pp. 503–519.

Jones, K. M. and A. de Brauw (2015) "Using Agriculture to Improve Child Health: Promoting Orange Sweet Potatoes Reduces Diarrhea", *World Development*, Vol. 74, pp. 15–24.

Joy, E. J. M., Kumssa, D. B., Broadley, M. R., Watts, M. J., Young, S. D., Chilimba, A. D. C. and E. L. Ander (2015) "Dietary Mineral Supplies in Malawi: Spatial and Socioeconomic Assessment", *BMC Nutrition*, Vol. 1, No. 1, pp. 1–25.

Kabunga N. S., Dubois T. and M. Qaim (2014) "Impact of Tissue Culture Banana Technology on Farm Household Income and Food Security in Kenya", *Food Policy*, Vol. 45, pp. 25–34.

Kassa, H., Ayalew, W. and Z. Habtegabriel (2003) "Enhancing the Role of Livestock Production in Improving Nutritional Status of Farming Families: Lessons from a Dairy Goat Development Project in Eastern Ethiopia", *Livestock Research for Rural Development*, Vol. 15, p. 6.

Kassie, M., Shireraw B. and G. Muricho (2011) "Agricultural Technology, Crop Income, and Poverty Alleviation in Uganda", *World Development*, Vol. 39, No. 10, pp. 1784–1795.

Kennedy, G. L., Pedro, M. R., Seghieri, C., Nantel, G. and I. Brouwer (2007) "Dietary Diversity Score is a Useful Indicator of Micronutrient Intake in Non-Breast-Feeding Filipino Children", *Journal of Nutrition*, Vol. 137, No. 2, pp. 472–477.

Kerr, R. B. and M. Chirwa (2004) "Participatory Research Approaches and Social Dynamics that Influence Agricultural Practices to Improve Child Nutrition in Malawi", *EcoHealth*, Vol. 1, pp. 109–119.

Kidala, D., Greiner, T. and M. Gebre-Medhin (2000) "Five-Year Follow-up of a Food-Based Vitamin A Intervention in Tanzania", *Public Health Nutrition*, Vol. 3, No. 4, pp. 425–431.

Kikulwe, E. M., Kabunga, N. and M. Qaim (2012) "Impact of Tissue Culture Banana Technology in Kenya: A Difference-in-Difference Estimation Approach", No. 117. Courant Research Centre: Poverty, Equity and Growth-Discussion Papers.

Kumar, N., Hariss, J. and R. Rawat (2015) "If they Grow it, Will they Eat and Grow? Evidence from Zambia on Agricultural Diversity and Child Undernutrition", *The Journal of Development Studies*, Vol. 51, No. 8, pp. 1060–1077.

Lambrecht, I., Vanlauwe, B., Merckx, R. and M. Maertens (2014) "Understanding the Process of Agricultural Technology Adoption: Mineral Fertilizer in Eastern DR Congo", *World Development*, Vol. 59, pp. 132–146.

Larsen, A. F. and H. B. Lilleør (2017) "Can Agricultural Interventions Improve Child Nutrition? Evidence from Tanzania", *The World Bank Economic Review*, Vol. 31, No. 3, pp. 767–785.

Lindner, R. K., Pardey, P. G. and F. G. Jarrett (1982) "Distance to Information Source and the Time Lag to Early Adoption of Trace Element Fertilisers", *The Australian Journal of Agricultural Economics*, Vol. 26, No. 2, pp. 98–113.

Manzeke, G. M., Mtambanengwe, F., Nezomba, H. and P. Mapfumo (2014) "Zinc Fertilization Influence on Maize Productivity and Grain Nutritional Quality Under Integrated Soil Fertility Management in Zimbabwe", *Field Crops Research*, Vol. 166, pp. 128–136.

Masset, E., Haddad, L., Cornelius, A. and J. Isaza-Castro (2012) "Effectiveness of Agricultural Interventions that Aim to Improve Nutritional Status of Children: Systematic Review", *British Medical Journal*, Vol. 344, pp. 1–7. https://doi.org/10.1136/bmj.d8222 (Published 17 January 2012)

Mathur, S. and R. Gaiha (2003) "Impact of Agricultural Research on Rural Poverty — A Review of Some Analytical Issues for Agricultural Development", Chapter 2 in *Agricultural Research and Poverty Reduction — Some Issues and Evidence*, eds. S. Mathur and D. Pachico, CIAT.

Mekonnen, D. A., Gerber, N. and J. A. Matz (2017) "Gendered Social Networks, Agricultural Innovations, and Farm Productivity in Ethiopia", *World Development*, Articles in Press.

Mellor, J. W. (2014) "High Rural Population Density Africa: What are the Growth Requirements and WHO Participates?" *Food Policy*, Vol. 48, pp. 66–75.

Mokwunye, U. (2010) "Regional Research of Africa's Agricultural Research and Development", GCARD.

Moser, C. M. and C. B. Barrett (2006) "The Complex Dynamics of Smallholder Technology Adoption: The Case of SRI in Madagascar", *Agricultural Economics*, Vol. 35, No. 3, pp. 373–388.

Muller, C. (2009) "Do Agricultural Outputs of Partly Autarkic Peasants Affect Their Health and Nutrition? Evidence from Rwanda", *Food Policy*, Vol. 34, No. 2, pp. 166–175. DOI:10.1016/j.foodpol.2008.10.010.

Palacios-López, A. and R. Lopez (2014) "Gender Differences in Agricultural Productivity: The Role of Market Imperfections", Department of Agricultural and Resource Economics, The University of Maryland, Mimeo.

Pandey, M. K. (2018) "Africa's Food Insecurity and its Determinants", in *Hunger and Malnutrition as Major Challenges of the 21st Century,* ed. R. Jha, Singapore: World Scientific Press.

Proctor, F. and J. V. Lucchesi (2012) "Small-Scale Farming and Youth in an Era of Rapid Rural Change", London: International Institute for Environment and Development.

Quisumbing, A., Meinzen-Dick, R., Raney, T. L., Croppenstedt, A., Behrman, J. and A. Peterman (eds.) (2014) Gender in Agriculture: Closing the Knowledge Gap. FAO.

Rajendran, S., Bekunda, M. and P. J. Lukumay (2014) "Does Crop Diversity Contribute to Dietary Diversity? Evidence from Integration of Vegetables into Maize Based Farming Systems in Tanzania", Contributed Discussion Paper prepared for presentation at the 88th Annual Conference of the Agricultural Economics Society, Agro Paris Tech, Paris, France, April 9–11.

Raitzer, D. A. (2003) "Benefit-Cost Meta-Analysis of Investment in the International Agricultural Research Centers of the CGIAR", CGIAR.

Robinson, E., Nwuneli, N., Henson, S. and J. Humphrey (2014) "Mapping Value Chains for Nutrient-Dense Foods in Nigeria", *IDS*, March.

Robinson, E., Akinyele, I. O., Humphrey, J. and S. Henson (forthcoming, 2014) *Policy Options to Enhance Markets for Nutrient-Dense Foods in Nigeria*, IDS Evidence Report, Brighton: IDS.

Ruel, M. T., Alderman, H. and the Maternal and Child Nutrition Study Group (2013) "Nutrition-Sensitive Interventions and Programs: How Can They Help to Accelerate Progress in Improving Maternal and Child Nutrition?" *The Lancet*, Vol. 382, No. 9891, pp. 536–551.

Saltzman, A., Birol, E., Bouis, H. E., Boy, E., De Moura, F., Islam, Y. and W. H. Pfeiffer (2013) "Biofortification: Progress Toward a More Nourishing Future", *Global Food Security*, Vol. 2, pp. 9–17.

Seck, P. A., Touré, A. A., Coulibaly, J., Diagne, A. and M. C. S. Wopereis (2013) "Africa's Rice Economy Before and After the 2008 Rice Crisis", in *Realizing Africa's Rice Promise*, eds. M. C. S. Wopereis, D. E. Johnson, N. Ahmadi, E. Tollens and A. Jalloh, Wallingford, UK: CAB International.

Sibhatu, K. T., Krishna, V. V. and M. Qaim (2014) "Production Diversity and Dietary Diversity in Smallholder Farm Households", *Proceedings of the National Academy of Sciences of the United States of America*, Vol. 112, No. 34.

Simtowe, F., Kassie, M., Asfaw, S., Shiferaw, B., Monyo, E. and M. Siambi (2012) "Welfare Effects of Agricultural Technology Adoption: The Case of Improved Groundnut Varieties in Rural Malawi", Selected Paper prepared for presentation at the International Association of Agricultural Economists (IAAE) Triennial Conference, Foz do Iguaçu, Brazil, August 18–24.

Stewart, R. L., Silva, N. D., Muchiri, E., Zaranyika, H., Erasmus, Y., Randall, N., Rafferty, S., Korth, M., Madinga, N. and T. de Wet (2015) "The Effects of Training, Innovation and New Technology on African Smallholder Farmers' Economic Outcomes and Food Security: A Systematic Review", 3ie Grantee Final Review, London: International Initiative for Impact Evaluation (3ie).

Sumberg, J., Anyidoho, N. A., Leavy, J., te Lintelo, D. J. and K. Wellard (2012) "Introduction: The Young People and Agriculture 'Problem' in Africa", *IDS Bulletin.*

Suttie, D. (2015) "Youth Employment and Agriculture in Sub-Saharan Africa", *Food and Business News Platform*, November 19.

Tadele, G. and A. A. Gella (2012) "'A Last Resort and Often Not an Option at All': Farming and Young People in Ethiopia", *IDS Bulletin*, Vol. 43, No. 6, pp. 1–11.

Thirtle, C., Lin, L. and J. Piesse (2003) "The Impact of Research Led Agricultural Productivity Growth on Poverty Reduction in Africa, Asia and Latin America", Contributed paper for the 25th conference of the International Association of Agricultural Economists Durban, August.

Timmer, C. P. (1981) "Is There 'Curvature' in the Slutsky Matrix?" *The Review of Economics and Statistics*, Vol. 63, No. 3, pp. 395–402.

Timmer, C. P. (2015) *Food Security and Scarcity: Why Ending Hunger is So Hard*. Philadelphia: University of Pennsylvania Press.

UN Women, IFAD, FAO and WFP (2015) Technologies for Rural Women in Africa, Policy Brief.

Vanlauwe, B., Descheemaeker, K., Giller, K. E., Huising, J., Merckx, R., Nziguheba, G., Wendt, J. and Zingore, S. (2015) "Integrated Soil Fertility Management in Sub-Saharan Africa: Unravelling Local Adaptation", *SOIL*, Vol. 1, pp. 491–508.

von Braun, J., Johm, K. and D. Puetz (1994) "Nutritional Effects of Commercialization of a Woman's Crop: Irrigated Rice in The Gambia", in

Agricultural Commercialization, Economic Development and Nutrition, eds. J. von Braun and E. Kennedy.

WHO (2016) *Vitamin and Mineral Nutrition Information System*. World Health Organization (www.who.int).

World Bank (2007) *From Agriculture to Nutrition: Pathways, Synergies and Outcomes*. Washington, DC.

World Bank (2015) *Africa: Youth Employment in Sub-Saharan Africa*. Washington, DC.

Yokouchi, T. and K. Saito (2016) "Factors Affecting Farmers' Adoption of NERICA Upland Rice Varieties: The Case of a Seed Producing Village in Central Benin", *Food Security*, Vol. 8, pp. 197–209.

Chapter 11

Rethinking Agricultural Transformation and Food Security in Africa

Abbi M. Kedir*,‡ and George Kararach†,§

**Sheffield University Management School (SUMS), Conduit Road, Sheffield S10 1FL, UK*
†United Nations Economic Commission for Africa, Addis Ababa, Ethiopia
‡a.m.kedir@sheffield.ac.uk
§kararach@un.org respectively

Abstract

Food security has eluded much of Africa over many decades. Despite remarkable GDP growth figures, millions of African suffer from both income and food poverty. Rapid population growth and climate change pose major threats and lie at the heart of many of the structural and developmental problems of the continent such as persistently low agricultural productivity, recurrent food shortages and malnutrition. Scanning the historical landscape covering the period from 1960 to 2015, we draw attention to the role of technology and research in transformation of the agricultural sector in Africa. We argue that science and technology strategies play a critical role and are the key to future improvements in agricultural productivity, diversification and food security in Africa. These desirous improvements and strides do not come cheap, and hence necessitate major, contextualized, strategic and sustained technological investments (e.g. in R&D). The economic history of successful regions of the world reinforce the case for investment in technology for sustained reduction of the high rates of poverty and food insecurity that stubbornly plagued the continent for centuries.

Keywords: Food security, climate change, agricultural productivity, technology, Africa.

1. Introduction

Despite remarkable macroeconomic or GDP growth figures, food security has eluded much of Africa over many decades. The continent is faced with two broad tendencies: a rapidly rising population implying a rising demand for food. The other feature is one where farmers in African countries are subject to a variety of risks resulting from, inter alia, droughts, floods and other natural calamities that undermine agricultural productivity and sustainable food production. The major focus of this study is agricultural transformation and food security in Africa and our study broadly covers the period from 1960 to 2015. We will emphasize the role of technology and research in African agriculture in a bid to transform the sector, raise its productivity and secure food availability. Science and technology strategies are essential to improve agricultural productivity and food security in Africa (InterAcademy Council, 2004). Minten and Barrett's (2008) research clearly indicated the need to support technological investments for improved agricultural production as one viable source of economic diversification and as an important part of any strategy to reduce the high rates of poverty and food insecurity that stubbornly plagued the continent for many decades. Many years of growth research tells us that the high returns are associated with Research and Development (R&D) investments in terms of growth and poverty reduction. Robert Solow won the Nobel Prize in economics in 1987 for his discovery that technical change is the engine of growth. Apart from the fundamental inputs to production such as land and labour, investment in science, technology and agricultural research is what brings technological change and structural transformation of agriculture with interlinkages with other sectors of the economy. For agricultural productivity, food security, poverty reduction and its transformation in Africa, there is an increasing recognition of the necessity to invest in technology and research backed by commitment. This is very true given the predominant rural nature of poverty in Africa and the persistently low levels of R&D investment in the continent particularly in agriculture. The 2008 World Development Report (WDR) calls for increased investment in agriculture in the developing world if the Millennium Development Goals (MDG) targets of halving extreme poverty and hunger by 2015 were to be achieved. Only 4% of Official Development Assistance (ODA) flows went to agriculture even if 75% of the world's poor lives in the agricultural sector or rural regions such as Africa (World Bank, 2008). Despite the recent high level and intensified effort to support agriculture in Africa, agriculture is still heavily taxed and only 4% of the national budget is devoted to it for many decades. There is a huge capacity challenge with regard to smart investment in technology and research. India has 8% more agricultural researchers than Sub-Saharan Africa (SSA) taken together. In absolute terms it has 5,000 more PhD graduates as agricultural researchers than SSA. According to the recently compiled authoritative and reliable African Science and Technology Indicators (ASTI), about 1/3 of the 32 countries surveyed have less than 100 agricultural researchers while 2/3 of them have less than 200 researchers. This simple example illustrates the enormous challenge. Agreement on Agriculture (AOA) was introduced in 1995 to help poor countries in their agriculture but did not improve the competitiveness of Africa's agriculture in a noticeable way.

The chapter has six parts. The second, third and fourth parts focus on defining food security and importance of nutrition in development, the role of technology and research in the transformation of African agriculture and food security, respectively. The fifth part discusses lessons from within and outside Africa on successful technology and research, and explores policy options. Among others, we critically discuss the role of technology and research in the last 50 years, trends in agricultural R&D expenditure, capacity challenges in agricultural technology research (both physical and human), political economy of biotechnology and the role of technology and food security. One important issue is linked to regional integration to benefit African nations from the recently proposed WTO agricultural trade policy reforms (e.g. not complete but partial and reluctant removal of subsidies by rich countries). There is also an argument for a technology focus in Africa in relation to the same WTO reforms. Simulation and other empirical studies indicate that WTO reforms via the Doha Development Agenda (DDA) are not going to benefit/transform the agriculture of smaller developing countries in Africa as opposed to large ones such as Brazil and China (Nuetah *et al.*, 2010; von Grebmer, 2008; Anderson and Valenzuala, 2007). Part six forms our conclusion.

2. Food Security and Nutrition in African Development

The notion of food security embodies the changes in the policy and programme-related perspectives among stakeholders. It focused on addressing the challenges facing the agriculture sector in various parts of the world. It is not surprising that there are a number of definitions for food security sprawling the literature. For example, the 1996 World Food Summit of 1996 defined food security as a situation "*when all people, at all times, have physical and economic access to sufficient, safe and nutritious food that meets their dietary needs and food preferences for an active and healthy life*"(8). Food security exists when all people at all times have access to sufficient, safe, nutritious food to maintain a healthy and active life (Boyer, 2010; Sowman and Cardoso, 2010), and fit their dietary needs and food preferences (Scanlan, 2001). This definition implies at least four dimensions: sufficient quantities of food of appropriate quality; access by individuals to appropriate foods for a nutritious diet; utilisation of food with adequate diet, clean water, sanitation and healthcare to reach a state of nutritional well-being where all physiological needs are met; and equality across populations, households and individuals to have access to adequate food at all times (Kararach, 2014). The economic dimension is an additional critical aspect that exhibits itself often with limited or complete lack of purchasing power by households suffering from sporadic and chronic bouts of food security in many parts of Africa.

A household or population is said to be food secure when it can have reliable access to food in a quality and quantity sufficient for all the members to have a healthy and active life. Access, however, can be determined by extra-economic factors well beyond the market dynamics. For instance, it is plausible for individuals in food-secure households to suddenly become deficient or have unbalanced diets due to political economy and cultural dynamics that affect access (Benson, 2004). Equally, they might as well be food secure marginally with strong propensity and vulnerability to fall to food poverty traps that arrest them in food insecurity and be a subject of social protection and safety net interventions and constant appeals by multilateral organizations and non-governmental humanitarian entities.

Malnutrition results when an individual's diet does not have adequate calories and protein for growth and maintenance, or if the individual is unable to fully utilize the food they eat due to illness. It is a direct consequence of food insecurity. Although one may have enough calories, this does not guarantee adequate intake of essential micronutrients — vitamins, minerals and trace elements. Insufficient calorie intake often goes hand-in-hand with micronutrient malnutrition. Nutrition security is thus achieved when secure access to food is coupled with good sanitation, adequate health services and knowledgeable care to ensure a healthy and active life for all household members and the general population (*ibid*).

Food insecurity and malnutrition has many consequences for health and development, with women and children being the most vulnerable to the devastating effects. Malnourished women risk dying at childbirth and of delivering low-birthweight babies who fail to survive infancy. Equally, undernourished babies often suffer stunting and shorter lives. Children are vulnerable to food insecurity and malnutrition because of their physiology and high calorie needs for growth and development. For instance, malnutrition is the underlying cause of death of more than 2.6 million children each year, a third of under-five deaths, and a third of total child deaths worldwide (Black *et al.*, 2008).

Von Grebmer *et al.* (2015) notes that Sub-Saharan Africa still has the highest 2015 Global Hunger Index (GHI) score globally, at 32.2, despite the recent strong economic growth performance (UNCTAD, 2014). There have also been advances in public health with importance outcomes for overall morbidity and mortality (AVERT, 2014; WHO, 2013). The levels of conflicts have significantly reduced since the 1990s making the continent politically relatively stable and consequently hunger levels have fallen. We note that the causes of hunger are complex and cannot be attributed to conflict alone and a comprehensive analysis of the root causes of hunger needs to be explored.

Africa has seen slow progress in reducing stunting. The figure dropped slightly from 42.3% in 1990 to 32.0% in 2014 (UNICEF, WHO and World Bank, 2015). Although the prevalence rates of stunting in pre-school children in Africa fell by 10.3% between 1990 and 2014, the absolute number of stunted pre-school children has actually increased by 23%. Hence, the battle against chronic food insecurity is far from over. The number of stunted children rose from 47 million in 1990 to 58 million in 2014 — projected to reach 64.2 million in 2020 due to food insecurity and demographics. Given the heterogenous nature of the continent, any effort to reduce the level of chronic malnutrition on the continent must target these countries. Because of the acute/chronic food crises in the Sahel, an estimated 1 million children under the age of five are at risk of severe acute malnutrition (de Onis *et al.*, 2011).

Some noticeable progress has been made in Africa over the past 15 years in addressing micronutrient deficiency diseases. This is because the solutions to address these deficiencies are relatively inexpensive to implement and associated with the levels of public health education. These solutions include salt iodisation, fortification of commonly consumed commercial foods, and supplemental doses of vitamin A and iron for women and children (UNICEF and MI, 2004). Educational campaigns that promote the importance of a balanced diet will go a long way to accelerate the progress made so far and sustain associated gains. Good nutrition is a strong driver of progress towards and dependent on each of the Sustainable Development Goals (SDGs). For example, good nutrition status reduces poverty by boosting productivity throughout the life cycle and across generations (Goal 1), ending hunger, achieving food security and reducing malnutrition (2), leading to improved educational outcomes (Goal 4), empowering women (Goal 5), reducing child mortality by over

50% (Goal 4), supporting maternal health (Goal 5), and slowing the onset of AIDS in HIV-positive individuals and increasing malarial survival rates all of which creates the basis for productive lives and sustainable growth (Goals 8, 10, 16) and reduces the risk of diet-related chronic diseases (related to Goals 1, 4 and 16). Ensuring availability and sustainable management of water and sanitation for all (Goal 6), access to affordable, reliable, sustainable and modern energy for all (Goal 7), taking urgent action to combat climate change and its impacts (Goal 13), conserving and sustainably using the oceans, seas and marine resources for sustainable development (Goal 14); protecting, restoring and promoting sustainable use of terrestrial ecosystems, sustainably managing forests, combating desertification, and halting and reversing land degradation and halting biodiversity loss (15); promoting peaceful and inclusive societies for sustainable development, providing access to justice for all and building effective, accountable and inclusive institutions at all levels (16); and strengthening the means of implementation and revitalizing the global partnership for sustainable development (Goal 17) reinforcing themselves to bring food security and sustainable food production systems.

The costs of food and nutrition insecurity in Africa constrain efforts to foster sustained economic growth and improve general welfare (Conceição *et al.*, 2011). It is no surprise that of the 187 countries with a Human Development Index (HDI) for 2014, the 34 lowest ranked were in Africa. Among the 30 countries ranked at the bottom, only Afghanistan and Haiti are outside the continent (UNDP, 2015). The link between agriculture, food security and growth has been explored by many authors. Delgado *et al.* (1994) show that an initial increase in rural incomes in a set of African countries is amplified through growth multipliers averaging 2.0 and higher. Furthermore, agricultural multiplier estimates obtained by other authors (for example, Haggblade *et al.*, 1989) range from 1.5 to 2.7 and are comparable to estimates for Asian countries which range from 1.5 to 2.4. The relationship between food security and human development can be traced back to the seminal work of Amartya Sen on poverty and famines (Sen, 1981, 1982) and his subsequent work with Jean Dreze on public interventions to avoid hunger (Dreze and Sen, 1989). Sen's work was based on a new analytical framework in which hunger (and broader destitution) is seen as a consequence of "entitlement failure," or the inability of people to access and command food through legal means. This analytical framework was in contrast with the prevailing explanations. Bresciani and Valdes (2007) investigate four important transmission channels between food production and food security: rural labor markets, farm incomes, food prices, and linkages to other economic sectors.

Improving domestic infrastructure, particularly roads and communications, and increasing international trade could improve market access and thereby provide incentives to augment food production and reduce yield gaps. But, unrestrained global trade in food mostly facilitated by commercial farms and big businesses could bypass the most vulnerable communities. Arguably resolving the food insecurity and malnutrition challenges in Africa provides a path towards making under-development not be an issue on the continent. We thus need to examine the notion of food sovereignty.

Following Ehrlich and colleagues (Ehrlich *et al.*, 1993, p. 3), one can argue that a nutritionally secure society provides its entire population with diets adequate to sustain work and other normal daily activities. By implications, individuals and the wider society have protection against inadequate harvest or supplies. Food sovereignty is the success in protecting local livelihood strategies to guarantee access to sufficient and nutritious food at the household or family level for a healthy life (Devereux and Maxwell, 2001).

The notion of food sovereignty emerged in the 1990s as a reaction to the perceived failures and weaknesses in the approach to attaining food security (Arthur, 2011). There was growing concern — especially by international civil society that the knowledge, priorities and aspirations of small-scale producers, and other citizens whose livelihoods depend on food provisioning, were rarely included in policy debates on the future of food, farming and development (Edelman, 2003). This evolved in the various attempts to reform global governance. The idea of food sovereignty was driven by the global farmers' movement and transnational coalition, *La Via Campesina*. A notion of food sovereignty, which adopts a rights-based cum political economy approach, prioritising access to productive resources (Windfuhr and Jonsén, 2005), and associated factors such as conflict and social exclusion that contribute to food insecurity, hunger, malnutrition and undernourishment (Boyer, 2010). The need for food sovereignty in Africa has received a lot of attention as it provides the basis for local decision-makers and professional organizations to regain leadership in defining and directing agricultural and food security policies. The Nyéléni Declaration of 2007 (issued at the International Forum for Food Sovereignty at *Sélingué*, Mali) defined food sovereignty as the right of people to have healthy and culturally appropriate food produced through ecologically sound and sustainable methods and the right to define their own food and agricultural system. Operationally, food sovereignty restores sectoral policies and public intervention in the agricultural sector, as well as places food producers at the centre of the agricultural system rather than the demands and expectations of the big businesses and corporations, the market, and international forces (Boyer, 2010). This process would demand that states and society redefine the policy making framework by opening it up for greater participation and accountable-governance as part of the broader development agenda. Food governance in its widest sense is at the core of food sovereignty.

There is a growing acknowledgement of an emergent middle class in Africa (Ncube and Shimeless, 2013). This income shift is likely to generate change in dietary patterns, following rapid increases in income, along an Engel curve type of response function. The change in diet is increasingly associated with rise in the consumption of fast foods. Most of these foods have high sugar and fat content which has implications for obesity and, further down the line, for non-communicable diseases. This dietary transition is already taking place at a rapid rate and has several costs attached to it. Popkin *et al.* (2001), for example, discuss the health implications of the shift in dietary intakes toward higher fat and lower carbohydrate content in India and China. In 2014, almost half of all overweight children under 5 lived in Asia and one quarter lived in Africa. Indeed, the number of overweight children under 5 in Africa has nearly doubled since 1990 from 5.4 million to 10.3 million in 2014 (UNICEF, WHO and World Bank, 2015).

The dietary changes speak to broader dynamics in society that may undermine food security and healthy lives. The importance of transforming agriculture — especially enhance agro-productivity as part of wider food security and fighting malnutrition cannot be overstated (FAO, 2004). The world food crisis of 2007–2008 demonstrated Africa's vulnerability to a market and donor-based solutions to food security. Prior to the crisis, the region saw the largest cereal-grain imports per capita in the world as a result of Africa's own agricultural policies and the role of foreign aid. Masters (2009) argued that despite over two decades, prior to the crisis, of steadily declining agricultural aid per capita in Africa and the rapid growth in continent's production of cereal grains per capita, the price hikes hit the continent hard. The price rise needed to be complimented by continued improvements in trade policy, particularly if combined with interventions to recognize and scale up the new technologies now being adopted by African farmers. Enhancing investment in agricultural technology is one sure way of increasing productivity and reducing poverty among farmers (Minten and Barrett, 2008).

Block (2014) estimates of cross-country agricultural productivity growth in Sub-Saharan Africa confirms the importance of R&D in agricultural transformation. The results show that Total Factor Productivity (TFP) growth in African agriculture has accelerated dramatically since the early 1980s. By the early 2000s, average annual TFP growth in African agriculture was over 4 times faster than it had been 25 years earlier. The success is qualified by the finding that much of this acceleration represents a recovery from the substantial decline in TFP growth rates during the 1960s and early 1970s. The reasons provided to explain the turnaround in fortune includes increased investments in R&D, macroeconomic reforms and sectoral policies that enhanced agricultural incentives. For our purpose, the findings demonstrate the importance of technology and research in agricultural transformation. Africa needs to prioritize more investments in science and technology as part of the wider agricultural development strategy (Borlaug and Dowswell, 1995).

3. The Role of Technology and Research in the Transformation of African Agriculture

There is a strong link between agriculture and nutrition in Africa. Over two-third of the region's population depends on agriculture for income and livelihood, including more than 90% of the region's extreme poor (O'Sullivan *et al.*, 2014). However, agricultural productivity levels in Africa are the lowest of any region in the world. As part of the fight against hunger, organizations and governments at all levels are seeking ways to improve agricultural productivity, along with dietary diversity and environmental sustainability, in order to benefit the most vulnerable. The continent is rethinking the role of technology in efforts to transform agriculture.

The history of investment in both public and private sector in R&D in African agriculture for many years has been one that has not inspired confidence in the sector given the generally low levels of budgetary commitments (Beintema and Stads, 2006; Block, 2014; Qaim, 2005). Countries vary in the degree to which they have developed R&D and used biotechnology and the associated systems governing its use (Omamo and von Grebmer, 2005; Mnyulwa and Mugwagwa, 2005). This reality should be exploited to ensure that all countries attain a minimum level of technical and regulatory capacity, especially for monitoring the development and use of genetic modification technologies and their resulting products. African countries have to recognize their interdependence in the context of the regional integration and the current global economy and the need to monitor the movement of materials across borders (Omamo and von Grebmer, 2005). The Maputo Declaration has provided countries with the impetus to invest more in R&D and in agriculture broadly (Kararach, 2014). The African impetus is welcome as modern agricultural biotechnology has been adopted rapidly at the global level, including in several developing countries (Qaim, 2005).

There is ample empirical evidence that demonstrates agricultural R&D investments have greatly contributed to economic growth, agricultural development, and poverty reduction in developing regions over the past five decades (World Bank, 2007; IAASTD, 2008). Effectively disseminated new technologies and crop varieties resulting from R&D investments have enhanced the quantity and quality of agricultural produce, at the same time increasing sustainability, reducing consumer food prices, providing rural producers with access to markets, and improving gender-based allocations and accumulations of physical and human capital within households. Given important challenges, such as rapid population growth, adaptation to climate change, increasing weather variability, water scarcity, and the volatility of prices in global markets, policymakers are increasingly recognizing the value of greater investment in agricultural R&D as an essential element in increasing agricultural productivity in Sub-Saharan Africa (SSA) (Beintema and Stads, 2006).

In the face of climate change and other pressures on food production, Africa needs to use smart or precision technology, enabled by genomic, as the pathway to global food security and sustainable agriculture (Roling, 2010; Juma, 2011). The World Bank notes that "the direct use of biotechnology for plant propagation and breeding could drastically raise crop productivity and overall food production in developing countries". This argument is reinforced by those of Juma (2011), Ackello-Ogutu (2011), Sowman and Cardoso (2010, p. 285) as well as Puplampu (2011) who contend that new technology, especially biotechnology can play a significant role in addressing food security challenges in Africa since it can help in increasing food (Puplampu and Essegbey, 2004) and livestock productivity (Noyes *et al.*, 2011), and ultimately deal with increasing poverty and also enhance nutrition. Juma (2011) argue that modern technologies, including biotechnology and investment in geographical sciences for improved natural resource management, can contribute to agricultural productivity by bringing about technical efficiencies in production. Improvements in seed technology enable farmers to create better products that meet specific needs and within shorter periods of time (Puplampu and Essegbey, 2004). It is against this backdrop that Kijima *et al.* (2011) argue that in an effort to boost food security in Africa, there is no substitute or alternative to the Green revolution, which enhances crop yield per unit of land. This revolution for them was evidenced in the successful adoption in Uganda of the New Rice for Africa (NERICA) varieties. These high yielding up-land varieties which are suitable for the African environment were developed by the Africa Rice Centre (WARDA). Despite its success in Uganda, Kijima *et al.* (2010) argue that in order to achieve a wider dissemination of NERICA and to realize a rice Green revolution, the extension system must be strengthened with regard to teaching farmers how to grow rice. This is especially true in the appropriate timing of planting to avoid crop failure. Kiggundu (2006) documents similar adoption outcomes with respect to fish farming in Uganda.

Smale *et al.* (2006) reviewed the applied economics literature on the impact of transgenic crop varieties in non-industrialized agricultural systems. They note four categories of impact analysis with respect to farmers, consumers, industry and trade. For example, Ismael *et al.* (2002a, 2002b) found that farmers who grew biotechnology cotton had both higher yields and lower pesticide costs than those who did not, outweighing the higher seed costs. They estimated the difference in gross margins at 11% in 1998/99 and 77% in 1999/2000. Whether or not growing such cotton variety is associated with reduced pesticide use has since been questioned by researchers. Reduced pesticide use can lead not only to lower production costs and labour savings, but lower exposure of farmers and the environment to hazardous chemicals (see Hofs *et al.* (2006) as an example).

Qaim (2005) argues that some distinction must be made between current biotechnology — especially Genetically Modified (GM) technologies and those associated with previous crop innovations, such as the High-Yielding Varieties (HYVs) of the Green Revolution. These differences arguably influence the patterns of technology adoption. The major differences the author notes are: First, while traditionally the supply of improved seeds to smallholder farmers in developing countries was dominated by the public sector, GM crop development and commercialization are driven by the private sector — mostly rich country multinationals. As a result, intellectual property rights (IPRs) have gained in importance in shaping adoption. Second, GM crops have raised new concerns about environmental and health risks, requiring new regulatory procedures at national and international levels. Uncertainty and risk aversion have defined the limited public acceptance and cautious public policy approaches in many countries including those in Africa. Third, modern biotechnology permits a separation between the act of developing a specific crop trait and the breeding of locally adapted germplasm. Unlike previous HYVs, the outcome of GM research is not a particular new variety, but a transformation event, or a GM trait, which can be used for backcrossing into numerous locally adapted varieties. Many studies suggest the benefits of biotechnology may be context specific. With these issues in mind, a number of partners are also investing in agro-technology research in Africa — especially under the umbrella of CGIAR (AfDB, 2011).

There have been attempts to quantify the rate of R&D and innovation in any economy. The Global Innovation Index seeks to summarize R&D efforts across countries (see Table 1). Of the 128 countries surveyed in

Table 1. Global Innovation Index 2016 rankings: African countries surveyed against other major economies.

Country/Economy	Score	Rank	Income	Country/Economy	Score	Rank	Income
Mauritius	35.86	53	UM	Switzerland	66.28	1	HI
South Africa	35.85	54	UM	Sweden	63.57	2	HI
Morocco	32.26	72	LM	United Kingdom	61.93	3	HI
Tunisia	30.55	77	UM	United States of America	61.4	4	HI
Kenya	30.36	80	LM	Finland	59.9	5	HI
Rwanda	29.96	83	LI	Singapore	59.16	6	HI
Mozambique	29.84	84	LI	Ireland	59.03	7	HI
Botswana	28.96	90	UM	Denmark	58.45	8	HI
Namibia	28.24	93	UM	Netherlands	58.29	9	HI
Malawi	27.26	98	LI	Germany	57.94	10	HI
Uganda	27.14	99	LI	China	50.57	25	UM
Ghana	26.66	102	LM	Russian Federation	38.5	43	HI
Tanzania	26.35	105	LI	India	33.61	66	LM
Senegal	26.14	106	LM	Brazil	33.19	69	UM
Egypt	25.96	107	LM	Yemen	14.55	128	LM

Côte d'Ivoire	25.8	108	LM
Ethiopia	24.83	110	LI
Madagascar	24.79	111	LI
Mali	24.77	112	LI
Algeria	24.46	113	UM
Nigeria	23.15	114	LM
Cameroon	22.82	118	LM
Benin	22.25	121	LI
Burkina Faso	21.05	122	LI
Burundi	20.93	123	LI
Niger	20.44	124	LI
Zambia	19.92	125	LM
Togo	18.42	126	LI
Guinea	17.24	127	LI

Note: World Bank Income Group Classification (July 2015): LI = low income; LM = lower-middle income; UM = upper-middle income; and HI = high income.

2016, the bottom 20 poor performers excluding Yemen are African countries. Whether an African country is low income, lower-middle income, or upper-middle income did not determine its overall ranking in the innovation league table.

However, one of the most quoted R&D indicators is how much a country dedicates to research and experimental development as a percentage of its GDP.[1] The "one per cent goal for African countries" was endorsed by the Executive Council of the African Union in the Khartoum Decision (EX.CL/Dec.254 (VIII) on Science and Technology) (AU, 2006). This indicator is the gross domestic expenditure on research and experimental development (GERD). To estimate how much is actually spent on R&D in any country, it is necessary to have reasonably reliable data not only on GERD, but also on its components of R&D spending in different sectors of the economy as well as the aggregate level of economic activity — something that Africa needs to improve on (Morten, 2013). The Frascati Manual (OECD, 2002) recommends data be collected for four sectors: the business enterprise sector (irrespective of ownership), the government sector, the higher education sector and private non-profit organisations (PNP). The sum of expenditure for the four sectors is thus equal to the GERD. Ten of the African countries participating in the ASTII programme have collected data (through surveys) on R&D expenditure. However, three of these countries have not yet collected data for the business enterprise sector, while two countries have no data for the PNP sector, and one lacks data for the higher education sector (NEPAD, 2010).

Absolute levels of public agricultural R&D spending and staffing varied considerably across the 32 ASTI countries. In 2008, Nigeria, South Africa, and Kenya invested $404 million, $272 million, and $171 million, respectively, on agricultural R&D, whereas a further 11 countries spent less than $10 million each, all measured in inflation-adjusted purchasing power parity (PPP) dollars. Some countries reported such low investment levels that they were unlikely to have a sustainable impact on rural development and poverty reduction. Figures 1 and 2 show the latest picture of R&D in agriculture in Africa. Nigeria, South Africa, and Kenya

[1] Sometimes the ratios of research personnel in various institutions are used.

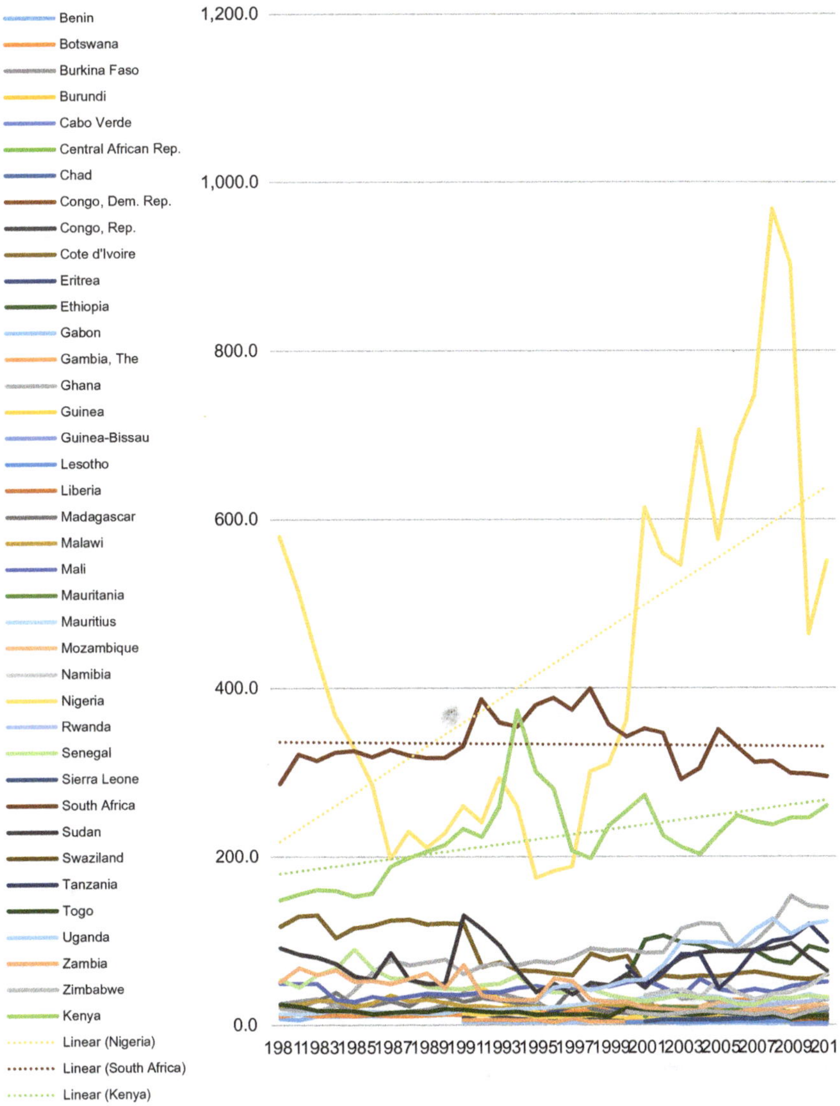

Figure 1. Absolute levels of agricultural R&D spending as share agro-GDP total 1980–2011 (million constant 2011 PPP dollars).

Source: ASTII database 2016.

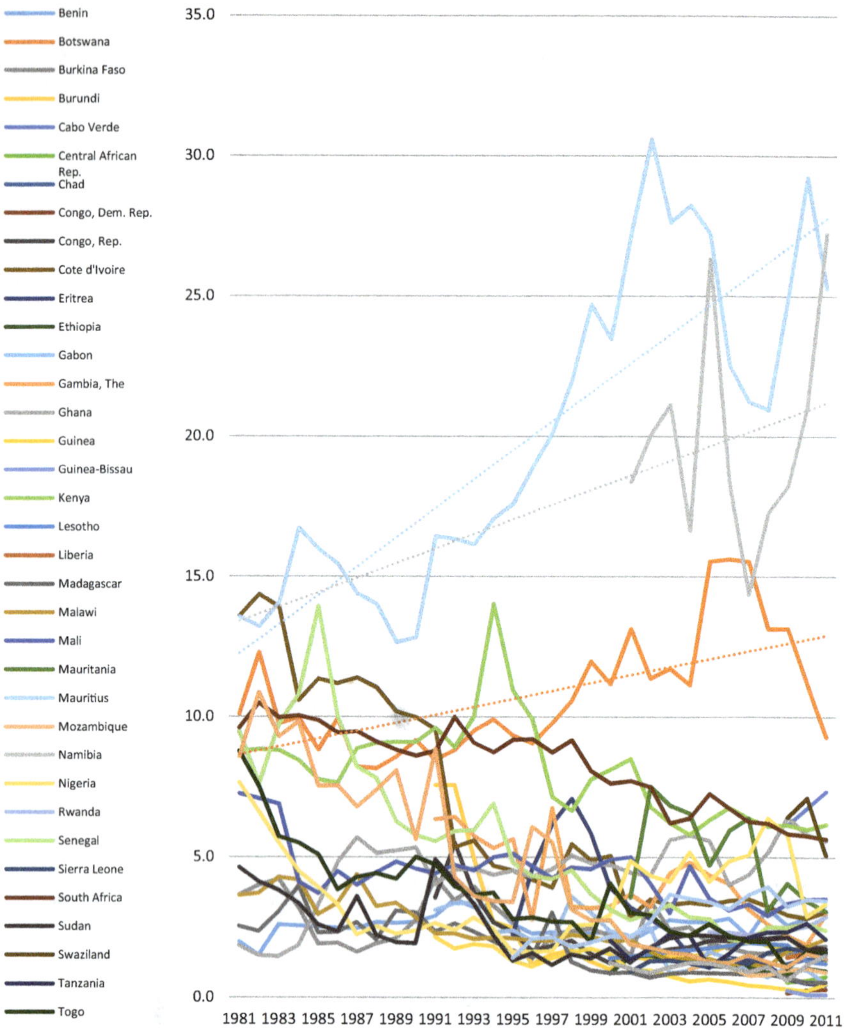

Figure 2. Spending, total (million constant 2011 PPP dollars per million population).
Source: ASTII database 2016.

dominated the scene when innovation is assessed in terms of agricultural R&D spending as share of agro-GDP total for the period 1980–2011.

Analyzing absolute levels of research expenditures explains only so much. Another way of comparing the commitment to public agricultural R&D investments across countries is to measure total public agricultural

R&D spending as a percentage of AgGDP. This relative measure indicates the intensity of investment in agricultural research, not just the absolute level of spending.

From Figures 1 and 2 it is clear that countries have invested in diverse ways in the R&D capacity on the continent. Focusing on West African countries, Nuetah *et al.* (2010) argue that "*regional leaders should raise agricultural budgetary allotment above the minimum 10% which the Maputo declaration called on African governments to provide annually for agricultural development, and further intensify regional agricultural research*". They also underscore the importance of supply-side factors such as infrastructure, farmer incentives, farm inputs and innovative technologies. Kararach (2014) argue that regional integration has enormous potential mainly in the context of making food availability sustainable — a huge step in the quest for food security in Africa.

However, there are a number of issues that create barriers to adoption of the "gene" revolution (FAO, 2004) as means to resolving problems of food insecurity in Africa. In spite of biotechnology bringing in much needed solution to Africa's food insecurity, critics note that not only is the impact of biotechnology, which is equated to genetic engineering, uncertain, but also it poses a danger to human health and the environment (Puplampu and Essegbey, 2004). Biotechnology has attracted some controversy because it might be seen as "interfering with the workings of nature and creation", which involve some unknown risk taking for commercial gain (Omiti *et al.*, 2002). Possibilities of environmental hazards from new products of biotechnology have raised concerns that companies may use African and other developing countries as "test sites" for their products. Some of the potential environmental risks concern plant pests, where genes escaping from Genetically Modified Organisms (GMOs) could result in increased weediness in sexually compatible wild species. GMOs could also inadvertently produce toxins and allergens. Thus the need for appropriate legislation and setting up of regulatory bodies for all aspects of bio-safety in Africa. Finally, GMOs are seen by farmers' movements as part of the economic and ecological logic of intensive agriculture and a US- and corporate dominated food system that threatens to undermine health, environment, and cultural specificity (Edelman, 2003, p. 212). Despite the controversy and varying perspectives and arguments, the debate about biotechnology should not be necessarily whether or not the continent needs biotechnology but rather how biotechnology can be promoted, supported and applied in safe and sustainable ways that contribute to improved agriculture and livelihoods (Puplampu, 2011). Biotechnology will perhaps affect even the most isolated villages on the African continent thus changing the configuration of farming systems the way we currently know them (Juma, 2011). It may be neither wise nor justified for Africans not to pursue effective participation in this revolution. African nations must balance the expected advantages with due recognition of related dangers or risks of biotechnology. Developing policies that encourage investment, education, collaboration, and technology access will promote technology transfer and access to biotechnology products that can improve livelihood and food security in Africa (Omiti *et al.,* 2002).

While biotechnology can assist African agriculture, that optimism should not be taken as inevitable since technological innovation does not function in a vacuum, but rather in a socio-cultural, political and economic context (Puplampu and Essegbey, 2004; Puplampu, 2011). Institutional support and infrastructure as evidenced in a number of African countries such as Ghana, South Africa, Kenya, Zimbabwe, Nigeria and Egypt to assist the biotechnological sector are important. Biotechnology development should involve institutional support by research agencies and institutions in order to effectively harness the technology. Attention by policymakers should focus on institutional and organizational mechanisms that would enable researchers to engage in technology and bring about its expected political, social and economic benefits (Puplampu, 2011). Incentive framework, funding, access to foreign technology, infrastructure and the supply of human capacity and human capital are critical. Infrastructure is critical not only in terms of enhancing connectivity to markets but also combating long-standing problems in African agriculture such as post-harvest waste, pests and water shortages.

Spencer (1994) notes in particular that rural infrastructure, comprising rural roads, markets, irrigation systems, water supply, health and educational facilities, is basic to quality of life in rural areas, and is an important facilitator of economic development (see also Ahmed and Donovan, 1992). Many types of infrastructure have critical roles to play in any agricultural development strategy for Africa (Cleaver, 1993). However, a detailed review of all aspects of rural infrastructure is outside the scope of this paper, so we concentrate on rural transport and irrigation systems. These are fundamental factors that influenced the success of the green revolution in Asia. The importance of rural transport infrastructure for agricultural development has been well established (Devres Inc., 1980; Ahmed and Donovan, 1992; Platteau, 1993). Evidence from Asia shows that in villages with better access to roads, fertilizer costs were 14% lower, wages were 12% higher and crop output was 32% higher (IFPRI, 1990). In Africa, rural road construction has been found to be associated with increases in agricultural production, especially in non-food export crops, expanded use of agricultural credit, increases in land values, proliferation of small shops and expansion of rural markets (Anderson *et al.*, 1982).

Colonial legacy has not only left the continent with poor infrastructure but also ensured that most African economies are locked into an innovation trap. Relatively, South Africa has a national innovation system with a structurally different base from the rest of the subcontinent and the continent as a whole. The relationship of the South African economy with the non-African global economy still positions it as a peripheral trader, with a competitive advantage in the primary sector, but importing commodities that require a high intensity of skills and knowledge to produce than the rest of the continent. The global trading system rarely promotes the development and productivity of African agriculture. The degree of diversification among African economies is low and affords limited opportunities for intra-African trade in comparison with trade flows between the continent and the rest of the world. Indeed, some countries even have zero-level of intra-regional trade. This reality is mitigated to some extent by the entry of the post-apartheid South African economy as a legitimate member of the African Union — that is: operating in a sanction-free trading arrangement. As a result, South African investment across Africa has risen remarkably since 1994, as have its exports of skills and knowledge-intensive goods and services to the rest of the continent. Within the subcontinent and Africa as a whole, South Africa has therefore assumed a central economic position as a driver of R&D and innovation. However, this asymmetry creates problems for the integration of economies in Africa due to concentration of gains of integration.

This similarity in economic structures, in the narrow export base and in competitive capabilities based on natural-resource endowments, limits the scope for complementarities in innovations, R&D production and consumption. This partly explains why South Africa, with its relatively highly diversified production base, has rapidly assumed a dominant role as the major R&D hotbed and exporter across Africa, particularly in Sub-Saharan Africa. The general similarity of economic structures in most African states thus severely constrains the potential for trade and cross-border investment, except for a small group of economies (Leke *et al.*, 2010).

African governments need to rethink how best they encourage the penetration and adoption of R&D. Some of the issues that need special attention include but are not limited to: the use of social networks and Mobile technology (farmer-to-farmer supply/demand of/for information), marketing and crop insurance information. Bandiera and Rasul (2006) show that farmers' decisions to adopt a new crop relate to the adoption choices of their network of family and friends. They found the relationship to be inverse U-shaped, suggesting social effects are positive when there are few adopters in the network, and negative when there are many. In addition, the adoption decisions of farmers who have better information about the new crop are less sensitive to the adoption choices of others. Finally, adoption decisions are more correlated within family and friends than religion-based networks, and uncorrelated among individuals of different religions. Conley and Udry (2005) confirm the importance of farmers' communication patterns as defined by each individual's information neighbourhood. In their study of the diffusion of a new agricultural technology in Ghana, the duo show that farmers adopt successful neighbours' practices, conditional on many potentially confounding factors including common growing conditions, credit arrangements, clan membership, and religion. The relationship of these input adjustments to experience further supports their interpretation as resulting from social learning. Strengthening social networks as learning is thus crucial for enhancing agricultural sector transformation and productivity.

4. R&D and Food Security Respectively

Despite declining foreign aid, productivity increases have been registered in Africa over the last two decades. It is encouraging to witness increasing R&D investment in some African countries despite tight budgets in the wake of the global economic slowdown. However, there is need to investigate whether green revolution in Africa is a lost cause or is an opportunity to be seized given the technology transfer from key emerging economies such as Brazil and China to the continent. What steps can be taken to improve the sustainability of agriculture and enhance the competitiveness of the smallholder agriculture? Indeed, there are controversial issues such as Genetically Modified (GM) seeds, High Yielding Varieties (HYVs) and fertilizer use that countries need to address. Given the non-negligible agricultural productivity in Africa in recent years, important lessons must be learnt as to how existing positive developments can be sustained into the near future and beyond. The key will be identifying key technology and research capacity which can be deemed feasible for the potential sustainable development of agriculture and food security situation in the continent.

In the previous section, we presented and reviewed the evidence on the analysis of R&D spending and human resources capacity in African countries (Beintema and Stads, 2011; IFPRI, 2004). In addition to the role of social networks (Bandiera and Rasul, 2006; Conley and Udry, 2001) for technology adoption in Africa, there is need to address the important issue of institutional innovations which create the enabling environment for agricultural growth and its competitiveness. By innovations we mean innovation for accessing finance, insurance coverage and efficiency in input/output markets (e.g. the use of mobile phones) to acquire technology, sustain and upgrade agricultural development. These issues are crucial because the Structural Adjustment Programmes (SAP) of the 1980s and early 1990s dismantled the public provision of credit, insurance (e.g. weather indexed/crop/livestock insurance), land, improved seeds and other key inputs to farmers such as fertilizer credit schemes. This is a vast area of focus in its own right but, for brevity, we focused our discussion on the "technology and research" theme. Illustrative examples include the institutional failure associated with a smart cotton technology studied by Gouse (2005) and the organizations arrangements that benefit agriculture discussed by Ochieng (2007).

5. Challenges and Lessons

Before any lessons can be drawn, there is need to recap the major challenges to food security and agricultural transformation in Africa. It is generally acknowledged that challenges in the fight against food insecurity and malnutrition are enormous and dynamic, thus the need for versatility by the African countries. While fertility trends around the world will decline between 2010 and 2050 worldwide, women in Africa will still give birth to children in larger numbers compared to women in other parts of the world. "During this period, Sub-Saharan Africa's Total Fertility Rate (TFR), on average, will still be the highest in the world and will account for a 60% increase in its childhood population below age five" (Thomas and Zuberi, 2012). At the same time, more people will migrate to the cities, thereby increasing the demand for food and good nutrition. Total cereal demand in SSA is projected to almost double to 317 million metric tons by 2050; 24% of the increase is expected for maize, 20% for millet, 19% for wheat, 18% for sorghum, 14% for rice and 5% for other grains (*ibid*). With rapid urbanisation, city dwellers have fewer opportunities than rural people to produce their own food and so must rely on purchases and the cash economy to eat.[2] This trend will partly increase food prices and have a large impact on people who rely almost entirely on cash income, especially the poor.

Firstly, climate change and erratic weather patterns will be a major challenge for the future food security in Africa. Climate change affects the spatial and temporal distribution of vector borne diseases such as malaria. Most of the projected climate-related disease burden will result from increases in diarrheal diseases and malnutrition (*ibid*). Drought represents a constant threat to world food security and ranks as the single most common cause of severe food shortages, particularly in African countries that

[2]There is need to give serious thought to the role of urban agriculture (see D'Allessandro *et al.*, 2013 for a discussion).

depend on rain-fed agriculture, and represents one of the most important natural triggers of malnutrition and famine (*ibid*).

The role of the state in all matters affecting the society cannot be overemphasized. Although, individuals arguably should be responsible for their own nutrition security, improved nutrition is a public good and may not be achieved by market-based solutions. Therefore, the responsibility for ensuring that individuals are able to attain food security must ultimately lie with the nation state. Hence, proactive and sound policies need to be put in place if African countries are to eliminate food insecurity and malnutrition. To tackle climate causes of food insecurity, African countries need to shift from a reactionary approach to a more proactive approach by providing forecasting mechanisms and social safety net measures to absorb effects of unfavourable weather patterns.

As we noted earlier, broad-based agricultural development remains a major route to long-term food security; policy effort should be made by governments and development partners to encourage agricultural research and technology assisted food production. African governments must also have agricultural policies that give incentives to farmers to produce in large scale in order to meet the food needs of future generations. Concurrently, the best way to relieve pressure on the region's natural resources is through proactive population policy. Governments, Non-Governmental Organisations (NGOs) and civil society groups should encourage family strategic planning practices, especially among the region's poorest populations to exploit any demographic dividends.

Secondly, securing peace and security are also important conditions for progress to be made in the fight against food shortage in Africa. When wars, civil unrest, insecurity, large numbers of refugees and warlords dominate the scene, no sustainable and socially-inclusive development can be achieved (*ibid*). The relationship between famine and conflicts in Africa suggests attention should be given to refugees and Internally Displaced Persons (IDPs). A conscious effort should be made by regional organisations like the African Union to resolve regional conflicts and have a means of stable livelihood.

Thirdly, infrastructure in terms of adequate energy and water/irrigation supplies, high-speed communications, and seamless transportation systems connecting areas of high production with centres of high consumption remain crucial in safeguarding food security. Because of differing locations of activities along the food supply chain, their economic relationship is based on efficient connectivity and logistics. These are essential to ensure sustainable access to basic food products. Moreover, the development of regional infrastructure that can contribute to food supply and price stability will have a decisive impact on the overall level of consumption and on food security.

In Africa, agricultural resources are unequally distributed across national and subregional territories because of the disparate endowments and potentialities of different countries (ACBF, 2011; UNDP, 2012). Domestic policies are also crucial players in determining households' access to essential inputs. The inadequacy of connective infrastructure between deficit and surplus areas for the production, collection, and distribution of food heightens food insecurity in all subregions. This vulnerability is accentuated by a lack of high-tech infrastructure (including refrigerated storage) for national and regional trade of food products — which are, by definition, generally seasonal and highly perishable.

Transportation infrastructures are paramount for distributing agricultural inputs to farmers to improve productivity, but are equally critical in transporting large volumes of produce from areas of production to those of processing, storage, marketing, distribution, and consumption. For transportation to be cost-effective, it needs to be reliable and delivered at low-cost, which is problematic for a continent with challenging economic geography. Furthermore, increasing urbanization and migration to cities means that more and more people are relying on rural manpower and increased agricultural productivity to meet their nutritional needs. Information and Communication Technology is also critical for dissemination of market information and removal of the constraints associated with poor information flows necessary for productive activities. Across the food supply chain, efficient infrastructures of transportation, telecommunications, and energy facilitate cheaper long-distance product flows as well as enhance commercialization and trade between complementary regions. Regional infrastructure generates economies of scale by opening up larger markets, thereby lowering transaction costs.

Fourthly, demography and migration will continue to influence food security dynamics. The money received by migrant households is used for daily household consumption, and among other things, for food purchase. For example in Kenya, between 13 and 14% of remittances are reportedly spent on food (World Bank, 2006). Remittances therefore contribute to ensuring the food security of migrant households not just through direct food purchase but also contributing to investments in the agricultural sector. This seems to be particularly true in less economically favoured rural areas. Unfortunately, urban migration seems to favour the adoption of bad food consumption habits, the so-called "junk food" common in cities. However, more research needs to be undertaken on this. This issue is still widely neglected by students of migration who mainly focus on development and poverty impacts. Equally, the implications of money transfers on food security have received insufficient scrutiny.

There is a received belief among economists from the Lewis model about the limited effects on food security due to migration impact on agricultural productivity in rural areas. Also, no case study points to any sizeable influence of migration on labour markets and land use in rural areas. In Kenya, in capital-rich/labour-poor areas (cash-crop and granary areas such as Western Province and Rift Valley areas), emigration has been offset by the recruitment of workers from other parts of the country. Indeed, farming on smallholdings does not require a large workforce and emigrants are usually replaced by other family members (the spouse). Only cash-crop areas attract seasonal workers from other parts of the country. Arguably, migration may have a more negative impact insofar as women have to oversee every aspect of household reproduction in the event that their male partners migrate.

Fifth, technology adoption has been known to experience different types of barriers. Eicher *et al.* (2006) case studies unearth a number of unexpected scientific, legal, economic and political barriers to the development of GM crops and long delays in developing and implementing national biosafety regulations and guidelines. We conclude that most GM crops are at least 10–15 years or longer from reaching smallholder farmers in Africa. During this time special attention should be given to strengthening conventional plant breeding programs in NARS (National Agricultural Research Systems), African universities and the CGIAR.

Biotechnology approaches must be nested and integrated into plant breeding programs. Special attention should also be given to raising public awareness of biotechnology, mobilizing political support and commitment to strengthening African capacity in biotechnology, biosafety, food safety and IPR (Intellectual Property Rights) and mounting long-term training programs to train the next generation of African plant breeders and GM crop specialists.

Finally, African countries must assume full responsibility for eliminating food insecurity by ensuring such conditions as good governance, health and educational services and the empowerment of their populace. As we argued earlier in this chapter, the linkages between poverty and food insecurity are unambiguous, thus poverty alleviation efforts must play a major role in securing access to food and proper nutrition for all. A rights-based approach to food security elevates freedom from hunger as a fundamental human right to be implemented by national Governments and international development partners as stipulated in relevant instruments. African countries need to develop socio-political systems for protecting those in immediate need and must create a safe and enabling environment for sustainable livelihoods. Similarly, effective social safety nets will remain a critical element of comprehensive food policy (Thomas and Zuberi, 2012). Equally, educational campaigns that promote the importance of balanced diet will go a long way to accelerate the progress made so far. Indeed, the efforts must also have a regional lens whenever necessary.

Despite the challenges above, there are homegrown lessons within Africa that can be of use to others lagging behind in transforming and improving agricultural productivity (Gisselquist, 2002; Kiggundu, 2006). We will review a range of lessons from countries to learn how they got it right and also outline alternative policy options cautiously without playing down the important peculiarities of each country. Ghana managed to reduce hunger by 50% in recent years and farmers were taught to use best technological practices in irrigation and fertilization to increase yields (Kufour, 2011). One important area, for instance, is dissemination of existing technologies. There are lessons that we review based on technology uptake and scaling up evidence from Uganda, Kenya, Tanzania and Democratic Republic of Congo (Duruma, 2010). A striking example is the recent technological advance which might lead to enormous saving to African farmers by tackling one of the diseases attacking livestock. Africa loses an estimated US$ 5billion a year due to the livestock disease "*sleeping sickness*". Recently, scientists discovered two genes in cattle that may help African farmers improve their livelihood by preventing this disease, but they pointed out the difficulty of disseminating the technology to farmers (Noyes *et al.*, 2011). This is a fundamental capacity gap that needs urgent attention (see ACBF, 2012).

African countries need to enhance their governance of biotechnology products to harmonisation of appropriate protocols and regulation. Mugwagwa (2012) analyses the roles of three supranational organizations (SNOs), the African Union (AU), New Partnership for Africa's Development (NEPAD) and Southern African Development Community (SADC), in the development of cross-national policy, regulatory and administrative systems for managing modern biotechnology, also referred to as biosafety systems, in southern Africa. The desire for convergence of these systems is not an uncontested issue. Therefore, in seeking to understand the feasibility of this policy agenda, this paper traces how the three SNOs are contributing towards coalescence of the many contending issues. One of the major arguments presented by the paper is that the policy footprint of the SNOs has varying intensity across the biosafety terrain of the region, leaving one wondering whether this is by design or by accident, and what impact this has on the countries that see the SNOs as rallying points for regional aspirations.

There is also evidence that biotechnology may cause greater social differentiation. Indeed, gender reinforces the way R&D outcomes are absorbed. Doss and Morris (2001) provide empirical evidence from Ghana suggesting that gender-linked differences in the adoption of modern maize varieties and chemical fertilizer result from gender-linked differences in access to complementary inputs. This finding has important policy implications, because it suggests that ensuring more widespread and equitable adoption of improved technologies may not require changes in the research system, but rather introduction of measures that ensure better access for women to complementary inputs, especially land, labour, and extension services.

Equally important is the need to rethink the role of market-based solutions to Africa's agriculture and food security problems. Some of the policy difficulties arise from its treatment of markets (Woodhouse, 2009). While acknowledging widespread market failure in "agriculture-based" economies, particularly in input supply, credit, and research and innovation, there remains a strong presumption of not only the desirability, but also the feasibility, of making such markets work to the benefit of the poor. One evident assumption here is that "the poor" have command of land and labour that will enable them to take advantage of such inputs. It is often the case, however, especially in those rural areas (with good accessibility and high rates of immigration) with large numbers of poor, that the poorest have very little land and earn much of their living from rural employment in agriculture or a variety of other low-paid natural resource-based work (fishing, herding livestock, wood-cutting, etc.) (Barrett *et al.*, 2006; Start, 2001). The recent land grab drive mainly facilitated by the need to attract big multinationals and investors in the agriculture sector makes the access issues more complex and the share of land available to the needy and the voice of the poor limited. Some of these issues require countries to undertake land administration reforms based on strong institutional arrangements (Deininger *et al.*, 2007). For example, without strong governance framework, land titling efforts may trigger attempts at land grabbing by local elites and bureaucrats and end up disempowering the poor who were expected to benefit from these programs (Jansen and Roquas, 1998) with deleterious consequences for livelihood sustainability and food security.

African countries also need to build sufficient capacity to tackle problems that dog the agricultural sector. Deininger *et al.* (2007) show how strong capacity was critical to ensuring land registration procedures in Ethiopia were run smoothly — especially where update information needed improvement by (i) redesigning registry books and ensuring that no new certificates were given out without cancelling old ones; (ii) defining institutional responsibilities to eliminate gaps and time lags which currently are a potent source of possible inconsistency; and (iii) spelling out protocols to ensure broad and public access to information. First, lack of updating could create problems particularly in commercial areas with higher transaction frequencies and jeopardize trust in the overall system. Second, although considerable effort is expended for first-time registration of individual holdings, this has not resulted in better registration system.

6. Concluding Remarks

Poverty and food insecurity are major development challenges facing Africa. Enhancing food security through the widespread adoption and impact of appropriate agricultural technologies has been discussed as the continent's development priority. Recent history has seen the emergence of technologies that are able to increase agricultural productivity, and improve food, nutrition and income security. Unfortunately, the adoption of many of these technologies remain very low for a wide range of reasons including poor infrastructure, weak institutional capacities, concerns about biosafety, limited financing and restrictive intellectual property right regimes. The limited uptakes have resulted in the perpetual low agricultural productivity and insecure livelihoods. There is therefore need to rethink technology generation and dissemination methodologies to enhance adoption. A number of factors need to be taken into account in this regard including the increasingly complex and dynamic world economy, different risks including climatic conditions, market and economic unpredictability and social change. The heterogeneous needs of farmers and associated partners mean that innovation and knowledge could originate from many different sources and therefore agricultural research and development of equal complexity is required. African countries have to work with diverse stakeholders, at different levels and scales, sometimes simultaneously to develop effective R&D framework to transform agriculture and combat food insecurity.

In addition, African policy makers need to acknowledge the problems associated with market-based access in "agriculture-based" economies, particularly to input supply, credit, and research and innovation. Policy designs must move beyond the strong presumption of not only the desirability, but also the feasibility, of making such markets work to the benefit of the poor. The reality is that "the poor" have limited control over land and labour to enable them to take advantage of such inputs. Widening access to and adoption of new technologies accompanied by guaranteed property right over key productive assets such as land will go a long way in transforming African agriculture, enhancing food security and reducing poverty.

References

ACBF (2011) *Africa Capacity Indicators 2011*: *Capacity Development in Fragile Environment in Africa*. Harare: ACBF.

ACBF (2012) Africa Capacity Building Indicators 2012: Capacity Development for Agricultural Transformation and Food Security in Africa.

Ackello-Ogutu, C. (2011) "Managing Food Security Implications of Food Price Shocks in Africa", *Journal of African Economies*, Vol. 20, No. 1, pp. i100–i141.

AfDB (2011) *Closing Africa's Infrastructure Gap: Innovative Financing and Risks. Africa Economic Brief*. Vol. 2, No. 1, Tunis, Tunisia: African Development Bank.

Ahmed, R. and C. Donovan (1992) *Issues of Infrastructural Development: A Synthesis of the Literature*. Washington, DC: IFPRI.

Anderson, G. W., Vandervoort, C. G., Suggs, C. M. and C. Clapp-Wincek (1982) "Rural Roads Evaluation Summary Report", AID Program Evaluation Report 5. USAID, Washington, DC.

Anderson, K. and E. Valenzuala (2007) "Do Global Trade Distortions Still Harm Developing Country Farmers?", *Review of World Economics*, 32(2009), 3(03), pp. 351–384.

Arthur, P. (2011) *Food Security and Food Sovereignty in Africa*: *The Issues, Policy Challenges and Opportunities*. Africa Capacity Indicators Report (ACIR) 2012 Background Paper — Number 4. Harare, Zimbabwe.

AU (2006) Decision on the Report on the Conference of Ministers of Science and Technology — Doc. EX.CL/224 (VIII), Addis Ababa.

Bandiera, O. and I. Rasul (2006) "Social Networks & Technology Adoption in Northern Mozambique", *Economic Journal*, Vol. 116, No. 514, pp. 862–902.

Barrett, C., Marenya, P., McPeak, J., Minten, B., Murithi, F., Oluoch-Kosura, W., Place, F., Randrianarisoa, J. C., Rasambainarivo, J. and J. Wangila (2006) "Welfare Dynamics in Rural Kenya and Madagascar", *Journal of Development Studies*, Vol. 42 No. 2, pp. 248–277.

Beintema, N. and G. J. Stads (2011) *African Agricultural R&D in the New Millennium: Progress for Some and Challenges for Many*. Washington, DC: IFPRI.

Beintema, N. M. and G. J. Stads (2006) *Agricultural R&D in Sub-Saharan Africa: An Era of Stagnation*. Washington, DC: International Food Policy Research Institute (IFPRI).

Benson, T. (2004) "Africa's Food and Nutrition Security Situation: Where are We and How did We Get here?" International Food Policy Research Institute 2020 Discussion Paper.

Block, S. (2010/14) "The Decline and Rise of Agricultural Productivity in Sub-Saharan Africa Since 1961", NBER Working Paper, 16481.

Black, R. E. *et al.* (2008) "Maternal and Child Undernutrition: Global and Regional Exposures and Health Consequences", *Lancet,* Vol. 371, pp. 243–260.

Borlaug, N. and C. Dowswell (1995) "Mobilising Science and Technology to Get Agriculture Moving in Africa," *Development Policy Review*, Vol. 13, No. 2, pp. 115–129.

Boyer, J. (2010) "Food Security, Food Sovereignty, and Local Challenges for Transnational Agrarian Movements: The Honduran Case," *The Journal of Peasant Studies*, Vol. 37, No. 2, pp. 319–351.

Bresciani, F. and A. Valdes (2007) "The Role of Agriculture in Poverty Reduction: A Synthesis of the Case Studies", In: *Beyond Food Production: The Role of Agriculture in Poverty Reduction,* eds. F. Bresciani & A. Valdes. Rome and Cheltenham: Food and Agricultural Organisation & Edward Elgar. pp. 3–40.

Cleaver, K. M. (1993) "A Strategy to Develop Agriculture in Sub-Saharan Africa and a Focus for the World Bank", World Bank Technical Paper 203. World Bank, Washington, DC.

Conceição, P., Horn-Phathanothai, L. and A. Ngororano (2011) "Food Security and Human Development in Africa: Strategic Considerations and Directions for Further Research", Paper is drawn from the proposal for the 2011 African Human Development Report on "Food Security for Human Development".

Conley, T. G. and G. Udry (2001) "Social Learning Through Networks: The Adoption of New Agricultural Technologies in Ghana", *American Journal of Agricultural Economics*, Vol. 83, No. 3, pp. 668–673.

Conley, T. G. and C. R. Udry (2005) "Learning About a New Technology: Pineapple in Ghana", *Proceedings*, Federal Reserve Bank of San Francisco.

de Onis, M., Blossner, M. and M. Borghi (2011) "Prevalence and Trends of Stunting Among Pre-school Children — 1990–2020", World Health Organisation. Available at: http://www.who.int.

Deininger, K., Ali, D. A., Holden, S. and J. Zevenbergen (2007) "Rural Land Certification in Ethiopia: Process, Initial Impact, and Implications for Other African Countries", World Bank Policy Research Working Paper 4218. Washington, DC: World Bank.

Delgado, C. L., Hopkins, J. and V. Kelly (1994) "Agricultural growth linkages in Sub-Saharan Africa: A synthesis", in *Agricultural Growth Linkages in Sub-Saharan Africa*. Report submitted to the United States Agency for International Development by the International Food Policy Research Institute, Washington.

Devres Inc. (1980) "Socio-economic and Environmental Impacts of Low-Volume Rural Roads: A Review of the Literature", AID Program Evaluation Discussion Paper 7. Bureau of Program and Policy Evaluation, USAID, Washington, DC.

Doss, C. R. and M. L. Morris (2001) "How Does Gender Affect the Adoption of Agricultural Innovations? The Case of Improved Maize Technology in Ghana", *Agricultural Economics*, Vol. 25, No. 1, pp. 27–39.

Dreze, J. and A. Sen (1989) *Hunger and Public Action. WIDER Studies in Development Economics*. Oxford University Press.

Duruma, Z. (2010) "Dissemination of New Agricultural Technologies in Africa", CGIAR and CIMMYT.

Edelman, M. (2003) "Transnational Peasant and Farmer Movements and Networks," In *Global Civil Society Yearbook 2003*, eds. M. Kaldor, H. Anheier & M. Glasius. London: London School of Economics, Centre for the Study of Global Governance, pp. 185–220.

Eicher, C. K., Maredia, K. and I. Sithole-Niang (2006) "Crop Biotechnology and the African Farmer", *Food Policy*, Vol. 31, No. 6, pp. 504–527.

Ehrlich, P. R., Ehrlich, A. H. and G. C. Daily (1993) "Food Security, Population, and Environment," *Population and Development Review*, Vol. 19, No. 1, pp. 1–32.

FAO (2004) "From Green Revolution to Gene Revolution", FAO, Rome.

Gisselquist, D., Nash, J. and C. E. Pray (2002) "Deregulating the Transfer of Agricultural Technology: Lessons from Bangladesh, India, Turkey, and Zimbabwe", *World Bank Research Observer*, Vol. 17, No. 2, pp. 237–265.

Haggblade, S., Peter, H. and B. James (1989) "Farm-Non Farm Linkages in Rural Sub-Saharan Africa," *World Development*, Vol. 17, No. 8, pp. 1173–1202.

Hofs, J.-L., Fok, M. and M. Vaissayre (2006) "Impact of Bt Cotton Adoption on Pesticide Use by Smallholders: A 2-year Survey in Makhatini Flats (South Africa)", *Crop Protection*, Vol. 25.

IAASTD (International Assessment of Agricultural Knowledge, Science and Technology for Development) (2008) Synthesis Report. Washington, DC: Island Press.

InterAcademy Council (2004) *Realizing the Promise and Potential of African Agriculture. Science and Technology Strategies for Improving Agricultural Productivity and Food Security in Africa*. Amsterdam, The Netherlands: InterAcademy Council.

International Assessment of Agricultural Science and Technology for Development (IAASTD) (2007) *Global Report*. Washington, DC: International Assessment of Agricultural Science and Technology for Development (IAASTD).

International Food policy Research Institute (IFPRI) (1990) Annual Report, 1990. IFPRI, Washington, DC.

International Food Policy Research Institute (IFPRI) (2004) *Agricultural Science and Technology Indicators*. Washington, DC.

Ismael, Y., Beyers, L., Thirtle, C. and J. Piesse (2002a) "Efficiency Effects of *Bt* Cotton Adoption by Smallholders in Makhathini Flats, KwaZulu-Natal, South Africa", in *Economic and Social Issues in Agricultural Biotechnology*, eds. Evenson, R. E. Santaniello, V. and D. Zilberman. Wallingford: CABI Publishing.

Ismael, Y., Bennett, R. and S. Morse (2002b) "Farm-level Economic Impact of Biotechnology: Smallholder *Bt* Cotton Farmers in South Africa", *Outlook on Agriculture*, Vol. 31, No. 2, pp. 107–111.

Jansen, K. and E. Roquas (1998) "Modernizing Insecurity: The Land Titling Project in Honduras", *Development and Change*, Vol. 29, No. 1, pp. 81–106.

Jenkins, J. C. and S. Scanlan (2001) "Food Security in Less Developed Countries, 1970–1990", *American Sociological Review*, Vol. 66, pp. 718–744.

Juma, C. (2011) *The New Harvest: Agricultural Innovation in Africa*. New York: Oxford University Press.

Kararach, G. (2014) *Development Policy in Africa: Mastering the Future*? Basingstoke: Palgrave Macmillan.

Kiggundu, R. (2006) "Technological Change in Uganda's Fishery Exports", in *Technology, Adaptation and Exports: How Some Developing Countries Got it Right*, ed. V. Chandra. Washington, DC: World Bank.

Kijima, Y., Otsuka, K. and D. Ssreunkuuma (2011) "An Inquiry into Constraints on a Green Revolution in Sub-Saharan Africa: The Case of NERICA Rice in Uganda," *World Development*, Vol. 39, No. 1, pp. 77–86.

Kufour, J. A. (2011) *Ghana's Transformation*. Washington, DC: IFPRI.

Leke, A., Lund, S., Roxburgh, C. and A. van Wamelen (2010) "What's Driving Africa's Growth", The McKinsey Quarterly, June, McKinsey and Company, New York.

Masters, W. A. (2009) "Beyond Food Crisis: Trade, Aid and Innovation in African Agriculture", *ATDF Journal*, Vol. 5, Nos. 1, 2, pp. 3–13.

Minten, B. and C. B. Barrett (2008) "Agricultural Technology, Productivity, and Poverty in Madagascar", *World Development*, Vol. 36, No. 5, pp. 797–822.

Mnyulwa, D. and J. Mugwagwa (2005) "Agricultural Biotechnology in Southern Africa: A Regional Synthesis", In *Biotechnology, Agriculture, and Food Security in Southern Africa, IFPRI*, eds. S. W. Omamo and K. von Grebmerpp, 13–36.

Morten, J. (2013) "Poor Numbers: How We are Misled by African Development Statistics and What to Do about It". Cornell Studies in Political Economy.

Mugwagwa, J. (2012) "Multiple Meanings, One Objective: The Case of Biotechnology Policy Convergence in Africa." *Asian Biotechnology and Development Review*, Vol. 14, No. 3, pp. 31–48.

Ncube, M. and A. Shimeless (2013) "The Making of the Middle Class in Africa", African Development Bank Working Paper.

NEPAD (2010) African Innovation Outlook 2010, AU–NEPAD, Pretoria.

Noyes, H., Brass, A., Obara, I., Anderson, S., Archibald, S., Gradley, D., Fisher, P., Freeman, A., Gibson, J., Gicheru, M., Hall, L., Hanotte, O., Hulme, H., McKeever, D., Murry, C., Oh, S., Tate, C., Smith, K., Tapio, M., Wambugu, J., Williams, D., Agaba, M. and S. Kemp (2011) "Genetic and Expression Analysis of Cattle Identifies Candidate Genes in Pathways Responding to *Trypanosoma Congolense* Infection", *Proceedings of the National Academy of Sciences* (*PNAS*), Vol. 108, No. 21.

Nuetah, J., Zuo, T. and X. Xin (2010) "Agricultural Export Subsidies and Domestic Support Reform under the WTO system: What does it mean for Welfare in West Africa?" Working Paper, College of Economics and Management, China Agricultural University.

O'Sullivan, M., Rao, A., Banerjee, R., Gulati, K. and M. Vinez (2014) *Levelling the Field: Improving Opportunities for Women Farmers in Africa.* Washington, DC: World Bank Group.

Ochieng, C. (2007) "Revitalizing African Agriculture Through Innovative Business Models and Organizational Arrangements", *The Journal of Modern African Studies*, Vol. 43, pp. 143–169.

Omamo, S. W. and K. von Grebmer (2005) *Biotechnology, Agriculture and Food Security in Southern Africa.* Washington, DC: IFPRI.

Omiti, J., Chacha, R. and M. S. Andama (2002) "Biotechnology can Improve Food Security in Africa", *African Journal of Food and Nutritional Sciences*, Vol. 2, No. 2, pp. 14–21.

Platteau, J. (1993) "Sub-Saharan Africa as a Special Case: The Crucial Role of Infrastructural Constraints", Research Series No. 128, Facultes Universitaires Notre-Dame de la\Paix, NAMUR, Belgium.

Popkin, B. M., Horton, S., Kim, S., Mahal, A. and J. Shuigao (2001) "Trends in Diet, Nutritional Status, and Diet-related Noncommunicable Diseases in China and India: the Economic Costs of the Nutrition Transition", *Nutrition Reviews*, Vol. 59, No. 12, pp. 379–390. https://doi.org/10.1111/j.1753-4887.2001.tb06967.x.

Puplampu, K. P. (2011) "Science-Society Relations and Biotechnology Revolution: Policy and Institutional Considerations for African Agriculture". Africa Capacity Indicators Report (ACIR) 2012 Background Paper — Number 3. Harare, Zimbabwe.

Puplampu, K. P. and G. Essegbey (2004) "Agricultural Biotechnology and Research in Ghana: Institutional Capacities and Policy Options", *Perspectives on Global Development and Technology*, Vol. 3, No. 3, pp. 271–290.

Qaim, M. (2005) "Agricultural Biotechnology Adoption in Developing Countries", *American Journal of Agricultural Economics*, Vol. 87, No. 5, pp. 1317–1324.

Roling, N. (2010) "The Impact of Agricultural Research: Evidence from West Africa," *Development in Practice*, Vol. 20, No. 8, pp. 959–971.

Scanlan, S. J. (2001) "Food Availability and Access in Lesser-Industrialized Societies: A Test and Interpretation of Neo-Malthusian and Technoecological Theories", *Sociological Forum*, Vol. 16, No. 2, p. 231.

Sen, A. (1982) "The Food Problem: Theory and Policy", *Third World Quarterly*, Vol. 4, No. 3, pp. 447–459.

Sen, A. (1981) *Poverty and Famines: An Essay on Entitlement and Deprivation.* Oxford University Press.

Smale, M., Zambrano, M., Falck-Zepeda, J. and G. Gruere (2006) "Parables: Applied Economics Literature About the Impact of Genetically Engineered Crop Varieties in Developing Economies", Environment & Production Technology Division (EPT) Discussion Paper 159. Washington, DC: International Food Policy Research Institute (IFPRI).

Sowman, M. and P. Cardoso (2010) "Small-Scale Fisheries and Food Security Strategies in Countries in the Benguela Current Large Marine Ecosystem (BCLME) Region: Angola, Namibia, and South Africa," *Marine Policy*, Vol. 34, pp. 1163–1170.

Spencer, D. S. C. (1994) *Infrastructure and Technology Constraints to Agricultural Development in the Humid and Subhumid Tropics of Africa*. Washington, DC: International.

Start, D. (2001) "The Rise and Fall of the Rural Non-Farm Economy: Poverty Impacts and Policy Options", *Development Policy Review*, Vol. 19, No. 4, pp. 491–505.

Thomas, J. A. and T. Zuberi (2012) "Demographic Change, the IMPACT Model, and Food Security in Sub-Saharan Africa," UNDP Regional Bureau for Africa Working Paper, 2012.

UNDP (2015) Human Development Report.

UNICEF and MI (United Nations Children's Fund and the Micronutrient Initiative) (2004) *Vitamin and Mineral Deficiency: A Global Damage Assessment Report*. New York and Ottawa. Available at: http://www.wsahs.nsw.gov.au.

UNICEF, WHO (World Health Organization) and World Bank (2015) 2014 Joint Child Malnutrition Estimates: Levels and Trends (September 2015 update). Accessed April 17, 2016. http://data.worldbank.org/child-malnutrition

von Grebmer, K. (2008) "The Challenge to Hunger: Global Hunger Index", *International Food Policy Research Institute*, IFPRI, Washington, DC.

von Grebmer, K., Bernstein, J., de Waal, A., Prasai, N., Yin, S., and Y. Yohannes (2015) *2015 Global Hunger Index: Armed Conflict and the Challenge of Hunger*, IFPRI.

Windfuhr, M. and J. Jonsén (2005) *Food Sovereignty: Towards Democracy in Localized Food Systems*. Warwickshire, UK: ITDG Publishing & FIAN.

Woodhouse, P. (2009) "Technology, Environment and the Productivity Problem in African Agriculture: Comment on the World Development Report", *Journal of Agrarian Change*, Vol. 9, No. 2, pp. 263–276.

World Bank (2006) *Global Economic Prospects*. Washington, DC: World Bank.

World Bank (2007) "World Development Report 2008: Agriculture for Development". Washington, DC.

World Bank (2008) "World Development Report 2008: Agriculture for Development". Washington, DC.

Chapter 12

Nutrition, Health and Productivity in Africa: Evidence from Ethiopia

George Kararach[*,‡] **and Abbi M. Kedir**[†,§]

[*]*United Nations Economic Commission for Africa, Addis Ababa, Ethiopia*
[†]*Sheffield University Management School (SUMS), Conduit Road, Sheffield S10 1FL, UK*
[‡]*kararach@un.org*
[§]*a.m.kedir@sheffield.ac.uk*

Abstract

Ethiopia has been faced with major food insecurity problems over the last 4 decades with recurrent droughts affecting millions of households. This chapter examines the link between nutrition and productivity among urban residents who are differentiated by gender using a comprehensive panel urban household survey data collected covering the period from 1994 to 2000. Controlling for endogeneity of schooling and allowing for heterogeneity of returns to human capital investment, our estimated results showed the presence of significant and positive link between nutrition (e.g. BMI and height) and productivity, as well as schooling and productivity. The link is robust and significant under all specifications. In agreement with evidence elsewhere in the developing world, we got significant returns to schooling investment. Our findings can be used to highlight the importance of improving children's nutrition from a policy point of view as it has productivity implications when children are adults. Improving access to food (e.g. food price subsidies), investment in health and ensuring agricultural productivity growth should remain a policy priority.

Keywords: Nutrition, health, schooling, agricultural productivity, Ethiopia.

1. Introduction

This study attempts to examine the link between nutrition and productivity among urban residents who are differentiated by gender in Ethiopia using a panel urban household survey data collected in 1994, 1995, 1997 and 2000. The specific way in which the poor participate in growth tends to be through increased or more productive use of "their most abundant asset", labour (Kanbur and Squire, 1999). The link between human development (say proxied by adult nutrition consumption and health) and economic growth can be ascertained if one finds robust and significant relationship using data on nutrition, health and wages.[1] Therefore, identifying factors that significantly enhance productivity (often measured in wages) is crucial to assist the intellectual effort that attempts to understand the mechanism through which human capital investments at the household level contribute to overall economic growth.

The link between productivity and consumption and its impact on wages was first explored, among others, by Leibenstein (1957), Stiglitz (1976), Mirrlees (1976), Bliss and Stern (1978) and is now commonly referred to as "efficiency wage theory". For instance, Deaton (2003) pointed out that the nutritional wage model provides an account of how inequality affects both health and earnings while explicitly recognizing that health and earnings are simultaneously determined. Dasgupta (1993) has eloquently argued that nutritional wage models can account for persistent poverty and destitution in poor countries.

[1] We will augment a standard wage equation we estimated in another application (Girma and Kedir, 2005) including key variables (our variable of focus) such as nutrition and health.

Among macro- and microeconomists, there emerged an unusual consensus that recent periods of sustained growth in Total Factor Productivity (TFP) are dependent on improvements in a population's nutrition, health, education and mobility (Shultz, 1997). Many studies of nutrition, health and labour mobility have sought to measure the effect of these forms of human capital on the productivity of workers and hence on economic growth. However, these studies did not show the effects of human capital investment on different groups of people such as men and women.

The investigation of the link between nutrition and productivity is crucial (e.g. for understanding causes of poverty traps) (Kedir and Girma, 2007). For instance, Dasgupta (1997) shows the mechanism by which inequality determines malnutrition through the nutrition-productivity link. Jha *et al.* (2009) empirically tested and found the presence of Poverty Nutrition Trap (PNT) using Heckman's sample selection techniques using data from India. Therefore, a careful estimation of the link addressing all the outstanding empirical issues contributes towards a deeper understanding of the link and provides us the basic tools that are important for policy making to stimulate returns to human capital stocks such as adult nutrition, adult health, schooling, child nutrition, etc.

A non-convex relationship between labour supply and consumption underlies the argument about the link between nutrition and productivity on the one hand and the persistence of poverty on the other. Due to this non-convexity multiple equilibria are possible.[2] At the lower end of this spectrum of equilibria lies a low nutrition-low productivity point where people stay unemployed involuntarily. At the other extreme lies the high nutrition-high productivity equilibrium where people enjoy high levels of productivity and better nutrition. Because of the fixed requirements, individuals could be trapped in the low equilibrium point where they stay poor with little chance of getting out of the poverty. Not surprisingly, it is households without assets that are trapped in the low equilibrium point. Those who have access to non-labour income can secure some level of consumption while the poor require employment to finance the same level of consumption. Ironically, the quality of labour that is supplied depends upon the level of caloric consumption. From the

[2]Assuming others things being constant (e.g. technology), the equilibrium concept we adopt here is a partial one.

employers point of view, hiring the poor is therefore expensive, because the poor require a wage high enough to be able to consume what is required for Basic Metabolism Rate (BMR) (Dasgupta, 1993) plus additional amounts needed to undertake external work. Those who own assets, however, can partly finance their consumption even without having to work. Hence, a wage level below what is required by the poor would enable those with assets to supply the quality of labour that the poor cannot offer (Ayalew, 2003).

2. Related Literature: What Has Been Done so Far?

It is theoretically conceivable and empirically supported to state that investments in nutrition and health increase the lifetime productivity of individuals and thereby contribute to economic growth, socio-demographic development and hence lower poverty (Jha *et al.*, 2009; Shultz, 1997). At the macro level, research has been focusing on establishing a link between GDP per capita and daily calorie intake. Easterly (1999)[3] finds that daily calorie intake increases with GDP per capita. He estimated nutrition equation in first-differences (in order to control for unobserved, time invariant, country-specific effects)[4] and instrumenting GDP per capita lagged two periods (in order to control for random measurement error or potential endogeneity). Others have essentially reversed the causality and attempted to uncover the contribution of nutrition to the growth of GDP per capita (Arcand, 2001).

At the micro or household level, there are a number of studies touching various aspects of nutrition and food security. Using the intra-household literature as a framework, Basudeb and Gautam (2006) investigated how the relative position of some household members (i.e. women) is related to nutrition outcomes of children in Pakistan. Children nutrition outcomes (both short-term and long-term measures) are used as dependent variables. In this study, we do quite the reverse. First we use data on

[3]Easterly used a multitude of other indicators of quality of life such as health, education, transport and communications, etc.

[4]This is what is often referred to as unobserved heterogeneity in the econometrics literature.

adults wages and their nutritional position. We focus on uncovering the impact of nutrition (health) on the labour productivity of individuals using a unique household data. We do this both for the adult female and the male sub-samples in the data and draw broad policy implications of our results. Therefore, we focus on the microeconomic link among these crucial variables of economic development. Apart from its technical focus which is outlined below, this study will serve as a policy input and would attempt to give insight in to what constitutes effective intervention to fight adult malnutrition and ill health at the household level with an ultimate aim of promoting productivity, growth and poverty reduction.

Chronic and widespread malnutrition at the household level has been one of the major impediments of child schooling, adult employment and overall economic development in much of Sub-Saharan Africa (SSA) and Ethiopia is no exception.[5] Macro and micro level nutrition-health-productivity link has been extensively investigated over the years using data from developing countries. One of the established links between investments in human capital (say via good nutrition and hence improved health) and its impact on increases in productivity (as measured by wages) has been based on examining farm level data (Strauss, 1986; Deolalikar, 1988; Haddad and Bouis, 1991).

There are similar attempts using household survey data from rural Ethiopia (Ayalew, 2003; Croppenstedt and Muller, 2000; Kim *et al.*, 1997). Croppenstedt and Muller (2000) estimated the impact of health and nutritional status on the efficiency and productivity of cereal growing Ethiopian farmers. They specify a stochastic frontier production function that enables them to examine the effect on efficiency as well. They reported both indicators of health (measured in travel time to the daily source of water) and nutrition (measured in terms of weight for height of the household head) have significant effects on farm production. Since they used cross-sectional data all the limitations identified by Strauss (1986) apply to their study. Ayalew (2003) went one step further by using a panel data set

[5]Rather unfortunately, Ethiopia has been suffering from severe food insecurity over a long period of time. Regardless of the malnutrition measure used, the incidence of underweight children has been consistently around 45%, much larger than the average incidence of 33% underweight children in SSA in the 1990s (Christiensen and Alderman, 2004).

collected from the same rural localities investigated by Croppenstedt and Muller (2000).

Except for few applications in developing countries, most studies ignored the impact of nutrition and health on productivity of urban residents (Thomas and Strauss, 1997; Kedir, 2006). To the best of our knowledge, in Ethiopia no study has shown how investments in nutrition and health increase or affect productivity of individuals (i.e. for males and females separately) for urban households. Some attempts have been made to estimate earnings functions with a focus on uncovering the private returns to schooling without any explicit attempt to incorporate the impact of nutrition and/or health indicator variables (Girma and Kedir, 2005).

The innovative aspect of this study is the estimation of the nutrition-health-productivity link using a unique panel household data set which has been collected from 1500 households in 1994, 1995, 1997 and 2000. Each household has an average of 6 household members and most of them are in the economically active age group and they form the focus of our analysis in this chapter. In addition, we focus on an integrated approach because we examine the link not only using nutrition but also health indicator variables. We investigate the impact of adult nutrition and health on productivity of workers and hence economic development. Even if there are five different types of human capital (see footnote below), the focus of this study is to analyse the impact of only adults' current health and nutritional status (which is proxied by weight-for-height squared or Body Mass Index (BMI)) on labour productivity using a panel data set.[6] We use both panel data and quantile regression model estimates to report our final results.

The study has both a technical as well as policy focus. On the technical side, we adopt recent parametric techniques that handle the thorny empirical issues of econometric estimation in the presence of endogeneity and heterogeneity of returns. On the policy side, we will identify possible policy implications of the results of our estimation to inform development policy makers in Ethiopia.

[6]Broadly speaking, there are five types of human capital (Shultz, 1997), viz, childhood nutritional status, schooling, migration, fertility and adult's current health and nutritional status.

3. Data and Econometric Methodology

This study is based on four waves of panel/longitudinal data for 1994, 1995, 1997 and 2000 which were collected under the supervision of Department of Economics of Addis Ababa University (Ethiopia) in collaboration with Economics department of Gothenburg University (Sweden) and Michigan State University (USA). The survey covers 1500 households in each round, with the intention of resurveying the same households in subsequent rounds. In each round, household and individual level information had been collected over a period of four successive weeks during a month considered to represent average conditions covering seven major cities in Ethiopia — Addis Ababa (the capital), Awassa, Bahar Dar, Dessie, Diredawa, Jimma and Mekele. The sample of households surveyed is intended to be representative of the main socio-economic characteristics of the country's major towns. The total sample was distributed over the selected urban centres proportional to their populations, based on Central Statistical Authority's (CSA) 1992 population projections.

The use of panel data is useful for a number of reasons. If individual heterogeneity is an important determinant of human capital investments by parents and society, then panel data on individuals may be particularly useful for the estimation of individuals' fixed effects models (Strauss and Thomas, 1995). These panels may also permit more systematic treatment of measurement errors in anthropometric measures of health and nutrition (Shultz, 1997). Most studies that attempt to establish the relationship between labour productivity and nutrition are contaminated by *simultaneity* between calorie intake and labour productivity. The causation of the relationship could go in either direction. Variables that affect earnings or production affect nutrition consumption via the associated effect on income, in which case consumption is rendered *endogeneous* (Ayalew, 2003).

BMI affects the current productivity of the individual, particularly at low levels of calories and for energy-demanding tasks. This indicator of nutritional status among adults, as argued by Shultz (1997), should be treated as simultaneously determined with increased current expenditures on nutrition and the performance of more demanding jobs. However, it is also likely affected by nutritional intake over a substantial length of time but with significant implications for individuals' current health as well as productivity. Unbiased estimates of the one-directional effect of improved adult nutrition on wage or self-employment productivity requires valid instruments that predict current nutritional intakes or BMI and that are uncorrelated with the error in the wage equation.

One systematic study using data from Sierra Leone (again using a rural data set) tried to addressed the potential simultaneity problem using an instrumental variables (IV) estimation technique. The study found a statistically significant effect of calorie intake on farm productivity. However, the effect is not linear and the marginal effect on productivity falls as calorie consumption rises, but remains positive. Yet, the emphasis of the study on Sierra Leone is on the effect of the flow of nutritional status measured by caloric intake. Caloric intake, however, also affects the stock of nutritional status, namely the body mass which is directly related to productivity as noted above. This relationship is very important especially when individuals can adapt to short-term changes in caloric intake by drawing from the stock of nutrition without any significant reduction in their productivity. Moreover, as Strauss acknowledges, failure to control for time persistent household effects (e.g. managerial ability) may lead to biased estimates. The bias could go in either direction depending on the relationship between caloric intake and the omitted time persistent variables. Both of these shortcoming are addressed in Deolalikar (1988).

So far, there have not been empirical attempts to allow for heterogeneity in returns to productivity of human capital investments such as height (proxy for long-term health) and BMI. Therefore, we estimate quantile regression equations that give us heterogeneous returns to nutritional investments as opposed to a single marginal return in the case of a typical panel data model setting whether or not we fit a model with or without instrumenting. A quantile regression framework allows variations of the returns to investments in nutrition and health at different quantiles of the earnings distribution (Koenker and Basset, 1978).[7]

The following gives a brief overview of the econometric framework we adopt. Let y_i denote the log of hourly wage of worker i and let X be

[7]We use STATA 14 for the estimation of our model.

the vector of covariates which consists of nutrition, schooling and the full set of gender, ethnicity (as proxy for personal connections), year and location dummies.

The θth quantile of the conditional distribution of y_i given X is specified as

$$Q_\theta(yi \mid X) = \alpha(\theta) + X_i'\beta(\theta), \quad \theta \in (0,1). \tag{1}$$

where $Q_\theta(yi \mid X)$ denotes the quantile θ of log earnings conditional on the vector of covariates. Following Koenker and Basset (1978), the θth quantile estimator can be defined as the solution to the following problem:

$$\min_\beta \frac{1}{n}\left[\sum_{i:yi \geq x'\beta} \theta \left|y_i - X_i'\beta_\theta\right| + \sum_{i:yi \prec x'\beta} (1-\theta)\left|y_i - X_i'\beta_\theta\right|\right] = \min_\beta \frac{1}{n}\sum_{i=1}^{n} \rho_\theta(u_{\theta i}), \tag{2}$$

where $\rho_\theta(\cdot)$ is known as the "check function" and is defined as $\rho_\theta(u_{\theta i}) = \theta u_{\theta i}$ if $u_{\theta i} \geq 0$ and $\rho_\theta(u_{\theta i}) = (1 - \theta)u_{\theta i}$ if $u_{\theta i} < 0$. The minimization problem can be solved by using linear programming methods (Buchinsky, 1998). Like standard OLS estimates, a quantile regression estimate can be interpreted as the partial derivative with respect to a particular regressor at the relevant quantile.

Therefore, our estimation of the relationship between labour productivity, nutrition and health will be conducted in a framework of standard panel data model (e.g. random effects model), instrumental variable panel data model (i.e. two stage generalized least squares) and quantile regression using panel data from urban households. All the estimators are intended to help us to arrive at coefficient estimates that allow for both endogeneity of human capital investment (i.e. adult's nutrition and health status) and possible heterogeneity in the impact of this investment.

For our application, we use individual data on wage/salary, age, gender, location, years of schooling, height and weight. The years of schooling variable is not directly observed but is constructed by converting the reported schooling cycles completed. As is common in many anthropometric surveys, data on height and weight are subject to reporting error. We cleaned the data by removing prohibitively high values of height and weight.

We briefly describe a model of health, productivity and labour force participation, in which all three outcomes are treated as endogenous (see Thomas and Strauss (1997) for a static version of this model). This model is used to identify the effect of health on productivity in a panel data context.

Suppose we have a latent labour supply function of individual i at time t, h_{it}^* which depends on a vector of exogenous individual time-varying and time-invariant characteristics (x_{it}); community level characteristics (x_{ct}) such as prices, local demand; and infrastructure and productivity-related individual specific unobservables (μ_i)

$$h_{it}^* = h(x_{it}, x_{ct}, \mu_i). \tag{3}$$

An individual will choose to work if a wage offer is greater than the reservation or shadow wage in which case $h_{it}^* > 0$.

To examine the influence of our health indicators (height and BMI) on productivity, we consider a standard wage function (in logarithm form) which is conditional on both health x_{ith} and labour force participation $h_{it}^* > 0$

$$\ln(w_{it}) = w\left(x_{it}, x_{ith}, \overline{x}_{ct}, \mu_{it}\right); h_{it}^* > 0, \tag{4}$$

where $\overline{x}_{ct}$ is a subset of community characteristics x_{ct}.

Our results reported in Table 1 are based on the econometric framework outlined earlier. Equation (4) is the underlying structural relationship for the wage equation estimated.

Table 1. Average BMI by age and gender, all Waves 1994–2004.

Age group	**Gender**	**Mean BMI** (*N*)
15–29	M	20.6 (*N* = 4274)
	F	21.0 (*N* = 5135)
30 and above	M	22.4 (*N* = 3507)
	F	22.2 (*N* = 4618)

4. Results and Discussion

Before discussion of our regression results on the significant determinants of nutritional status, we present a descriptive distribution of the BMI variable for all the individuals surveyed by gender and age group. This information can be used as a general snapshot of the health of individuals via BMI and the risks associated with it. For instance, the nutrition literature states that an individual is overweight if her/his BMI is equal to 25 or above. And the individual is classified as obese if BMI is 30 or above. According to the average BMI figures reported in Table 1, none of the individuals surveyed in Ethiopia are either overweight or obese. Females in the age group 15–29 are slightly heavier than males, while for those aged 30 and above the average BMI figures between the sexes are similar.

The next set of results related to our regression estimates show the impact of schooling, gender and other correlates on BMI, which is our measure of nutritional status. Our regression results summarized in Table 2 show the estimates by location and age group. Our sample covers seven major urban centres, the capital city being the most represented in the data collection stage. Therefore, we split our sample between the capital city and those cities outside the capital for reporting the regression estimates.

Age has a positive impact in all specifications of the BMI equation except for age group 30 & above for the sample of individuals residing outside Addis Ababa. This is not surprising as older adults are most full grown and hence weigh more compared to the younger cohort of individuals in the age range of 15–29. Hence, the result should not be interpreted to mean that older individuals are necessarily prone to be overweight or obese which is not the case at least as the average figures reveal in Table 1. This is the most plausible explanation for the coefficient given that the average BMI in our sample is below 21 for all those living in the capital city (and the overall sample) and below 23 for individuals living outside the capital.

Parental schooling has no impact in our sample. This might be because we are not focusing on young children as our primary focus in this chapter is to examine the impact of nutrition or health on productivity

Table 2. Determinants of nutritional status: Random effects panel estimates.

	Addis Ababa		Outside Addis Ababa	
Variable	**15–29**	**30+**	**15–29**	**30+**
Log of age	3.4***	0.85**	3.23**	0.68
	(0.57)	(0.34)	(0.80)	(0.44)
Male	−0.36*	−0.30*	−0.12	−0.02
	(0.22)	(0.18)	(0.33)	(0.24)
Years of schooling	−0.01	0.15***	−0.04	0.11***
	(0.02)	(0.02)	(0.41)	(0.02)
Schooling of mother	−0.04	0.10	−0.5	0.03
	(0.04)	(0.08)	(0.07)	(0.14)
Schooling of father	0.02	0.06	0.04	0.09
	(0.03)	(0.04)	(0.04)	(0.06)
Oromo	0.23	−0.16	−0.54	0.55
	(0.29)	(0.23)	(0.45)	(0.34)
Tigre	−0.49	−0.22	−1.36***	−0.85***
	(0.45)	(0.38)	(0.44)	(0.31)
Gurage	0.02	−0.15	−0.33	0.60
	(0.30)	(0.26)	(0.60)	(0.54)
Other ethnic group	0.40	−0.36	0.16	0.71**
	(0.61)	(0.36)	(0.45)	(0.35)
Constant	10.95***	18.8***	11.58***	18.7***
	(1.78)	(1.38)	(2.41)	(1.76)
Wald chi-squared statistic (p-value)	43.9	79.4	33.3	48.2
	(0.00)	(0.00)	(0.00)	(0.00)
Number of observations	866	3836	884	908

Notes: *** significant at 1% level; ** significant at 5% level.

for the economically active population surveyed in the Ethiopian Urban Household Survey (EUHS). However, it is useful to note that the existing literature highlights the merits of education of parents (particularly maternal education) which is often found to be a statistically significant factor for the nutritional status of young children especially those under 5 years of age (Ickes *et al.*, 2015; Frost *et al.*, 2005).

The male dummy is negative and significant only for the Addis Ababa sample for both age groups (i.e. 15–29 and those aged 30 and above).

Meaning being a male is associated with a lower BMI but the estimated coefficient is significant only at 10%. Gender of the individual does not appear to matter to the BMI of individuals for all individuals in both age groups for those livings outside the capital city.

The schooling of the individual is positively and significantly associated with higher BMI as expected. However, this is true only for those aged 30 and above both in Addis Ababa and cities outside Addis Ababa. The ethnicity variable is an important variable that captures factors that can influence nutritional status due to heterogeneity in cultural norms surrounding food types eaten. Therefore, we also controlled for the ethnic group that individuals belong to and we make the Amhara the reference group. None of the ethnic group variables are associated with nutritional status in the Addis Ababa sub-sample and this is not surprising as none of the ethnic-specific food cultures are dominant in the capital city. However, for those living outside the capital city, belonging to the Tigre ethnic group is associated with negative nutritional outcome or lower BMI while being in the other ethnic group is positively associated.

Table 3 provides our core set of results based on panel data models and quantile regressions which address the potential empirical problems of endogeneity and heterogeneity of returns. The results provide the answer whether or not the nutritional/health status of individuals as captured by height and BMI has an influence on productivity (wage) with or without addressing the two econometric problems. The coefficient estimates of Random Effects (RE) Generalized Least Squares (GLS) estimator are given in the 2nd column as baseline estimates. They neither account for the endogeneity of schooling nor for the potential heterogeneity in the impact of BMI, height and other correlates. Therefore, in column 3, among a possible set of estimators for fitting panel-data models in which some of the right-hand side correlates are endogenous, we adopt the Balestra and Varadharajan-Krishnakumar estimator (i.e. G2SLS) (Balestra and Varadharajan-Krishnakumar, 1987). This estimator gives as a two-stage least-squares generalizations of a standard panel-data estimator. The last four columns of the table give us the quantile regression estimates and these will give us four different slopes or impacts of the right-hand variable hence allowing heterogeneity in return for key human capital investments such as schooling and health (captured here by BMI and height of the individual).

Table 3. Returns to height and BMI: Panel and quantile regression estimates.

Variable	Random effects GLS	G2SLS instrumenting schooling	25th quantile	50th quantile	75th quantile	90th quantile
Years of schooling	0.12***	0.15***	0.14***	0.12***	0.09***	0.08***
	(0.004)	(0.02)	(0.01)	(0.00)	(0.00)	(0.00)
Log of age	0.05	*–0.31*	*5.71****	*2.17**	*–1.28****	*–2.27***
	(0.56)	*(0.75)*	*(1.19)*	*(1.24)*	*(0.24)*	*(1.08)*
Log of age squared	0.17**	0.24**	–0.63***	–0.14***	0.33***	0.44***
	(0.08)	(0.11)	(0.16)	(0.18)	(0.04)	(0.16)
height	0.001*	0.001*	0.00	0.01*	0.01***	0.01***
	(0.00)	(0.00)	(0.00)	(0.00)	(0.00)	(0.00)
BMI	0.01***	0.01*	0.01***	0.01***	0.02***	0.02***
	(0.00)	(0.00)	(0.00)	(0.00)	(0.00)	(0.00)
Constant	1.78**	1.97*	–8.92***	–2.67	3.70***	6.08***
	(0.94)	(1.22)	(1.99)	(2.35)	(0.56)	(1.92)
Sigma u	0.69	0.66	—	—	—	—
Rho	0.59	0.60	—	—	—	—
Pseudo R-squared			0.29	0.28	0.22	0.17
Observations	*3432*	*2242*		*3432*		

Notes:

(i) G2SLS = generalized two stage least squares estimator of Balestra and Varadharajan-Krishnakumar implemented using xtivreg command in STATA version 14.

(ii) Standard errors which are corrected for clustering using bootstrap technique are reported in parentheses for all the quantile regression estimates.

(iii) *significant at 10%; **significant at 5%; ***significant at 1%.

Our results indicate the importance of the human capital variables (schooling, height and BMI) in the wage/productivity equation. All estimates show the statistically significant effect of schooling for the productivity of individuals. Empirical evidence so far from developing countries shows strong returns of schooling and this is supported by our results. The innovative aspect of our finding is the heterogeneity of returns for each of the variables and a control for endogeneity. We could not have captured this without the use of quantile regression and instrumental variable regression. After instrumenting schooling of the individuals by the schooling of their parents to control for potential endogeneity, we still have a significant impact of schooling on productivity but a stronger one as the estimate rose from a return of 12–15%. When we look at schooling returns from the quantile regression estimates, the coefficient is stronger for individuals at the lower end of the wage distribution. It is evident from the reported results that the returns show progressively declining returns as we move from the lowest (25th quantile) to the highest (90th) quantile. The returns of schooling for the 25th, 50th (i.e. the median regression equivalent return), 75th and 90th quantile are 14%, 12%, 9% and 8%, respectively. This suggests that schooling investment is well-paying for the less able or those at the lower end of the earning distribution (Girma and Kedir, 2005). However, schooling attracts a statistically significant productivity return for all Ethiopians at every point in the wage distribution even if some have better marginal returns in productivity than others for the schooling investment they make. In the quantile regression estimates, there is a nonlinear relationship between age and productivity as the life-cycle hypothesis suggests. Interestingly this nonlinearity takes two different forms for the various quantiles. For the 25th and 50th quantile, the nonlinearity is bell-shaped with wages rising with age and falling after a certain threshold while for the 75th and 9th quantile, the nonlinearity is U-shaped with wages falling with age initially and rising after a certain threshold. In the panel estimator with or without endogeneity correction, there is still a nonlinear relationship between age and wage, but only the quadratic term is positive and statistically significant suggesting a tendency of productivity at higher levels of age.

This heterogeneity is not only restricted to schooling but also to the returns from our health indicators (i.e. BMI). Height is a significant predictor of wages in all specifications (i.e. both in panel as well as quantile regression frameworks) and is positively and significantly linked to productivity. One notable observation is that the coefficients or the marginal returns are similar in the 2nd and 3rd column estimates (i.e. the panel data models). This is true also in the case of the quantile estimates (columns 5–7) with insignificant returns to height at the 25th quantile. But the marginal returns associated with height are stronger in the quantile regression estimates than in the panel data model estimates. The returns to height in the panel data estimates are 0.1% compared to 1% reported for the median, 75th and 90th quantiles. The strength of the impact of BMI for the panel data models and for the lower quantiles (i.e. 25th and 50th) are identical standing at 1% while the returns for the last two quantiles (i.e. 75th and 90th) are twice as much (i.e. 2%). BMI can be seen as indicator of bodily strength and its returns are higher for those individuals at the upper end of the wage distribution. However, one might expect to see higher BMI returns in the lower quantiles than in the upper quantiles because of the likely stronger significance of bodily strength for those earning lower wages. Most likely, those at the lower end of the wage distribution are engaged in low-skill and high labour-intensive jobs. However, such a pattern is not necessarily the case as the coefficients of the 75th and 90th quantiles show suggesting that bodily strength is important for the productivity of high earners too.

5. Conclusions

Ethiopia has been faced with major food insecurity problems over the last 4 decades with recurrent droughts affecting millions of households. According to a joint assessment of the Ethiopian government and development partners, about 10.2 million people were affected by the drought and needed emergency food and non-food aid by January 2016 (UN, 2016). Despite its impressive economic growth over the last decade, the country is still one of the poorest on the planet with enormous challenges such as poverty and food insecurity.

Hence, analysing the productivity impact of nutrition is critical to see the effect of human capital investment (i.e. in nutrition and health) on development outcomes at the micro level. This study attempts to examine the link between nutrition and productivity among urban residents who are differentiated by gender in Ethiopia using a comprehensive panel urban household survey data collected in 1994, 1995, 1997 and 2000. As argued in the introductory part of the study, the mechanism in which individuals especially the poor participate in growth tends to be through increased or more productive use of "their most abundant asset", labour (Kanbur and Squire, 1999).

Using Ethiopia as a case study and controlling for endogeneity of schooling and allowing for heterogeneity of returns of human capital investment, our estimated results showed the presence of significant and positive link between nutrition (e.g. BMI and height) and productivity, as well as schooling and productivity. The link is robust and significant under all specifications. This is true in baseline model that does not allow for endogeneity of schooling and heterogeneity and it is also true in the panel data model results with endogeneity correction and the quantile regression estimates that show the diversity of the impact of nutritional investment on productivity depending on the position of the individual in the wage distribution.[8] Therefore, identifying factors that significantly enhance productivity (often measured in wages) is crucial to assist the intellectual effort that attempts to understand the mechanism through which human capital investments at the household level contribute to overall economic growth.

This study provided evidence for the presence of a significant high-nutrition and high-productivity equilibrium using panel data on individuals from urban Ethiopia. In agreement with evidence elsewhere in the developing world, we got significant returns to schooling investment. We also note that the importance of BMI is more significant for those at the upper end of the wage distribution. Height is found to be significant in all regression except in the 25th quantile. Height is a cumulative measure reflecting both investment in nutrition during one's life (mostly as a child) and also, possibly, non-health human capital investment (Thomas and Strauss, 1997). Hence, our findings can be

[8]Note that our results in this study are based on augmenting a standard wage equation we estimated in another application (Girma and Kedir, 2005) by including key variables of focus such as nutrition and health (i.e. BMI and height).

used to highlight the importance of improving children's nutrition from a policy point of view as it has productivity implications when children are adults. In terms of potential policy implications, improving access to food (e.g. food price subsidies) in the current climate of local and global food price hikes seems an urgent priority. The policy makers in Ethiopia have critical challenges for decades in relation to food insecurity in the country. This is exacerbated by the recent drought that affected millions in the country making the extra needed investment in nutrition a more difficult task in the coming years. Ensuring agricultural productivity growth to provide secure access to food for millions of Ethiopians should remain a policy priority.

References

Arcand, J-L. (2001) "Undernourishment and Economic Growth: The Efficiency cost of Hunger", FAO Social and Economic Development Paper 147, United Nations.

Arias, O., Hallock, K. F. and W. Sosa-Escudero (2001) "Individual Heterogeneity in the Returns to Schooling: Instrumental Variables Quantile Regression Using Twins' Data", *Empirical Economics*, Vol. 26, pp. 7–40.

Ayalew, T. (2003) "The Nutrition-Productivity Link and the Persistence of Poverty", Discussion Paper, 2003–02. Belgium: Institute of Development Policy and Management, University of Antwerp.

Balestra, P. and J. Varadharajan-Krishnakumar (1987) "Full Information Estimations of a System of Simultaneous Equations with Error Component Structure", *Econometric Theory*, Vol. 3, pp. 223–246.

Basudeb, G.-K. and H. Gautam (2006) "Women's Status and Children's Food Security in Pakistan", Discussion Paper 2006/03. Helsinki, Finland: WIDER.

Bliss, C. and N. Stern (1978) "Productivity, Wages, Nutrition: Some Observations", *Journal of Development Economics*, No. 4, pp. 331–398.

Buchinski, M. (1998). "Recent Advances in Quantile Regression Models", *Journal Human Resources*, Vol. 33, pp. 88–126.

Christiaaensen, L. and H. Alderman (2004) "Child Malnutrition in Ethiopia: Can Maternal Knowledge Augment the Role of Income?", *Economic Development and Cultural Change*, Vol. 52, No. 2, pp. 287–312.

Croppenstedt, A. and C. Muller (2000) "The Impact of Farmers' Health and Nutritional Status on Their Productivity and Efficiency: Evidence from

Ethiopia", *Economic Development and Cultural Change*, Vol. 48, No. 3, pp. 475–502.

Dasgupta, P. (1997) "Nutritional Status, the Capacity for Work and Poverty Traps", *Journal of Econometrics*, Vol. 77, No. 1, pp. 3–37.

Dasgupta, P. (1993) *An Inquiry into Well-Being and Destitution*. Clarendon: Oxford University Press.

Deaton, A. (2003) "Health, Inequality and Economic Development", *Journal of Economic Literature*, Vol. 41, No. 1, pp. 113–158.

Deolalikar, A. B. (1988) "Nutrition and Labour Productivity in Agriculture", *Review of Economics and Statistics*, Vol. 70, pp. 406–413.

Easterly, W. (1999) "Life During Growth", *Journal of Economic Growth*, Vol. 4, No. 3, pp. 239–275.

Frost, M., Forste, R. and D. Haasc (2005) "Maternal Education and Child Nutritional Status in Bolivia: Finding the Links", *Social Science & Medicine*, Vol. 60, No. 2, pp. 395–407.

Girma, S. and A. M. Kedir (2005) "Heterogeneity in Returns to Schooling: Econometric Evidence from Ethiopia", *Journal of Development Studies*, Vol. 41, No. 8, pp. 1405–1416.

Haddad, L. and H. E. Bouis (1991) "The Impact of Nutritional Status on Agricultural Productivity: Wage Evidence from the Philippines", *Oxford Bulletin of Economics and Statistics*, Vol. 53, No. 1, pp. 45–68.

Ickes, S., Hurst, T. and V. Flax (2015) "Maternal Literacy, Facility Birth, and Education are Positively Associated with Better Infant and Young Child Feeding Practices and Nutritional Status Among Ugandan Children", *Journal of Nutrition*, Vol. 145, No. 11, pp. 2578–2586.

Jha, R., Gaiha, R. and A. Sharma (2009) "Calorie and Micronutrient Deprivation and Poverty Nutrition Traps in Rural India", *World Development*, Vol. 37, No. 5, pp. 982–991.

Leibenstein, H. A. (1957) *Economic Backwardness and Economic Growth*. New York: Wiley.

Kanbur, R. and L. Squire (1999) *The Evolution of Thinking About Poverty: Exploring the Interactions*. United Nations.

Kedir, A. M. (2006) Is Weight Linked to a Wage Premium in a Developing Country? Evidence from Quantile Regressions, mimeo, University of Nottingham, UK.

Kedir, A. M. and S. Girma (2007) "Quadratic Engel Curves and Measurement Error: Evidence from Ethiopia", *Oxford Bulletin of Economics and Statistics*, Vol. 69, No. 1, pp. 123–138.

Kim, A., Tandon, A. and A. Hailu (1997) "Health and Labour Productivity: Economic Impact of Onchocercal Skin Disease", Policy Research Working Paper 1836. Washington, DC: World Bank.

Koenker, R. and G. Basset (1978) "Regression Quantiles", *Econometrica*, Vol. 50, pp. 43–61.

Mirrlees, J. A. (1976) "A Pure Theory of Underdeveloped Economies", in *Agriculture in Development Theory*, ed. L. Reynolds. New Haven, Conn.: Yale University.

Shultz, T. P. (1997) "Assessing the Productive Benefits of Nutrition and Health: An Integrated Human Capital Approach", *Journal of Econometrics*, Vol. 77, pp. 141–158.

Stiglitz, J. E. (1976) "The Efficiency Wage Hypothesis, Surplus Labour and the Distribution of Income in LDCs", *Oxford Economic Papers*, Vol. 28, No. 2, pp. 185–207.

Strauss, J. (1986) "Does Better Nutrition Raise Farm Productivity?" *Journal of Political Economy*, Vol. 94, pp. 297–320.

Strauss, J. and D. Thomas (1995) "Human Resources: Empirical Modelling of Household and Family Decisions", in *Handbook in Development Economics*, eds. J. Behrman and T. N. Srinivasan, Vol. 3A. Amsterdam: Elsevier.

Thomas, D. and J. Strauss (1997) "Health and Wages: Evidence on Men and Women in Urban Brazil", *Journal of Econometrics*, Vol. 88, pp. 159–185.

UN (2016) Assessing the Cost of Drought in Ethiopia and the Case for Long-term Development Approach: Policy Note, Delivering as One, Addis Ababa, Ethiopia.

Index

CPSIA information can be obtained
at www.ICGtesting.com
Printed in the USA
BVHW011510311218
536665BV00007B/1/P

9 789813 239906